Our Society: Addiction and More Uncovered

Hear the voice of everyday people – collection of stories and experiences

by Gabriella Kőrösi, PhD, MN, RN

Front cover acrylic painting created by Andrea Mihaly October 2019

Our Society: Addiction and More Uncovered. Hear the voices of everyday people – collection of stories and experiences. Copyright @ 2020. 1st addition. By Dr. Gabriella Kőrösi

ISBN: 9798577493752

All rights reserved.

This book is dedicated to the memory of

Bagóczky József my uncle who died at age 19 – alcohol related car accident

and to everyone else who has been hurt or lost related to addiction

Many people had been supportive and inspiring to me so I could create this book. Both of my wonderful children told me, just write that book mom. My mom. I could have not done this without all the stories provided and the encouragement love and caring from my family and friends, nurses, doctors, counselors, teachers, professors, friends who are dealing with addiction and staying sober; and children, wives, husbands, mothers, fathers, sisters, brothers of people who are dealing with addiction currently. Thank you for speaking up, sharing your stories and life experiences. Thank you for all the people who read this book while in progress to provide feedback, ideas and encouragement for me to continue writing. I would like to say special thanks to my friends and family for believing me and encouraging me to go on.

Table of Contents

1. Hummingbird
2. My Uncle
3. Game of Life - Spirituality
4. The flow of things
5. Addiction- What is Addiction?
6. Mike's and Traci's story
7. Toni's story
8. Causes of Addiction
9. My Grandfather
10. Alcohol – Drinking
11. Kevin's story
12. Opiates
13. Bonnie's story
14. Marijuana
15. Joe's story
16. Smoking
17. Thomas's and Nicole's story
18. Sugar Addiction
19. Kristen's story
20. Happy Addictions
21. Dr. M's Story
22. Gambling
23. Lola's story
24. Technology - Social Media
25. Danny's Story
26. Suicide
27. Tammy's Story
28. Being the Provider

TABLE OF CONTENTS

29. HEALTHCARE – DO YOU HAVE A RIGHT TO BE CARED FOR?
30. VIOLET
31. GOVERNMENT
32. SOCIETY
33. INDIVIDUAL ROLE
34. DOUG'S STORY
35. THE CRIMINAL JUSTICE SYSTEM
36. SCHOOLS
37. FAMILY
38. LESLIE'S STORY
39. HAPPINESS AND JOY
40. STIGMA
41. DEBT AND CONSUMERISM
42. RESILIENCY AND PREVENTION
43. ROLE OF NUTRITION
44. HOMELESSNESS
45. SELF-PRESERVATION
46. REPRODUCTION
47. NEAL'S STORY
48. JAIL
49. HUMANITY
50. POSSIBLE SOLUTIONS
51. CREATING CHANGE
52. FINAL THOUGHTS
53. QUESTIONS
54. BOOK RECOMMENDATIONS

1. Hummingbird

Hummingbirds are amazingly beautiful and complex creatures. I have been really lucky the last few weeks to see a hummingbird every day. It is summer and they like all the flowers around the house. When they come, I just stand very still and watch them, enjoy the beautiful company. One of the favorite foods for them seems to be the Chinese lantern. The little birds are amazing, their colors are beyond words, the fast way they flap their wings and fly is spectacular. They make very beautiful bird songs as well. People love them. They are astonishing little beings. Well, so far, I have not met someone who does not like hummingbirds. Hummingbirds are very beautiful. Hummingbirds are very delicate creatures and have to fight to survive every day. It is truly amazing what their little bodies can endure. They have a very fast beating heart, extreme wing fluttering, have to drink nectar very frequently or they would starve to death. Many die during their first year. They are also able to control their temperature and heart rate which go down very low and slow at night and beat very fast during the day. It is a unique moment when someone can see them sitting on a branch. Hummingbirds also fight for their food and chase other hummingbirds away who are trying to get to the flower or the feeder. Hummingbirds and people dealing with drug and alcohol addiction have a lot in common. I believe all people are very beautiful, no matter what disease process, or habit-forming issue they have to deal with. Addiction is very a complex phenomenon. When someone is dealing with addiction, they have a strong urge and craving to get their next dose. Deep into addiction, people many times fall into a trap and all they know is how to live their addicted life. People told me that they kept using drugs because of the fear of what will happen to them if they don't. The fear included that they will die if they do not get their next dose or that they will get very sick. **Many people die of addiction within their first year of use.** Drugs and alcohol can increase and decrease a person's heart rate to a point many times that the heart cannot take it anymore and can result in fibrillation or heart attack. The heart can also slow down too much and can cause death. Getting to food for the hummingbird or the next fix for someone with addiction is the same process, a need to be filled. In both cases there is the knowledge that if this desire is not filled a person will become sick and start to withdraw. Withdrawal from substances can be very dangerous and could cause death. There is no choice in the matter. Life or death is at the stake. There is one major difference between a hummingbird and a person who is dealing with addiction. It is hard to see beyond the addiction and find the beauty in the human being. People won't judge a hummingbird, while people would judge someone who is dealing with addiction. Nobody wants to be addicted to anything especially if it is causes detriment to self and others. There are many addictions that people can get caught up in. These could include but not limited to smoking, vaping, using any device for smoking any harmful substance, food, gambling, sex, social media, gaming are some examples. People get caught up in a web that is hard to unweave. The goal of this book is to change some judgmental perceptions and uncover some false perceptions about addiction. This book will share my experiences and ideas with many others who I have interviewed including professionals from the addiction world, counselors, people from the medical world including but not limited to doctors, nurse practitioners, nurses, nutritionist, police, prosecutor, mothers of addicts, youth, priests, families and friends who know people with addiction as well as individuals who are currently addicted or have been addicted to any substance.

2. My Uncle

My uncle's name was Józsika. He always felt like a brother to me. Józsika had a twin brother his name is Attila. They stuck together and did a lot of things together.

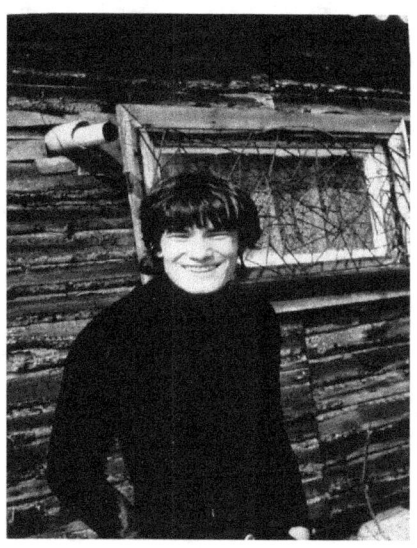

My Uncle Józsika, age 18, Hungary at Grandma's cabin in Pestezsébet

I really enjoyed spending time with them. I remember watching them playing cards with their friends, they would play in fillér it would be equivalent to play like in 1 cent, fillér does not even available in Hungary anymore, it is so small. It was in the circulation back when I was growing up in the 1970's - 1980's. It was always interesting to me that Attila had blond hair and Józsika had black hair. I had talked to multiple people in my family to try to provide an accurate picture of him. Mom found this picture of the three of us:

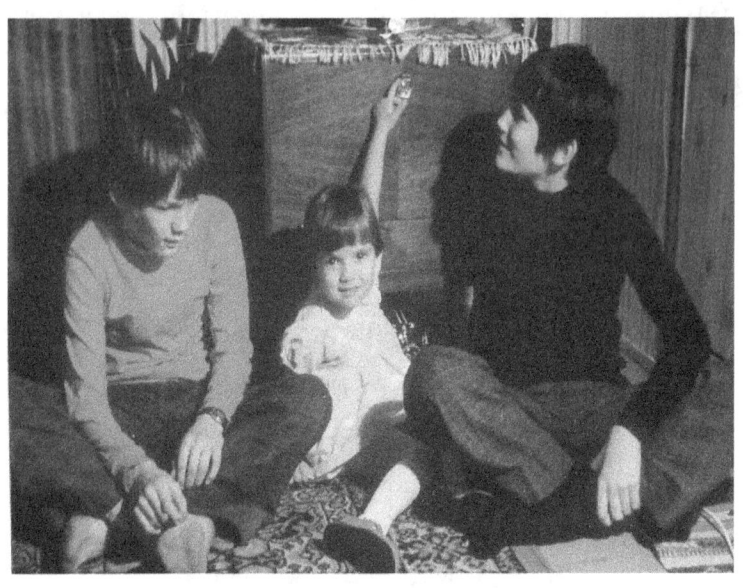

Attila, me and Józsika, Hungary, Budapest 1977, Jan 4th

    Talking to my dad, he recalls that when Józsika was 6 or 7 years old they played horse on my dad's knees. He recalls that the twins spent a lot of time together, they were inseparable. They were adorable little kids who loved to hang around my mom and dad. Józsika's death broke my heart when I was 10 years old. It was a huge loss for me and my family. Part of me always will miss him. Józsika had a father, but he was not there for him, Mom remembers, he did not stand by him. Mom said both the twins were great in sports but ended up not continuing in sports perhaps because of the missing father figure. Every sport they started they excelled in it. Shooting, running, water sports, no matter what it was. Józsika's story still creates waves of emotions for me. He did things like stealing flowers from someone's garden for my grandmother for Mother's Day. He was like a glue of love that pulled the family together. He would get into trouble sometimes, but he was so loving and kind that nobody could be mad at him for long. My mother mentioned to me that taking flowers is not stealing if they grew out in the street it is just a custom and that it is ok to pick them. The tradition was to get lilacs for Mother's Day. I can still see him bringing those dark purple flowers to my grandmother. He had a big heart for sure, Mom said. Once the boys grew up, my mom moved away, and I was born. Her brothers would come home to my mom after school. Close to the accident Józsika's brother was working outside of the country in Germany. Talking to Attila, he feels bad and sad because they used to fight as boys and before he left, they had a fight too and they actually beat each other up. Apparently, this was a regular occurrence. I had no idea. Attila tells me that at least once a month they beat each other up. I asked him what they were fighting about. He tells me it was a brother thing; they just would fight over little stupid things. Attila recalls that Józsika went to learn boxing in Újpest, Hungary when he was 14 years old. Then he would come home and show his brother the moves. He would say ok, this is what I learned, now defend yourself. Back then they would slap each other in the face. I burst out laughing at this point when he tells me this. I could just see it right in front of my eyes the two of them slapping each other. I asked if it was real fights or just goofing around. Attila said it usually started as being stupid and goofing around, but it could get a little tough and violent sometimes. Attila did not leave on good terms. He describes hatred from both sides when he left. Thinking back this was not the best thing. This still hurts Attila. Otherwise he tells me they always supported each other and stood by each other. Attila tells me that Józsika liked girls and he would brag about it too. Attila was always quieter about it. Attila tells me about Józsika's special loved one, her name is Kati. I remember her very clearly. Attila said the relationship was going on for 2-3 years off and on. Attila told me that Kati got pregnant and decided to abort the baby, and this was very difficult for Józsika. This happened very close to his death. Józsika also had some encounter with the police. I asked Mom about this and she said that Józsika was threatened by some people who stole a necklace from him if he testifies against them. Józsika had a gold necklace that he received when he had a surgery for chest expansion. Attila feels that a lot of bad things happened at once. Mom also told me recently that Józsika also got a notification to serve in the military. At that time every young man served 2 years. Mom felt that Józsika was probably lonely without his brother.

The Accident

Talking to my Mom she felt that the whole thing did not make much sense as they were all supposed to go down to lake Balaton that Saturday. The accident happened Friday to Saturday early morning coming back from Lake Balaton at 5am. The car was going 275 km/hr. There were 3 people in the car, but interestingly they found a 4th person's keys as well and someone anonymously called the police. Attila and mom went to the location. It was a long straightaway until there was a turn to the right. That is where the car hit a dich with the car's nose then flew off about 20 meters. If it had been 3 meters before or 5 meters after they would have just run off the road without major injuries, but on the spot, they flew off there was a ditch. The car cut 2 trees in half. Attila described the trees being the width of a thigh. He found the back-license plate on the scene when they were looking around and kept it for a long time. The accident happened on M7 road in Hungary coming from Lake Balaton to Budapest around 42nd kilometers. Mom was also telling me that when she and Attila was driving down the first time there was a road barricade that created a detour from the going down to Balaton lane to the oncoming lane that is coming from Balaton. She was wondering if they could have had a car coming from the opposite side when the accident happened. We will never know. First Mom went to the hospital and that is where she found out that her brother died and there were 2 other survivors. The first day my mom could not go to the morgue to see her brother because of the investigation. She went back the next day to see and identify him. I cannot even imagine how difficult it must have been for her to identify her brother. My grandmother was in no condition to do any of the things that needed to be done, Mom took over all the coordination for the funeral. Of the 3 people that we know for sure who were in the car; one person walked away with no injuries, one had a head injury and never fully recovered. Józsika died from internal bleeding, his aorta broke in his chest. He was blamed for driving, but our family never believed he could have driven with such a high content of alcohol level in his body. He had so much alcohol in his body that he had to be passed out. Not that we thought anyway. The police did think otherwise but could never prove he drove. Did he really drive? I don't know. There were two others in the car. Two men, in their 30's at the time much older than him, kind of makes me wonder what they were doing hanging out with this young man hand letting him get so drunk and allegedly drive. Nice friends, right? He was the only one who died, the others survived with only minor injuries. He did not wear a seatbelt and flew out of the car. Mom told me that there is no way he drove. He did not have a license. He would not even drive Mom's car; he was afraid something might happen. He did not like to drive at all. He also had some vision problems Mom recalls, and he did not like to drive because of it. Attila did not know the other two people who were in the car. He saw them at the court hearing. At court they were trying to say that Józsika drove, then it was proven that he could have not driven. Still in the newspapers it said that he drove. It is still painful to write about this. Just found out that the court case was because the car they drove was stolen. Mom was telling me Józsika had a fight with his girlfriend, he was a little down and this could have been a precursor of going down to Lake Balaton with buddies to drink. It was kind of unusual behavior for him. I was too young to get that he was really gone. Józsika always made everybody feel good, made us laugh. I was always happy to see my uncles. He was our family glue. I asked my Mom what it about Józsika was. She said his love; he was able to show affection and love so well. He liked to give hugs. Mom feels this was a huge miss for my grandmother after he was gone. Things were just never the same after he was gone. We never recovered. Mom was telling me today that we almost lost my maternal grandmother (Nagy Borbála) after he died too.

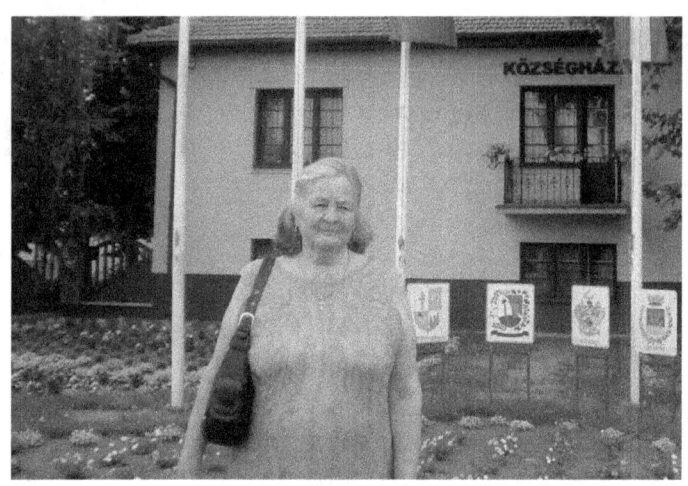

My grandmother Nagy Borbála, Jásszentlászló, Hungary 2011 – last time I saw her

I did not realize how sick my grandmother got. Thinking back, I remember now that she was not feeling well. Mom told me she had to be hospitalized in a psychiatric hospital for a while because of a nervous breakdown. I remember her crying and talking about my uncle a lot. It was hard to see, and I could not fully grasp the reality of it all. If I think of grandma now, I can still feel her pain, her loss. Loss of a child. I was in denial for a long, long time. I wanted my uncle back; I was angry for a long time why was he gone. He would do silly things like call my mom at 2 am to see if the windows need to be washed because he needed money. Mom said: "sure, come to wash the windows". It is amazing really how long a grieving process can go. It has been so long, and I am still grieving his loss. He was only 19 years old at the time. I still remember like it just happened, and this was over 34 years ago. I remember the funeral; my father took me. I remember Attila passing out during the funeral, he was as white as the wall. I went through the motions but did not really hit me until much later that he is really truly gone. Things like this do not just disappear from memory They stay and hang around for a long time. A loss of a child, a brother, a friend doesn't just rub off easily. There is a story to tell. A story about who József was, and what his life and death meant to all who have loved him and cared for him. I had a conversation with my Mom and asked her if she thinks there was anything, we could have done to prevent this accident. Mom said no. Once someone is dead their family will never have a chance to be part of that person's life. Mom felt like a contributing factor was that he was not able to continue school. My grandmother was raising the two boys on her own. She did not have enough money, so Józsika decided not to study but to go to work. Mom recalls a teacher coming by and asking my grandmother to send him back to school, he was so smart and a good kid. The teacher actually cried, begging my grandmother. Poverty. I did not realize that it hit my family, hit this close. Józsika decided to work to help out financially. He did labor work like doing packing and lifting boxes for big juice company. Even though school was free, money was not enough to pay for things. Their father did not help out at all at this point. My grandmother was starting to be sick and could not work as much as she did before. Mom really felt that a father figure would have helped a lot. She thinks that his death changed all of our lives significantly. Everything would be different if he would have lived. For a long time, I prayed and plead with God every day for some kind of sign that he is at peace or he is ok wherever he is. Then one day I saw him, in a dream, or vision. Since then I have more peace with his death, and I can feel his support and energy any time I need it. I think what happened to Józsika was a huge part of how I ended up working in addiction for so many years. Any loss of a family member is painful. It is like an and empty hole that can never be filled. Other parts of someone's life can be filled with love and joy, but that piece will always be missing.

3. GAME OF LIFE – SPIRITUALITY

Life and death. Spiritual beliefs. God. People we lose. Stories help paint a picture of what is happening to people who are dealing with addictions. My goal to raise awareness and create a conversation. Beth is a smart wonderful women, nurse, mother, wife, sister and daughter. She is great at taking care of others. Beth pays attention to details and makes sure everything is set for her patients and her family. I am very grateful for her for her willingness to share her story. Beth's brother Rick died from an overdose. He was way too young to die. Addiction can sneak up on anyone at any time. Beth was told that Rick died from drugs he got from his son's mother. This is so sad. His ex-girlfriend gave Rick the drugs. Beth feels very strongly about this and feels that Rick's ex should be held accountable for his death, accountable for murder. Should the person who is selling the drugs be held accountable? Is it the person who is selling or the person who is buying? Who is the responsible party for their own death? In addiction the brain is kind of hijacked and it is very difficult to think clearly and make good decisions. When a pharmacist or a doctor gives a wrong amount of medication, they are held responsible for a wrongful death. Should drunk drivers be held responsible for their own actions? The bartender is not getting in trouble for serving them with alcohol and letting them drive, nor the place they went for a party. It is difficult to decide who is ultimately responsible for Rick's death. The one who sold it to the ex-girlfriend? Rick's ex- girlfriend? The girl who was with him and did not call for help? Rick who took the drug? Others who knew he needed help, but did nothing? Drugs or alcohol, or any other substance that causes people harm can come out of nowhere and cause damage that is not reversable. There seem to be a new drug popping out frequently, for some people it is just a way to make money. Some get rich, some die. Beth she will never get her brother back. Life keeps throwing those curveballs at Beth. She tells me about her husband's drinking. Her nephew Larry is also into drugs, she had tried to help him. It did not work. She had to set up boundaries and does not have a relationship with Larry. Larry does call her grandmother, she bought him cigarettes before. Larry had lived with his grandmother before. Beth actually wrote out a contract with set rules and expectations if Larry was going to live there, included curfew, going to school or getting a job, doing chores, staying sober. Larry is on probation and he has always seemed to be in trouble. Did Larry ever really have a chance? His mother and father were both using drugs, his father died of an overdose. This is a lot to carry, a lot to grew up in and turn out ok, just think about the psychological effects. Larry still uses drugs. Beth does not trust him. He has been in and out of treatment. She still tries to support him. She feels she cannot make Larry better. It is very difficult when she tries to help somebody, and she can't. Beth describes heroin as being so powerful that she doesn't know how to help her nephew. Beth tells me that she would love to hear a success story of overcoming heroin addiction. That would give her hope that her nephew has a chance. The only time Larry talks to her is when he is in jail and wants money. As soon as he gets out, he disappears.

Beth's Older Brother

Beth also has an older brother Andrew who is homeless and has an addiction problem. Andrew used to be successful, he had his own business multiple times. Beth has no idea what drug Andrew uses. She can't reach him. She is scared for him. Andrew does not know how to cope, and Beth thinks when their younger brother died Andrew did not know how to cope with his death. She sometimes gets to see him, and they go for lunch. She describes Andrew as someone who has a very kind heart. Andrew does not talk about his use, but Beth knows he is using. Beth noticed how he has changed, the drugs changing him. She even offered to pay for treatment, but he denies he has a problem. It is very difficult to help someone who does not admit that they have a problem. How to help them? Beth would do anything to help her older brother. Her heart bleeds for him.

For some alcohol is just a game isn't it? It is really not. Sheila is an intelligent beautiful person. She described to me, she has many friends and family who are addicted to alcohol. One of her longtime friends becomes so aggressive and angry when he drinks that she had to cut ties with him and not to be around him anymore. She describes a relationship that is toxic, and even though she knows he could not control it became just too much and it really hurt her so that she had to stop seeing her friend. Avoiding him was very difficult for her for multiple reasons. It is hard to avoid a childhood friend. It causes pain for Sheila when she wanted to help but was not able to as her friend was not willing to change. It is very difficult to see a loved one destroying themselves. Many people might just think it is okay; they will just go home after work and have a nice relaxing evening with a glass of wine or a beer. This might actually work for some people but not all. There is a fine line between drinking occasionally, then drinking some nights, then drinking every night. Drinking can start very small and grow over time. I heard phrases like: "it makes me feel good". Additional comments I heard over the years included: "it helps me relax", or" everybody drinks". I was talking to a friend recently who told me that today's social norm is to drink alcohol and it is out of norm when someone does not drink. We went to a concert last weekend, there were drinks offered before the concert and during in the breaks and the lines were long. It was so weird, that having fun in a concert has to be associated with alcohol. Well, it probably it is "just fun" for a while at least, then reality kicks in again. During conversations with other people many of them felt that it is difficult not to drink when everybody else is drinking. All the reasons why people feel stressed, anxious, restless and want to relax with the use of alcohol or drugs will be still there the next hour the next day, the next month. The sad thing is that those reasons do not worth losing a life or becoming addicted. In the end of the day being grateful for what we have is what we should focus on. Problems are always there and always will be there. Some days are harder, some are easier.

Rory's Story

Spirituality. I was talking to Rory through a skype meeting that he invited me to attend with him for this interview. We talked around lunch time. He tells me a perspective that I did not really think about before. God and spirituality bring different things into different people's lives. Talking to Rory he does not believe in any Gods that are out there because he is gay and the religions that he describes do not like people who are gay. Rory rejects the higher power. Rory feels rejected by any God or belief because of who they are. Being rejected can send someone down all kinds of unhappy paths. Rory describes that all the organizations used some kind of spirituality that rejected him because he is homosexual and they told him what he is, a gay man, is wrong. Because of all this he had only the mental health side to support him in his recovery from stimulants.

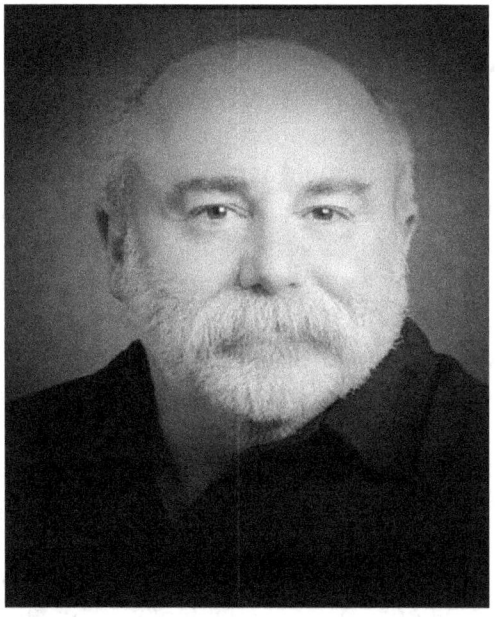

Rory in 2016, Oregon

Rory had been also diagnosed with so many mental health conditions that he did not even list them all. He told me: "you name it I had it". He saw his first psychiatrist when he was 8 years old. His parents were concerned that he will turn out to be homosexual. We laughed. Surprise, surprise he said. Still makes me smile. Let's look at some of the diagnoses he got: Bipolar disorder, bipolar rapid cycling, major depression, different anxiety disorders, personality disorders. He describes how with these diagnoses come a mountain of medications. He does not think that there is a medication that he did not put in his mouth. He laughs again. The medical and mental health system failed him, starting at such a young age. Wonder why? Starting at 8 years old. He was stuck, nobody helped him. The only way out at this point was to help himself. Rory went back to graduate school, learned psychology and educated himself. He learned about trauma, childhood history and how that affects how we feel about ourselves. He mentions Gabor Maté, MD and how much he likes him and talks about how he mentioned that all addictions are rooted in trauma. Rory describes that everyone he sits down with who was dealing with addiction had a trauma history and there is a connection. He feels like people can be in control of their lives and choose to be sober. He used the mental health system to support his sobriety. He feels like he does not want to be part of a group that does not support individual power and moving on, living their life and making their own choices. I asked Rory how he got clean. He said using just got boring. **Dope as he calls it did not get him high anymore, he called it "nope" so what is the point.** No more buzz, no more fun. No kick to it. Rory feels that for him it was not so much the drugs as the people. The people who were around drugs and alcohol took him back while "normies" did not. He describes: "hospitalized again, oh no problem". He felt comfortable around people who were just as wounded and hurt as he was. He fit in. He was so afraid of being alone, being lonely that drove him to even suicide multiple times. Rory feels he did dope because it kept people around. People would hang out with others if they had dope, he said. He was not alone anymore. He talks about growing up in the 70's and 80's in the culture where sexual encounters were counted, and amphetamines were the "street Viagra". He had been homeless, but he was ok with it. He does not feel that his story is sad or devastating. He survived all this. So many things could have gone wrong. He made it out. He tells me that when he was out on the street and homeless, he stopped using because he was afraid of being caught. He did not want to be stopped by the cops and being caught, while when he was in a house, home alone, the windows are closed, no one can see what is going on inside. Let's party he said.

  Fuchsia is a young energetic woman who visits me at our house, we sit on the porch and have a wonderful conversation. She tells me that she had a conversation with a friend who told her she feels that organized religion has a purpose and structure for those people who don't have the ability to question things or pursue things on their own. There are people who are not afraid to have their own thoughts and people who need to believe in something else; and for those people there is structure in religion. Fuchsia feels that there is so much judgment about addiction and people think that their way is right, and other ways are not. Fuchsia tells me about a friend who is struggling with this and has been repressing her sexuality because a promise they made to God when she was a child. Now she realizes she does not believe in judgement and why would she believe in a God who judges her for who she is.

Bill is a charismatic man who helps a lot of people in his community. I meet him in his office in a nice summer afternoon. He tells me that through his work he encounters people who deal with addiction issues or the effects of addictions all the time. People come to him looking for assistance. People usually know he does not have the way to help them break their addiction and doesn't have the physical means to help them separate from the behaviors, but they hope that it will be a safe place to tell their story, to be heard and process rather then look for an avenue to suppress or forget, or deny that addiction exists for them. People who walk into his office seem to have no visible means of support. They lack emotional and physical means to take care of themselves. Bill feels impotent when all he can do is give a listening ear and a few bucks. All that is available for him. He had volunteered in places like the warming centers and soup kitchens where people deal with addictions. We talked about loss and grief related to addictions. He explained to me that loss goes further than loss of life when it comes to addictions; it can be loss of relationships, property, freedom, self-esteem for example. Loss is a big part of addiction.

4. The Flow of Things

When someone looks at a river, one day it flows very smoothly, another can be deadly. Some places it will show down, some places it will speed up. Some places it will narrow and fall becoming a beautiful waterfall that also can be deadly to some, other places it will widen and open up to welcome another creek, river or the ocean. Riverbanks can be smooth with beaches and rough with deadly cliffs. Our everyday lives can be like a river some days, it is nice and flows without any issues and problems, then on other days it can be a hurdle of all kinds of stuff going on. Every day struggles can cause stress, anxiety, distress, hopelessness that create a ground for emotional pain and suffering. Everyone wants to feel good. Even if not all the time, but at least sometimes. This creates a great conflict and some people drink or take medications to feel better. Medications that are used and abused without a prescription. People also use and abuse prescription medications as well. This is all fine to do to smoothen the river, and when someone have to do it every day and starts to control their life it becomes a huge problem that goes out of control. Then every day becomes a deadly waterfall. Some days the river carries things floating on top, small branches are floating nicely with the river and do not cause any major problems. Bigger stumps are harder to move and might get stuck in places before they can move on again. Just like things in the river people can get stuck in certain places in their lives. It can be very difficult to break free from the mud and get moving with the river to enjoy the flow of life after being stuck for a long time. Judging the people who are stuck is also easy, helping them to dig deeper and trying to move branches of the big tree is much harder and might take months, years or the rest of one's life. Dealing with addiction and digging deep into our emotions is very difficult and painful work many times. It was difficult to see people who kept coming back to the hospital or coming back to treatment all the time. On the other hand, when they did not come back, we never knew what happened to them. Some patients would come back a year later or send a small gift to our unit or a card, so we would know they are ok. Those moments were the highlight of my day.

I talked to Kayla on the phone. She is a wonderful young woman who does great work to support her community. I asked Kayla how she feels about people who are dealing with addiction. She said her heart breaks for them. She wants to help all of them. Every single one. Could we just save everyone? We could give it our best shot. Are we doing it now? If it is another disease wouldn't we try everything we could to help? Kayla said: I wish I could bring people to see the light. She said:" just because someone is on the bottom right now, it does not mean that they cannot come back up". Give people support and provide hope. Just be there for them and don't give up. I recently talked to a wonderful writer and retired judge Neal Lemery, J.D. and he said the same thing, he wanted to make sure that I include in this book that **_HOPE IS THERE._** Neal wrote some wonderful books and there is one about mentoring young boys, the reference is at the end of this book.

5. Addiction - What is addiction?

What is addiction? What has been other people's experience? If someone would ask people randomly right now what addiction is what they would say? Beth told me she thinks addiction is when the body needs something, it's the brain signaling that it needs something that the individual cannot live without. Powerful, the brain is telling the person what to do. The individual affected becomes a whole separate person; the brain is in control. It can also be a genetic disease, something that people are were born with. She describes drugs as poison to the body. Beth also raised this during our conversation: **Does someone know that they have a problem if they are addicted to something?** She describes her drinking coffee and having chocolate. Is that an addiction? Do people know when they cross the line? I define crossing the line when an individual causes harm to themselves or others.

Having conversation with Sheila who has been working in nutrition. She said addiction is when people have an overwhelming need for something and are willing to do things that are not good for them, and it affects their social life, work life, or health. In any case, it is a negative effect for the individual. Sheila has been dealing with nicotine and sugar addiction in her life. She has now been nicotine free for 20 years, it has taken her many tries throughout the previous 20 years to stop smoking. Her husband is still trying to quit, and he has not been able to do so. Now she even hates the smell. She explained that smoking was extremely difficult to quit, and the motivation for her were her children. I am not here to talk about the professional definitions, anybody can look that up on the internet or in the dictionary. What does addiction mean to the person who is an addict? What does it mean to society? What does it mean to people whose life been touched by addiction or they know somebody who has addiction? It is a way different way to see someone in the street and say oh this is just a drunk; than having a father, mother or sister, brother, friend, grandparents; children suffer from alcoholism or any type of substance or drug addiction. There are of course many substances that are available for abuse today starting with food, cigarettes, vaping, different energy drinks and soda pops, alcohol, drugs including heroin, cocaine, methamphetamines, drugs used in anesthesia and that were banned, drugs that people can buy on the internet with a click of a button and many more coming in all forms types, sizes and shapes.

Edward works in a small rural community. He is passionate about helping others and making his community healthier. Talking to Edward he also mentioned that there are many different addictions, it is a broad topic, it goes beyond alcohol and opioids and some addictions might appear to be positive like running, sex, working, food, coffee, carbs, chocolate. It is a different level and continuum, but these addictions function in a similar fashion in the brain and it is important to have a discussion about it.

Substances can be abused in different ways, can be smoked, inhaled, snorted, injected, taped to the skin like Fentanyl, taken orally, rectally. Probably there are other ways too. Pills including prescribed opiates and benzodiazepines are easy just to pop in (as I have heard many times) or crush up and hard to keep count how many someone had taken when they are suffering from the disease of addiction. A pill might feel like all the pain in the world will go away. Then addiction kicks in and people just want one more and one more and one more. This is even harder when the medication is prescribed and the person thinks it is ok just to take one more, soon it will be more than just one extra pill. It will become two, three than even more, then prescriptions start to run out. Then what will happen, the doctor might or might not prescribe more so what the person will do when they are in pain and in distress and believe that need their medicine? They will do whatever means necessary to numb their pain. They will ask friends, buy off the streets. I was told by many people, the pills become too expensive and heroin or other substances are cheaper and the cycle begins. If this is all someone knows to numb the pain so of course the brain would say just take one more the pain will be better. They think that they will be happier. They will fall asleep, and do not feel what is going on in their life. Pain of living, any kind and anxiety, previous trauma, difficulty fitting in, mental health problems, stress can feel real. People who are trapped might not know that they are in a terrible cycle? Do they realize what is going on with them even if others tell them? Maybe they will, or maybe they will not, it is not easy to admit even if something is wrong. It is much easier to turn away and say: I am just fine. I just need my medicine to feel better. It is the person's truth even if others think they could deal with their pain in another way it is not their truth. It is very easy to say well why don't they do this or that.

Every day we can see the young and the old throwing their lives away deep into addiction. The shadows on the street that people do not want to see. They are there even if people pretend not to look. They are lost. All we can hope for that is we can touch their hearts and minds in some way that will give a drop of knowledge, hope for a future for them. Why should someone care? Should we just walk away? Should we show mercy? Can we just keep ignoring what is going on in our society? Can we ignore the pain? People sinking into the mud of addiction. What would they need to get out?

Mary is a passionate provider. She described her older brother to me as someone who has tried every drug there is to try. She was not sure if she would call him someone who is dealing with addiction. Mary also talked about a position where she provided direct service to people who dealt with addictions related to drugs and alcohol. Her clients were using substances to try to survive harsh living conditions. Something that had happened to them, living in a car, living with an abusive partner, or family member. Using substances become a tool to help them cope and mask the pain they endure. After a while this tool created more suffering and by then it is very hard to let go of the tool, the addictive behavior. People wanted to stop but were also scared of what they have to face once they stop. What is their trauma that they have to face on the other side? Many people Mary worked with were kind of stuck, so if somebody who is been drinking now let's say about 45 years old living in his car and tries to stop, have nobody to help or support, they are scared, what will happen when they stop. Their life will not just miraculously turn around. Mary felt many people felt pointless to stop they felt no hope for a normal life like having a job, having a house, it was out of their reach; so, then what is the point. People going through something like this feel absolutely alone and hopeless. They are already in pain, either before the addiction or now because of things they had done since they started using substances. Lack of hope.

Mary also tells me that she feels like addiction is a tool that people might start to use. Nobody thinks that they might start to use a tool then not be able to put it down. A tool to soothe the nervous system that has been hurt. Her analogy very interesting and thought provoking. People use this tool to try to navigate a difficult world when they have no access to other tools or skills. Lack of family support, lack of social support can create this when people are just trying to figure out how to be in this world. In the beginning Mary explained drugs and alcohol do make people feel more social, more confident, then addiction happens through the neuro-biological process. Then the process is being reinforced. Our brain is very complex as there are certain chemicals that play a role called dopamine, serotonin, natural opiates; these chemicals influence addiction, makes the choice to stop very difficult. Mary feels that people are being kept in a loop that different systems put around them.

    Addiction hurts a lot of people. I met a lot of people whose life was touched by the darkness of addiction. Even if they don't have someone in their family or friends, they hear about it, see it on the streets, and sooner or later they will know someone who went through addiction or currently dealing with it. There are many wonderful people out there who had been dealing with addiction or in the road to recovery. Addiction is a horrible disease affecting millions and billions of people around our globe. Addiction is everywhere. Our society is set up in a way that people in all of the classes are affected; even middle class and higher who have food on the table can become anxious and depressed over things; life is too much to handle for them at the specific time, or they just want to have fun. Prescription drugs don't help either. Many people become addicted after acute or chronic illness. It can be anyone at any time. People see medications around them for example in the advertisements, movies, shows, the neighbor's house. Some people want bigger and better even if they do not need bigger and better. There have been research studies that concluded more money and more things will not make people to be a happier person. Lack of community and support, seeking acceptance creates a major missing component in people's lives creating the anxiety and depression that moves them toward substance abuse. Many times, addiction can also be coupled with mental health problems where people self-medicate because they cannot get mental health care, or the side effects of the medications are intolerable to them. It does not help when the doctors start to prescribe benzodiazepines for anxious patients in the long term. Addiction touches many lives and as many of my patients told me opiates are making them feel good. Everyone wants to feel good. There is no harm in the beginning. Many people just feel good, still have jobs, have their family, house it is all good. But then of course those things will be lost if addiction continues. It is a lifelong journey, many had been down that road it is hard to come back, hard to resist and it is an everyday struggle.

Sheila describes addiction as an illness. Seeking happiness and acceptance and the fear of not being accepted by others creates a loop in many people's lives. Imagine it like a missing link that people will try to fill with whatever they can to feel better. It might not start that way in the beginning, but then pills and drinks will get out of control in time. Many people recognize that they do not want to take the pills, drugs or alcohol anymore, but also do not know how to stop. The brain is very powerful, once it knows what makes it feel good, it wants and wants more even if it causes distraction for the individual. No matter the cost. Craves and wants more and more frequently. Different social classes have anxiety and acceptance issues about different things, but anyone can end up with addiction. What could help? Every person is different and what motivates them could be different too. Additionally, social support to decrease social anxiety can be helpful; working on creating supportive communities, prevention, coping skills from a very early age. Environments where social connections are without substances at all levels of the social spectrum; and decrease the self-thought negative feelings could help decrease anxiety and fear in people thus decreasing the chance for addiction.

There are many questions relating addiction. Everybody's truth can be different. People might agree or disagree and that is fine. Why is addiction important? Why should we care? Why do people do what they do? Why do people who use substances hurt people? They are just homeless bums, aren't they? I heard this and similar comments so many times. Why don't people who deal with addiction appreciate life? How can they just throw away everything? Why do they hurt the people who love them? They don't want help; they just want to have fun. They go out and use the drugs don't care about anybody and anything. Are addicts as happy and careless people? Are drugs worth throwing their life away? Do they want to die? Why don't they know any better? Are people who use drugs, or any substances any happier? Not what I have seen, not what I have heard. People dealing with addiction have moments of happiness the same way we all have moments of happiness. All of us want to be happy. Being someone who is using substances is not fun at all. People can only think this is fun if they are a crazy careless human being who have no idea what they are talking about. Some people are and blinded by their own misperceptions and stupid interpretations of what addiction is. I have watched hundreds to thousands of people in the streets and patients in the hospital, in treatment, in clinics, in the community who struggle with addiction. Can people really think they can step into their shoes and know what is going on in their head? All of us are different. Can someone really know the entire trauma a person suffered? It is a true catastrophe; when someone's mind is being taken over by a substance so that they don't have a free will of self anymore. Imagine: Having a fight continuously between conscious life and unconsciousness. **A struggle between the** one place that should fight for someone; their brain turning against them and telling them that all they need is some more drugs to feel better. Sounds like so much fun and happiness. Addiction is a constant fight to survive and say no or yes for every day, from hour to hour, minute by minute for the rest of someone's life. **Only the person affected by addiction really knows their own horror and what they are going through in their disease process.** Why would anyone really want to be an addict? It is not a choice, it happens, then people get stuck in a terrible cycle and cannot get out. Does anyone wake up in the morning and say ok I want to be an addict now. This is my life goal. Does a child who had an addicted mother, father, aunt or a friend who started them on drugs or alcohol from conception in the womb or at age 5, 8 or 10 or 13 really have any choice? Yet, people judge, when they have no idea. How can someone look at a child who now become an adult suffering in the terrible cycle and tell them "well they are just an addict, they don't care; they are nothing"? How would they know any other life? If this has been their life since they can remember? Anybody who have not touched by addiction is privileged. People have no idea how lucky they are if they don't have any addiction problems. The people who are struggling with this disease are sick and need our help every day every hour every minute or they can and will die without support, love and caring. Many people have no choice and struggle every day, and many have no one to love of care for them. It is easy to move away and think this is someone else's problem. We live in this society together; addiction is everyone's problem. Please be kind. Think about the story behind the person. Help. Should anybody die just because they are trapped in a terrible disease? Is that justified? Is that fair? People could say: Why should we care? Society should care. Governments should care. Friends and family should care. The world should care. What can we do to stop this cycle?

    Talking to Mary she described to me that while most of her family had dealt with addictions from drugs to alcohol and she grew up in it and even tried some things, she never got caught up in the drugs. She just felt it was a waste of her time. Makes me wonder why some people are more susceptible to addiction then others. I was never drawn into drinking or trying anything that might alter my perception, the thought that I don't act like myself is scary to me. I have seen many people caught up in addiction, and they had no idea what they were talking about the previous day when they were under the influence of substances of drugs or alcohol.

    Edward was telling me that he is lucky in a way that there is no addiction in his immediate family or friends, some of his distant family he knows have had a problem with alcohol but does not know intimate details about the issue. He hears a lot about addiction at work but does not directly work with addiction. He hears a lot about the opioid crisis, that is a public health issue and needs to be addressed. Edward defines addiction when the physical body takes over the mental body overpowers it to become satisfied with whatever chemical it happens to be. There is very little control after that because it is more of the bodily or physical response then emotional or mental control. Had a discussion about this with Edward, he is thinking about the brain that is cognitive and logical. The brain that is usually in control, but not this time. Not during addiction. The brain gets hijacked when using drugs. Edward feels that some people have greater propensity to addiction then others, we also had a discussion about who is responsible to support the individual once the addiction took over. If the brain is hijacked, then is it really the individual's responsibility to try to get help? Would they even be able too?

Addiction can strike in many different ways, losing finances can be one consequence. Dr. Tedd Levin who has been a physician in family medicine was telling me a story about 2 people who spent $ 50,000 a year to support their cocaine addiction, and lost everything they had, including their home. He also describes a lot of overlap between mental illness and addiction. He had a lot of experience working with youth. Working as a center physician for Job Corps youth for 17 years he has seen lots of young people between 16-25 years old who have been in multiple rehabs for treatment of addiction, and multiple psychiatric hospitalizations. He describes that it is difficult to figure out if it is a drug induced psychosis or a primary mental illness that the patient is going through such as schizophrenia or bipolar disorder. Dr. Tedd Levin feels that all type of addictions are very tough to treat. We had a conversation about smoking and how smoking has been declining, but now a new thing coming up like vaping. There is always something new comes up. We discussed obesity and the consequences related to obesity. Addictions are tough no matter what the choice is alcohol, drugs, smoking or food.

Detachment. This is what Angel told me during our conversation. Addiction caused detachment in her family from both of her brothers. Even though now they are doing better the relationship was estranged because of addiction. The hardest part she said was watching her parents going through self-questioning what went wrong. They raised 4 children all the same way, two got touched by addiction the other two did not. She describes a nephew who is in prison right now for armed robbery because of a drug deal. He is 23 years old. Angel feels that she as many others feel that jail in not necessarily a bad thing because at least their loved ones are safe and not using. During our conversation I asked Angel what she thinks addiction is. She laughed. Not sure why but we both busted out laughing. Maybe because our conversation has been hard, and we just needed a laugh so we can go on. She said that this is so hard. It is so complex. She describes herself as a person who believes in moderation. She believes in a Bell-curve from biology, to be in the middle. She would enjoy a piece of cake but would not eat the whole thing. Addiction she notes slips into the extreme to either end either completely denying something or overindulging to cover something else up. Addiction is when alcohol, drugs, games, social media, eating, whatever it is, when that becomes the center point of someone's life and their decisions are made based on those things; that she felt is the moment when people get into those extremes. Angel described that when anything becomes the focal point of someone's life it becomes unhealthy even if it is their job. I asked Paige what addiction means for her. She said she thinks it is something someone cannot live without.

    Jason works at a police department. He had a lot of experience in his personal and professional life when it comes to addiction. He talked about his mom using alcohol and prescription drugs when he was growing up. He describes addiction as something that had killed his mother from inside out. He remembers her as a wonderful mother. It was difficult for the family, they worried about her. She had suicidal tendencies and Jason taking turns with his 4 other siblings took care of her. Jason thinks that seeing his mother dealing with addiction is what made him become a police officer. He feels that because of his personal experience he can understand and comprehend what the people with addiction and their families are going through. His mom passed away 15 years ago while in treatment due to a heart attack. She was 63 years old. Jason describes addiction as a sickness that can affect anybody. It can control someone's life and take over how they act. Including anger, stealing, lying that comes with feeding the habit of addiction. Jason recalls going to the doctor appointment with his mother and she would ask for more pain medication when she did not really need it. Kayla describes addiction as a lack of having something. Unhealthy series of behaviors. Getting to a certain point where someone is going to an extreme to find a certain feeling, mentality of physical state. Willing to do anything to get there.

    Addiction can be different for everyone. Rory who is currently works as a counselor and has his own practice went through different types of addictions himself. He describes it as being a person who was addicted to things on and off would use something, then become sober then use something else. He mostly used stimulants; he describes stimulants as something that was always very appealing to him. He had three DUI's (Driving under the influence of drugs or alcohol) as a consequence of using. Although he had friends that AA worked well for, he did not believe God and a higher power and rejected the idea of going to AA meetings. Rory defines addiction as a surrender of control. Something that is foundationally caused by trauma. He tells me a story about this. He was sexually molested when he was 8 years old by a 13-year-old boy. He did not understand at that time what was going on, neither did he feel ashamed. It was years later he understood how that was not appropriate. He was more afraid of what his mother would think that he is trying to fool around with an older boy. He still remembers his name. He wonders what his story was. He did not really understand what was going on and he was disappointed that this boy did not want to be his friend anymore after that incident. Rory also describes another story when he was 6 years old and his uncle came to live with them. His uncle was promoting sexual behavior among the neighborhood boys at a local fort. His uncle got into trouble for this before that is why he had to move away from his grandmother's house. Rory was exposed to a lot of sexual behaviors from a very early age. He describes that this exposure and amphetamines felt good. Felt better than the shame he felt growing up in a fundamentalist tradition as he describes that told him he will go to hell. He felt there was no hope. He felt that there was no hope since he was 8 years old. Then he said why not party if there is no hope anyway. Loss of control.

    Tracy describes addiction as when something else takes over. It takes over the mind, and the body. An addict can't stop, no matter what. Can't go anywhere else. People can be addicted to a lot of different things. She feels like we all probably have some kind of addiction. She describes her teens as playing video games, or with cell phones. Addiction just takes over; it changes who the person is. It takes people down on a negative path. Diana describes addiction as the inability to accept and act on life in a good and productive way, so people find another way to get through the day or a week and they turn to what seems the easiest. Then they are hooked, and it turns out not to be the easiest. Just trying to deal with daily lives does not work. Then people try to find something that they think will help them. No matter what others say that this isn't good, they will not listen and just follow what they know to feel good. She feels that the tendency it is in families. She worries about her grandkids because of this, hoping they don't fall into any addictive behaviors in the future. Chloe describes addiction as a compulsive need to do something over and over again. No strength to stop even if willingness is there. Michelle tells me that in addiction the body's needs for the chemical that is now being created. (by using whatever the person is using at the time) A force that is created that impacts what people do and the decisions they make. Addiction takes over that people don't have control over their life anymore.

    Ron talks about addiction in the little town he lives in now and asserts that for such a small rural touristy town there is a lot of addiction that can be found here. Ron works as a nurse at a clinic. He has never seen a small town with so many heroin and meth users. He supports marijuana use. He saw a lot of opiate addiction. It keeps surprising him how much is going on in a small town. He has a lot of friends from south Florida who used meth, cocaine and alcohol. He talks about a guy he lived with that he knew for decades. They were social friends. They ended up moving in together for a while. Everything was great for a while, then his friend started to get into the meth crowd. It was very popular then. This was around 2008-2009. Things started to go very "wonky". As time went by and his friend was doing more clubbing and using meth, he started to do very weird things. He started to get paranoid. He thought people are watching him and getting signals through the appliances in the house and the neighbor next door is one of "them". (whoever they are). Consequently, Ron said he found a way to get into the wall space between the two condos and he would spy on the neighbor. The neighbor could hear him walking in the space between the condos. One day he took the electric pencil sharpener apart and was showing Ron proof that "they" came into the house and reconfigured the electronics of the pencil sharpener. He was showing Ron how they are transmitting signals through it. Ron told him it looks like a pencil sharpener that was taken apart. He would get very frustrated with Ron because Ron did not see what he saw. His friends did not see it. He slowly thought his friends were watching him and doing things because they did not play along in his fantasy. It became more and more bizarre and less rational and stable; he began to have financial problems because he spent money on meth but not paying bills. Ron came home one day, and his friend handed him a battery charger that was Ron's; it was wet. Ron asked why is it wet? His friend said he had to throw it into the toilet, it was the only way they would stop sending signals. Ron was like, oh, this is bad. All this happened in south Florida where air conditioning is essential. It is hot and humid. Ron thought "we are on a rollercoaster now". He would come home and find his friend covering up the windows and doors with black tarp and plastic taped on. His friend thought that "they are" in the parking lot watching him. It was dark in the apartment. Ron, at this point started to plan to escape. Ron was one of the last one's he was not one of them yet. The circle of friends was getting smaller and now the inner circle of friends was even getting smaller. He was at the deep end. The friends tried interventions, but it did not work. He elected to keep doing meth. One-night Ron's date was afraid to stay over, because his friend was getting very weird. Ron was planning to move out as soon as he could. At night Ron when was sleeping his friend barged in woke him up and asked him who he was talking to. Ron said he was sleeping. He insisted Ron was talking to somebody. He told Ron: "I know that you are talking to them now". At that point Ron become one of them, he was fearing for his safety. He came home the next day, and his key wouldn't open the door. His friend locked him out and told him he cannot come back there anymore. He allowed him to come back on Saturday between 9-11 to get his stuff. Ron was actually glad to be out of there. This event made him move sooner than later. He went from a very good friend to a mentally disturbed person. His friend ended up selling the condo. He moved away and eventually got into rehab and got sober. Ron said we will always be fine. He had not heard from his friend now for about 7-8 years. He was one of those people who got wrapped up in this destroying lifestyle. Ron witnessed this transformation from someone normal with a lot of friends and being popular to this "monster". It was very sad. His friend took the refrigerator and the oven apart, took the air conditioner apart. Ron would tell others these stories and it sounded fictional, but it was not. He would go home and there was no air conditioning. Ron was glad he did not become one of "them" until the end. Ron was telling me a lot of people were dying at this time in South Florida from using meth, overdosing, committing suicide. Ron would talk to other people who confirmed what was common in meth use: voices in the walls, signals from appliances. Ron calls this story: "My roommate from hell". He can laugh about it now, it was sad, but also funny, the things he did was crazy, sad and funny at the same time. The recovery was very hard for his friend from being a meth addict to become a normal person again. It cost a lot of money. All his resources went to getting sober. He got so caught up in the addiction that he did not realize what was going on. He got into it because of the social community around him. It was a party scene town especially in the gay community. Coming from non-acceptance in family or the community. That group become a chemical community, sense of belonging, become a social activity that sucked people in. Ron felt that people got really wrapped up in the party drugs and sex. Sex was a big focus too.

Ron describes addiction as comfort food. It is a way for people to interact, belong, be supported. He compares escape to a peanut butter and jelly sandwich at night. I asked him what is the escape from? He said: pressures, sanity, responsibility. **It is easier for people he saw to be a meth using sex addict then to be a responsible person in the real world.** Joel describes addiction as beyond needing something to get by, losing control over a thought process where a person cannot make another choice besides to follow the addiction what they are driven by. Something that would create a detriment and exclusion of other things. Inability to think rationally about something.

Joel came to visit me in a nice sunny afternoon. She is a care provider. We had a discussion on wine, she describes not drinking much before she met her husband. Now, they have a bottle of wine every few days, that is his lifestyle she said. She does a check in with herself about this especially with the history of her family. It is a fear she has; she does not want to tip over to the addiction side. So, what is that mean? We talked about could she and he stop if they wanted too? Can they go a weekend without drinking wine? She is trying to self-evaluate what is this means for her. Is it a need to have it for things to function she asks? She talks about replacing it with something else maybe going to the gym in the morning instead and going to bed early. She feels like if someone stops doing something, they need to replace it with something else. Where is the point of no return? Having a glass of wine with dinner is ok Joel feels. We talked about food, bread and cheese, Joel was off of bread for a year, now she has some, she said she was strong then not as much now and she don't fit the clothes she wore last year. We talked about if we want to, can we stay off of it? Can we say no to bread for a week or longer? Do we absolutely have to have it, or can we survive without it?

    Janett feels like addiction is habitually doing something that is bad for the person. Physically, emotionally and/or also bad for our relationships with other people. This is the gauge Janett uses like with her aunt. It is affecting her health and relationships. It is an addiction. If people do too much of something sometimes it does not necessarily mean it is an addiction. If it is affecting our life and relationship with other people and they are continuing to do it then it is obviously out of control Janett asserts. She laughs and said any sane person would stop doing it if it affects those things.

    Talking to Bernadette, she describes a lot of addiction in her family. She had been dealing with addiction in her whole life. Both of her parents were dealing with addiction, lots of family members including her brother. Her father had been drinking a lot, he developed cirrhosis of the liver, he started to develop ascites in his abdomen and turned yellow, so he had to stop drinking or he would have died. He gave up alcohol, but smokes pot. He might do other things; Bernadette was not sure. Her mom was a binge drinker and smoker, become an alcoholic when she was about high school age, her mom was in her 30's. Bernadette's mom also smoked for 40 years, she started smoking in her teens. Her mom developed COPD (Chronic Obstructive Pulmonary Disease) had to be on oxygen all the time, when this happened, she stopped smoking and drinking. Later she developed lung and brain cancer. Bernadette recalls that drinking first was fun for her mother but not for long, alcohol stopped working and she became "pathetic" and hated herself, she had a lot of self-loathing. She would fall down drunk. This made Bernadette feel very sad, she just wanted her mom not to do this to herself and not to hate herself. Bernadette was angry and mad at her mom in the beginning, then she accepted that if her mom wants to drink and smoke and that is how she wants to die, it is her choice. At that point she would get mad when her mom was lying or manipulating. Her mom would say she is not smoking then stuff cigarette buds down the toilet and clog the toilet. Bernadette calls this a very teenage behavior. She really wanted her mom not to hide what was going on and not lie. Her mom would not show up and lie that she had pneumonia when she was hung over. She would say she was sick when she was not. She just wanted her mom to be honest and not lie to her. Talking about it is still upsetting for Bernadette, I can hear it in her voice. She also spent the majority of her career working with people who were addicted to substances, she has been severely affected by addiction. Her brother is deep into addiction, so she lost contact with him for a while. Last year they had to connect because their mother was dying of brain cancer. This was the fourth time. This is when she learned that her brother drank his way through the marriage he had, he is been a binge drinker and was hiding it. He was a youth pastor at a Baptist college. He was living a double life. He was verbally and emotionally abusive to Bernadette when their mom was dying. She did not know her brother was capable of the things he did. He was abusive and accusative in person, in e-mails, in texts. He was telling lies and doing bizarre things like attacking his sister. She describes him as having a cocky personality coupled with being super religiousness. Bernadette had been in Al-Anon for 23 years dealing with the addiction her parents had and from previous relationships. She had relationships with people who were active alcoholics. Because of her experience in Al-Anon she was able to figure out her brother's behavior pretty quickly when it was happening. The behavior got really bad, she had to block him on her phone and social media. This made Bernadette feel pretty alone, it was just him and her left from the family. At her work Bernadette saw families having a hard time with their loved ones dealing with addiction. She saw sadness, hopelessness, sadness. In an education setting she saw students trying to get better. Other students who use substances stop coming to class. A good motivation she saw for college students to get sober is just wanting to be better parents for their kids, or finally just decided to address their lives to get better. Bernadette tells me about her parents, they are from a small town. She tells me that many times in small towns kids just drink, because there is not much else to do, she lives in a small rural community now too, and people drink a lot. Lots of people she knows whom her parents age would drink themselves to death. Lack of opportunity. She describes addiction as the inability to quit. If someone is an alcoholic it is a first drink that gets them drunk.

Chelsea is an inspirational and caring person. She describes addiction as any type of behavior that is done in excess. It is causing distraction in someone's life or causing bad outcomes. Albert feels addiction is hopelessness mostly, numbness. It seems to Albert that a lot of people he talked to after they are clean for 2-3 months, they are surprised about all the feelings they are having. Albert feels they buried their feelings before to mask things. He sees a lot of people coming back after 2-3 months and saying they could not handle all the feelings and other stuff they were dealing with so now they are in trouble again, back in the system. I asked Albert why they could not handle it what had happened, do they tell him? He tells me sometimes people get overwhelmed, coming out of numbness now they have to deal with recovery and learn how to function in society again. It is hard. If someone is not used to that and are out of it for a while and now have to do it again people get overwhelmed and slip back sometime. Albert also tells me that he believes that there are some people out there using drugs for just fun, but it is also really easy to spiral down from that when things go bad. Era describes addiction as a habit combined with emptiness or something that is missing from inside, something that is lacking in someone's life and turns into habit. She describes addiction as a branch on the tree. A person might think they can pull themselves up, they can't. They get into deeper and deeper every day. One day the branch breaks and they can lose everything financially, spiritually. They lose their family.

Dr. Frazier Beatty describes addiction as a loophole state, or a chronic disease. He tells me that we cannot look at someone and tell that they have diabetes. He feels that addiction is one of those things that had been missed, misdiagnosed neurologically or in the brain. He feels like the tendency to addiction is to fill that void that is missing in the person. He was not sure. He definitely felt that addiction is more of a disease, that gets misdiagnosed or misdescribed because he does not think it is a chemical that causes a problem but a neurological issue. He describes to me people feeling a certain way about themselves then using a drug to numb the pain. Dr. Beatty describes that he met people who had a lot of mental health problems that caused shame, and a lot of people use substances to make them feel better. It can also be a reckless sexual behavior as well, that could be someone's drug he adds. Brenda tells me she sees addiction as a behavior that becomes prominent in a person's life. The person gets some type of benefit from the addiction. It might not be positive, but a benefit regardless. The benefit can be a "high", dealing with anxiety, it becomes encompassing in their life where to be able to get whatever they are addicted to them, they are willing to make poor choices that affect relationships and their own lifestyle.

Susan describes addiction when someone is not able to enjoy life the way it is, hide from something. She feels that people get so into it that they can't see that that is why they are doing it. Then they can't remember what life is without substances. They just keep falling more into it. Susan had a little uncertainty about how to describe addiction. Dolores feels addiction is an unhealthy reliance on substances to get a person through the day. She tells me that the unhealthy part is the issue, it affects people's life in a negative way. Dolores tells me about chemical reactions in the brain that occur when someone take any addictive substances. The brain will continue to promote to keep taking those substances and do those activities. She mostly thinks about addictions as drug and alcohol.

Sitting on the porch with a nice August afternoon I have a conversation with Bob. He tells me he has seen changes of behavior of co-workers and people around him when they drink or use other substances. I ask him what the changes were that he noticed. He noticed agitation, shorter attention span or just being short with other people. He tells me that can be frustrating in a workplace. He feels peer pressure can be a big thing, something people do in a group in bars, parties, he feels it is pretty engrained. I ask him how he feels about that. He said it is too bad that it is the way it is. I ask Bob what addiction means to him based on his experiences. He thinks about it a bit. Then he tells me doing something that is a mistake that people know it is a mistake, yet the person still is having some compulsion to keep doing it again. He tells me it even can be a good thing, just if it is done excessively. I ask him what he means. He gives me some examples. He tells me we need carbs to survive but too much can lead to obesity or diabetes. He talks about general addiction to sugary things. We take a moment to acknowledge that this can be very hard in our society today. It can be anything he said. He knows some people who are dealing with addiction. He could tell from people's behavior. He feels that they are in a loop. Bob also tells me that people might be using drugs and substances to cover up deep trauma and pain. Interestingly when I ask Bob why he thinks people would use substances to cover up things, he tells me he imagines it being more exciting than being at home and taking a pill. People are able to go out and party or hang out with friends. More sociable, more enjoyable especially if someone is depressed. We discuss coping skills. He also feels like that some people are using drugs and drinking because all this had been done through generations and that is the coping they know.

6. MIKE'S AND TRACI'S STORY

I went to Mike and Traci's house on a nice summer evening. We had been texting and calling back and forth for a while to arrange the time. When I got to the house, I received a wonderful welcome by Traci, her temporary foster child Alexi and their puppy. Mike was not home, yet he works as a Paramedic and was getting home any moment. While waiting for him Traci invited me into the kitchen where she and Alexi were preparing dinner. I was sitting and watching by the kitchen counter, listening to light music and Traci was asking me questions about the book, the purpose of the book and some of my experiences so far. She was also teaching Alexi how to properly cut with a knife. It was very nice and relaxing to watch them and we had a wonderful discussion. Mike arrived within 20 minutes or so and we all sat around the dining room table. This was the first time when I sat down with more than one person at the time to discuss their experiences. It ended up being a wonderful and amazing experience. We would go back and forth sharing experiences. There was sadness, tears, happiness, laughter and even a prayer together. We all forgot dinner and talked for over 3 hours. I left their house just before 11PM. When I first asked about experiences in addiction Mike starts to tell me about his encounters. Mike grew up with his brothers being addicted to drugs, methamphetamines and pot, alcohol, they been through the whole gambit. Mike is the oldest of 5 brothers and a sister. I asked Mike more about his brothers. One of his brothers started smoking pot at a very early age 7-8 years old. Addiction started to progress from there. Mike assertively told me that nowadays people say that pot is not a gateway to addictions, but it is because it lowers inhibition. He feels very strongly about this. Mike never got into that scene. His brother was using pot, then alcohol; then he progressed into other stuff.

John's Story – Somalia

Mike's other brother John did the same thing, he got into meth. John was diagnosed being bipolar at an early age. The addiction did not bear its ugly head until John got back from Somalia. Mike describes a real change in him after he got back. He was in the Marine

Corp; he was 25 years old. John was there during the Black Hawk Down crisis in 1993. This was a horrible situation for everyone. Loss of lives, lots of injuries with a battle that was never supposed to happen, was never planned and happened anyway. Troops taking fire and John had no option but to fire back. Imagine the pressure that they had only seconds to decide to shoot or be killed. Traci asks Mike if John's turning to drugs was PTSD (Post Traumatic Stress Disorder)? It might have been Mike said, there were things that went down that his brother can never forgive himself. John had to make a very difficult choice and shot back. He was out on point and over there it is either shoot or be killed. He was being shot at and he had no choice but to shoot back. PTSD is inevitable in these situations, definitely. When John got back Mike continues, he dealt with the PTSD by going to alcohol and drugs. I asked Mike if John ever talks about his struggles with him. He does not. John was able to finally now get to a point where he is controlled with medications, he does not have those addictions anymore as far as Mike knows. I asked Mike how long it took John to get out of the addictions. Easily 15 years he said. He ended up in jail. He was in jail for 5-6 years. He straightened up in there. Mike helped him in the past. John came for help this last time after getting out of jail and Mike told him this will be the last time he helps. Mike and Traci outfitted him, took him where he wanted to go, dropped him off. They helped John go back to a base where he can start again. He lives in Oregon now and managing construction crews. John is now doing well. He was able to get out of his addition.

Mike's brother Rob's accident

Mike then tells me about his other brother Rob. Rob is still smoking pot and he lives in a trailer on Mike's sister's property. Rob has his alcohol and marijuana and that is his life. Mike sounded sad telling me this. He repeats it a few times. That is Rob's life, work, alcohol, marijuana. Rob had an accident where he took half of his face off when he was high on drugs around age 32 or 34. Mike was not sure. Rob was trying to prove a point. He was high on drugs and it did not turn out well. Someone told him he couldn't get a small tire on a big rim; he forced the small tire on the big rim to prove a point that it can be done. It became like a rubber band and shot the rim up into his face. Broke a big 8 by 8 beam that was 20 feet up in the air, shattered it. He lost his eye; he suffered a brain injury, so his mentality is now about of a 15-year-old. He can work. His mouth gets him into trouble Mike said, he has that adolescent mouth so there are no filters.

    Mike's dad also had addiction to alcohol. He has his own stories. It took a lot for him to sober up, until Mike's mom was threatening to walk out. He was addicted for the longest time to alcohol. He did not touch the hard stuff. Occasionally now he might have a sip of a beer but even that he does not tolerate any more. Mike tells me if his dad touches the hard stuff, he would not come back from it. I ask Mike how this affected him growing up? Being the oldest he tells me he became the young adult in the family. Mike tells me that he did not get a chance to be a kid. His voice changes here. There is resentment. He had to do things a certain way or there were consequences for him. His dad understands it now that that was not a right path, and Mike now calls him a great guy. His dad's story involves a car accident and a death. Mike tells me that there were multiple times where his dad should have been killed, but never did. He is a minister now. While all this going on with Mike's brothers John and Rob Mike is dealing with his own issues of abuse. Mike suffered emotional and psychological abuse from his ex-wife. He didn't go into a lot of what was happening to his brother. It did affect his relationship with his brothers. Mike does not want few of his brothers to know where he lives. It is very sad. They knew where Mike had lived in the past and he had stuff disappear. Things that were very important to Mike. I can see this still bothers him, things that his grandfather left him. Some of his weapons had disappeared. He does not want to go through that again. It is very unfortunate he tells me.

    Mike tells me his biggest thing when it comes to addictions is food. He tells me he loves food. We laugh and we all agree that we all love food and it is difficult to get away from food. It was a nice relief after hearing the tough stories about his brothers. Mike tells me is that is hard for him to try to figure out limitations with food. Figuring out what he can and can't eat as he gets older. He tells me he put on a little weight he points to his stomach; he makes me laugh. ***The biggest thing is knowing when to stop.*** We have a conversation about not eating foods that have sugar and corn syrup. The doctor recommended Mike and Traci to do the Keto food, not the Keto diet. He tells me that food is actually very good. They were doing it for a while. His favorite keto food is chicken cutlets or the pork. Traci laughs and tells me she likes all food. Makes me laugh again. The room sparkles for a moment. Traci likes vegetables, and/or a great steak. She loves vegetables. Mike tells me the thing is with the keto thing they cannot have corn, potatoes, bananas, starch, beans, or rice. We had a conversation about different diets, research and books. We talked about plate sizes in Europe, sizes of meat, having smaller portions. We all agreed that the more vegetables, fruits and nuts we eat the better for our body. Then Traci said it is also better for the planet. We laugh again. It was a very lively fun conversation, kind of lightened up the mood a little. People in general get excited about food. Mike thinks for him it would be easy to get pulled into alcohol because he likes it, and he could go without it, he tells me he does not need it. There are different bottles of alcohol in the home. They are in a small cart next to the dining room. Mike tells me it is nice to have it every now and then. Then Traci asks me if I want to know what she thinks his addiction is. Traci then said: TV and noise. Mike tells me he never thought about it. Traci adds that as soon as Mike walks in, he wants the TV on. He wants to fall sleep to the TV at night, he likes the noise. Traci feels like that is an addiction. Mike is a little taken back based on his reaction. He never thought about it this way. He tells me he can sit quietly but only up to a point then it "drives him insane". No, he can't Traci adds. He has to be on his Facebook. Sorry, Traci said to Mike:" I am telling on you". Another addiction he has is he wants to hear the news and wants to see all the stories that people post that he can immediately say, did you hear about Iraq? Did you hear about the shooting? Did you hear about that plane that went down? Did you hear? Traci said it drives her nuts. He wants to be in the know. Traci is not saying it is a bad thing, but she tells me it is hard for Mike to be anywhere and not to be on his phone or trying to get information from a source. Mike tells me he goes out to the barn and listens to music. At this point he seems a little puzzled and family reassures him that they love him. He tells me he has had earphones on to do yard work.

We have a discussion about music and positive benefits. Then we talk about social media and the youth.

Mike's Work Experience

In the last 20 years Mike has been in the EMS (Emergency medical Services) field and has been dealing with the results of drug use. He had also been teaching various classes about addictions. As part of being a paramedic he is also part of trauma nurses talk tough (an educational training). It is not supported in his current community because of money he thinks. People have been telling Mike he is too graphic with his material. At this point the whole house smells like garlic. It smells wonderful. We all acknowledge the wonderful smell of garlic. Mike continues; he feels he is not too graphic; this is reality. He tells people if they want their kids to grow up and understand consequences of their actions this is what they have to deal with. In his program he goes over alcohol addiction, drug addiction, meth use, pot use, safety, seat belt use, distracted drivers. He used to talk to the hospital for minors and possessions. He had a class for younger kids and one for the older kids. He would go through actual stories of people who made bad choices and consequences and how it affects the body. Kids would tell him that they can't get addicted and overdose on pot. He would tell them:" yes they can". His slides show that it is not just certain individuals, it is everybody, all classes. He tells me about one group of slides involving a nurse and a firefighter and their daughter who dies. He shows me a picture of a beautiful young girl. It affects everybody. Some stories come from personal experience. Mike adds that **the biggest thing about addiction is people think it is my problem, so it is not going to hurt anybody else.** He tells me that we know that that is not true. He talked to kids before prom in high schools. Some of the kids laugh, they think it cannot happen to them. Mike has seen lots of these attitudes, kids thinking it is not going to happen to them, until it does. Mike talks about who is affected by an emergency situation related to substance abuse. He tells me about effects on first responders, he has seen decapitations, he has seen impalements because of the choices people make. The first responder is deeply affected by these things, the police, the nurses, the fire department, mom, dad, brothers, sisters, cousins, grandma, grandpa, it affects everybody. EMS is the best job in the world, Mike loves it. The problem is that people do have their ghosts. The ghosts, he tells me are not the old people, it is the kids. He tells me some stories but does not want them in the book. Traci recalls a time when Mike was coming home crying. She wanted to help and take it away. It broke a little part of Traci, seeing the impact on Mike. It was hard to see him going through the pain. There was a little silence around the table. Mike shares that at work they had seen heroin overdose, meth overdose, alcohol overdose over and over again. He sees the families who are crying on the scene because there is nothing the paramedics can do as it has been too long. Then he tells me about the unintentional accidents that did not have to happen, but somebody chose to get behind the wheel when they were drunk. I share an accident that happened in front of my eyes coming home one day a car flipped on its side. I ran to help; people were able to climb out I looked in the car and saw a lot of alcohol bottles in the back. Luckily that time no one got hurt. Mike then tells me that when he teaches a class, he tells people it is not a matter of if it happens but when it happens. He tells people the actual accidents that happened. He shows me some pictures from accidents. It is not a pretty scene. People get upset when they see the slides. I ask about the kid in the picture. What happened to him? Mike tells me the story that him and three other kids were driving down Hwy 26 in Oregon by Hillsboro, drunk, high speed, no seat belt, they got ejected. One kid walked away, he landed in blackberry bushes. One kid ended up on the road and suffered a brain injury, he was brain dead. It is still hard for Mike to share his brother's story in the slides. Then Traci said something very important. She said: ***"A lot of lost potential"***. Mike then tells me about more on the teaching he has done, shows me some more slides he uses. He gets a lot of grief when he talks about marijuana. Traci had sat through some of Mike's lectures and she shares a story that impacted her more than other stories. There were a lot of friends who went out to party and they were trying to do the responsible thing and they had a designated driver. They got into the van and a lot of them were drunk and they all started to think that is very funny to block the driver's eyes. He hit a telephone pole and he was the one who was killed. That is awful and very scary. Traci gives me other examples when kids think it is funny to shift the vehicle back and forth that could also cause a wreck because of the way the weight shifts. It is all funny until the end result because of decreased inhibitions. Mike tells me about an experience when he got drunk, he does not remember a thing that happened. He had no idea. He had a blackout. Others were telling him he was hilarious, he was hanging his head out the door of the car, threw up all over the place. At home he was stumbling all over the place hit the walls and the door to the bedroom. Mike does not think that was funny at all. He did that once and never again. Alexi was trying to say something at his point she had a hard time finding the words. We all encourage her. Traci asked her how the stories we been talking about make her feel? She said it is between a heartbreak and a judgement. Why would people do those things? She tells us she is not good at this. Traci tells her she would like to hear her thoughts. She said it would be better to sit down and think about things, the consequences before people get drunk, some of these things are very hard to even think about. She tells us she does not plan on doing anything like that. It is not a very good thing to do it. It is not her choice she tells us. She tells us about her uncle who every morning wakes up with 3 beers. After 5 pm he is done for the day. She tells us about a day when he was on his motorcycle and he started swaying his motorcycle back and forth. Alexi was thinking to herself; it was a very stupid thing to do. Very mature from a young girl. She was in the car behind him. She does not think that is a safe thing to do. She tells us to think about things because they will have a consequence no matter what. Take a moment and consider the consequence. Mike then steps in and said the other thing to think about is what is the economic impact, who will pay for this is something should happen? Insurance covers only so much after that who is going to cover the cost? Time lost from work? Productivity? Mike sees addictions all the time, he fills like it is epidemic. I ask him why he think that is? Escape and thrill he tells me. I ask him escape from what? Reality he tells me. There is no perfect answer. It is hard not to be judgmental he tells me. He sees a lot of addiction in the homeless community, he knows it is not all just there, but that it where it is most visible. He sees this with interactions with other crew members and interaction in the hospitals. It is an unfortunate assumption he tells me that if people are homeless, they are addicted. He said it is hard to try to break that barrier. There are few people who are regulars, that is not a standard for everybody else. It is more on a forefront when someone is homeless, more visible for people to see. Mike feels that addiction is something that people are trying to get out of but not sure how to escape it. Mike feels we don't have enough resources in place to help people with addictions. People need to be ready to make the change to get out of addictions. He sees parents begging their kids to stop. They are hooked, they can't get out of it. Mike sees it in families. Genetics is a factor but that could be overcome with help, the environment is a huge factor, the biggest issue is peer pressure.

Traci

Traci been writing notes during the conversation. Traci feels that addiction is a sense of loss of control and trying to find some way to get some of that control back. Traci shares that she did not have a lot of self-worth for a long time. She had found that to compensate for that she become addicted to work. She felt like if she can do work well, she is successful, she is good enough, she was working insane hours and really running herself to the ground. She went into a deep depression a couple of times. Traci was admitted to the hospital for one of those times. Even after Mike and she got married up until the time of her accident it was work, work, work, never take breaks, don't take lunch, work late, go in early, bring home stuff to work on it on the weekend. She got a sense of her self-worth from work. She talks about the little rush with accomplishments or eating a piece of chocolate. Gain some control by eating, shopping or whatever it is, running for example, it gives a sense of control. She talks about someone in town who took exercise to an addiction level where it is even detrimental to the family. It is very hard to see it Traci asserts. Anything that can give a sense of control she said. She talks about someone she knows who was overweight, she had problems in her family, dealt with some losses. She started walking. It got to a point that every time she looked up, she would see her walking rain or shine, day or night to excess. It was impacting family time connections; it is still an issue today. Traci starts to talk about chocolate. She is still in therapy from an accident in February. She found that all sense control was removed. She found this in chocolate once she passed through physical pain and got to emotional pain. She got an addiction to chocolate and wanted to hide it. She felt like a loss of control about to losing control of her own decisions. Traci is still dealing with PTSD from the accident. It is incredibly hard to stop. There were times when she would only have chocolate all day long. She tears up. Alexi goes and gives her a hug. It is an awful feeling; she felt nauseated and still take the next chocolate. She feels lucky that she did not get into hard drugs, alcohol or tobacco. She asserts that chocolate is very much an addiction. It is hard to admit that she does not have control over that. We talk about moderation and how some people can do that or not. Traci feels either have it or not. Cannot do both. Food is very difficult. It is different for everybody, depends on how deep someone is into their addiction. Traci had a lot of help with therapy. Traci also tells me about child abuse in her youth. She has been shutting that part of her emotions down, as though she has been dealing with her 5-year-old self it feels like her 52-year-old self-talking to her 5-year-old self. The pain is still there. Traci is finding that as she is finding breakthroughs to help her 5-year-old self-heal, she does not have those cravings anymore. She is working through her trauma. We have a great conversation about childhood trauma. She feels that a lot of people who are dealing with addictions are dealing with past trauma. Traci feels that as human beings we want to be socially accepted. Part of it is peer pressure, people want to be accepted and want to feel good enough, doing what we feel others want us to do. Part of it is our brains and bodies and how it impacts things. Cover up sadness or pain to feel a little better even if it is for a moment. Hang out with friends like smoking with friends.

    Traci tells me about some experiences when she used to be at the sheriff's office. She started out as a junior in high school, she wanted to go fire guns at a gun range. She loved the officers and the work, she loved to help people. She tells me about two close friends who were highly impacted by addictions. One officer was responding to a code 3; lights and sirens at night to a call and he was heading into Seaside. A gentleman who was intoxicated with a very high level of

ETOH stumbled across the road in dark clothes, the deputy did not see him and ran into him. He did not survive, and the officer really blamed himself. He took that home with him. It affected everybody at the department, every single person felt like it could have been them. It had an impact on everybody. The deputy had a lot of trauma from this, he was trying to do everything right. He went through a lot of therapy and got better. There was a lot of sorrow for the person lost as well of course.

Painful memories – Butch's son

Traci tells me another story about another person at the police department who was like a father figure for her. His name was Butch. He went through something no parent should ever go through. He had a teenage son who with 5 friends were out in on old Hwy 30. An individual who was intoxicated come over the center line and run into them. All kids died. Butch was the first person on scene responding to this wreck. He had no idea his son was there. He went about his police business routine as a deputy to start checking people. When he took a look in the back his son was there, he did not have a scratch on him, and he was dead. He never recovered from that. Unimaginable trauma. All the boys were 16-17 years old. Traci tells me she cannot even imagine losing a child and losing a child with nobody being there for support. Butch would go into a deep depression on the anniversary. He would take time off and going into a drinking binge, he could not cope with it. We are not supposed to lose our children. It is just not right Traci said especially in such a senseless way. It made a huge impact on the entire community. There are so may emotions in the room at this time, so much sorrow and sadness.

The accident that changed Traci forever

Traci keep telling me stories and experiences. When she was a young reserve deputy, she went out on a call late at night for a wreck. They found a truck on the side of the road. It is very sad and devastating to hear about so much loss to alcohol and see the impact also that it had on people who had to respond to the scene. The story that Traci heard in the end that the kids two boys and two girls were out looping drinking and driving from place to place. Nobody had seatbelts on. The driver reached back to deal with a beer can that his friend put on the floor. He did not want a mess in his truck. He got off the road drove into a ditch and hit a tree. The driver got caught behind the steering wheel, the other three passengers got ejected from the car. The driver's girlfriend ended up getting ejected through the windshield and landed in a creek, she hit a rock in the river with her face. They think she died instantly. It took a few days and divers to find her. The girl from the back ended up under the vehicle on the ground. She hit something with such a force that she lost all her bone structure in her face. When Traci got there, she was still breathing but she was just gurgling blood. Traci was praying that she did not know what was going and she was not in pain, there was not much Traci was able to do for her when she got there, she had no medical training, Traci did not know what to do to help her and she felt very inept and lost, not knowing what to do. The boyfriend in the back got ejected from the truck and ended up being upside down pinned to the tree by the truck. He was coherent and was asking Traci to help him. It was very dark, Traci was trying to use the flashlight and trying to figure out what to do, it was going to be awhile before people show up. The story is still hard for Traci to share. I could see the pain in her eyes, and she takes long pauses and big sighs throughout the story. I see the hopelessness and the internal struggle of the situation as Traci tells me that she was trying to help this kid but was not sure how. Traci was trying to reassure the boy. He was begging Traci to get him out then he started to ask about his girlfriend. Traci did not know what to say. He was in so much pain. She went up the embankment to look at the situation and this boy looked like he was literally cut in half. His legs were kind of flopped over. It was a living nightmare. She felt like there is nothing she could do to make it better. People could not get there soon enough. Traci was trying to warm him up with her jacket, trying to talk to him and reassuring him. When the ambulance and the tow truck got there, they were trying to figure out how to get this vehicle off of this boy without finishing him off and how to keep the bleeding and the internal injuries under control, so he won't bleed out. It was a very weird angle even the tow truck was started slipping they had to hook it up to another vehicle. It seemed like a never-ending nightmare until they were able to get him out. They were trying to find the 4th girl kept searching for her all night. It was a very rough night for everyone. The driver ended up surviving and going to jail for many years for manslaughter. The kid who was pinned to the tree survived but could not cope with what happened and ended up becoming an alcoholic and drinking himself to death. Once they finished at the crash site they had to go to the hospital and talk to family and friends that had shown up at the hospital. They had to let the family for the girl who was under the car know that she had not survived. Traci ended up being the person had to do this. Traci remembers going up to this gentleman who was crushed and was looking for any glimmer of good news. He was in the hospital sitting in the hallway in a chair and Traci had to go up to him and had to tell him that his teenage daughter had died. I cannot withhold my tears. Traci never experienced ever before or after such a hatred that the father associated with her. He was so upset. Since then Traci had heard that his gentlemen had already lost another child to drinking and driving. Again, unimaginable pain. This pain is so great that it crushes a person. They cannot move, think or do anything. Life just stops. A pause, when someone's life changes, their heart breaks in half. A person can try to glue back the pieces. The crack will always be there. He never rebounded from this loss. Traci tells me that for about 20 years every time this gentleman saw her in the community, he looked her with a hatred so great that crushed Traci. She does not blame him; it was very hard to see this parent in so much pain. In the last 10 years or so he won't recognize Traci anymore. One beer can spill in the back-seat Traci said dramatically changed so many lives. All the 4 people in the truck were drinking that night. That accident changed Traci forever.

Toni's accident

There is one more very close incident for Traci and that is when her sister Toni was involved in a car accident. Toni also agreed to talk to me and her recollection of the accident you can also read about in the next chapter in the book. Toni and her boyfriend went to

Portland on a 4th of July. They been drinking and they were coming home at night when at Cornelius Pass, they rolled off the road at a sharp turn and ended up down by the railroad tracks. One of the railroad ties was sticking up out of the ground for some reason. The vehicle landed upside down and the tie went through the roof of the car and ended up in her sister. Toni's neck had a 365-degree break. Her boyfriend was able to get out of the vehicle and ran for some help. Toni was originally diagnosed as a paraplegic. Toni thought she was abducted by aliens and they are doing experiments on her. Toni got medications which helped not to remember a lot which Traci is very grateful for. This is hard for Traci to talk about. When she got the call, she got her mom and went up to the hospital. Toni was in ICU. They let Traci and her mom to go in and see Toni for a brief moment. Traci was literally brought to her knees. She can't even explain what it was like walking into the room and seeing her vibrant beautiful twin sister with a halo around her head, with weights pulling her head away from her body, so many tubes coming out of her body, bloody. She is still in tears now. Traci did not know if Toni was going to make it. Nobody knew. It was her twin sister from the womb, team T, always together, intertwined. Traci is crying. The family spent many days sleeping in the hospital. Traci spent all day long just praying for a miracle. The hospital had to wait days before the surgery to fix Toni. There was not enough metal in the area Traci explains to put Toni back together. The hospital had to fly metal in from all over the US. Toni's C6 and C7 was shattered in her spine. She had to learn how to brush her teeth, how to brush her hair, how to walk, how to write, speak. Everything she had to start over from scratch. In the beginning she could not even hold a toothbrush, they had to strap it to her hand. She had to try to get the general function of arm in the right position. Toni could not get comfortable she could not regulate her temperature. Her legs were hot. Traci would ice her hands in a bucket full of ice water and try to cool her sister's feet down, she would be hot 5 minutes later again. Traci would do this over and over again. Toni had a lot of nerve damage. Now she walks fine and drives. She is not taking any days for granted. Life is short and it can be taken away any moment. It is amazing that she survived and able to function. She can't turn her head, jog or run but can do everything else. Toni died a few times after the accident.

Mike said Toni died on the operating table. Traci describes Toni rose up above her body and had her boyfriend's grandfather; come and show her the grave site and showed her the gravestone then took her back and told her that she is not done. Traci remembers the doctors coming out after the surgery and telling the family that she died a couple times and they were not sure if she is going to survive. The doctors were struggling keeping her alive. Toni thought her family will think she is crazy when she told them about her experience. Toni did not know she died on the table; she was shocked to find out. Toni kept her bloody clothes for a long time, she kept them for years before opening the bag and letting go that part of her story. Her survival and the wreck impacted many, many people Traci asserts. Toni is into helping others. Traci is very adamant about drinking and driving and she knows the impact it can have firsthand on individuals, families, communities. It took Toni months to recover in the hospital. She was in a rehab facility and in a wheelchair for a long time and slowly recovered. At the time this happened one of Traci's job was as a cocktail waitress. She was always cognizant of cutting people off. After the accident she could not serve even one drink to anybody. She could not bring herself to serve alcohol anymore. She could not do it. She could not even serve alcohol in the restaurant. She had to stop. It impacted her life in every way. Her sister now lives in California. Traci did not know in the beginning that she had anything to add to this book. Now with all these experiences bubbling up there is so much to tell. The room is flooded with emotions. We had been talking for hours. We occasionally get up take little breaks I offer the family to eat, they don't. There is too much to say.

Traci's family

Traci tells me about addiction in her family. She had an aunt and an uncle who she never met but heard stories about. They were alcoholics. They had never left their homes. They had alcohol ordered by the case delivered to their door. They were so inebriated all the time that there would be fecal matter and urine all over the place. They could not feed themselves. They could not even go into the bathroom to defecate. This always scared Traci. Because of this Traci always had this rule that even if she is very sad or upset, she would not turn to alcohol. She was terrified of the genetic predisposition of alcoholism. She did not want to end up the same way. It always impacted her. She also had a grandfather and grandmother where it was a daily event to drink. It impacted many lives. Her grandmother would drink and maybe cook meals. Never figured out how to write a check or drive a car. That was her life. They came out once when Traci's parents were building a house. Their grandmother could not even step over a pipe without grandfather she become so reliant on him for everything. It made Traci very confused. There was a lot of co-dependence issues. Traci felt that this was the was her grandfather kept control. She hated to say this. Mike said it was manipulation. Her grandmother was drinking more than her grandfather, Traci said, still he definitely had a drinking problem. Traci decided when she saw the codependence one day that she will never be that person. She knew that will not be a path she will take in her life. The family for a long time did not realize her father's drinking problem and the extent of it. Her father would have big water containers in the back of the fridge, that were constantly filled with alcohol. It took them years to figure it out. Addictive issues always scared Traci and because of this being addicted to chocolate is been very hard. Traci wants to believe that she is stronger than that. Even though it is not alcohol or something else it still bothers Traci. It makes her vulnerable. Traci starts to tell me about her brother. He was really drinking a lot. He is doing well now, but for a long time they did not have a relationship. He was either a mean drunk or the life of the party. Traci could not handle that type of turmoil in her life. It was too much to put herself through it. It estranged them. He was drinking and driving with his young son in the car with him. Traci could not understand why he would do that. Drink and drive with his son in the car, it made Traci angry. Traci was worried about others in the road. Traci had an accident last year, her brother told her it saved the family, now everyone is communicating again. It woke everybody up. With addiction Traci feels people believe that it will not happen to them not just when it comes to drugs and alcohol but to gambling, sex or anything else. Traci asserts that it is so easy to think that it only happens to the other people, until it doesn't. She feels it is hard to get the perspective that it can happen until someone is impacted by it. This is especially hard to get for young people whose brain is still developing. At this point tears are flowing and Alexi all the sudden asks for everyone's hands and ask if we can pray. Traci said sure if she would like to. We sit around the table holding hands. It is late, after 10 pm at night, it is dark outside. None of us had dinner, kind of forgot while telling stories. It is quiet, only can hear the water circulating in the aquarium. Alexi said this prayer:

> *Prayer by Alexi: God, I hope that every time we drive or make a wise or a stupid decision, make sure to guide us to our believes and mis guidance's. God, I hope that this wonderful lady who I am holding hands with makes it home safely. And everybody to have a wonderful life. Jesus, Lord, Amen.*

Traci said to Alexi, that was very nice, thank you. I ask about the tree planted out in the yard. Traci planted a tree for Butch. He was like a father figure for her. Around the anniversary he really struggled. He drank excessively during those times. It impacted many aspects of his life and his ability to connect with people in a meaningful way. People loved him; his funeral was at the fairgrounds because there were too many people to have it somewhere else. Traci did not realize the extent of the impact of his live. Traci loved him very much. He was in his early sixties when he passed. He liked to be with other people. Traci feels it helped to hide all he went through. He hid the pain. Sunset maple is the tree they planted for him. Traci "lost it" when Mike come and told him about Butchs' death. She did not want his loss to be the end. She wanted to continue his life somehow. She picked the prettiest tree. It's been over 10 years. She loves the tree and looks at it and sees all the birds, the leaves, all the colors. She just loves the tree. Her face shows joy as she is talking about this tree. Traci had conversations after he passed with Butch's wife about all the loss and sorrow, they went through losing their son. Traci sent me a picture of the Butch memorial tree.

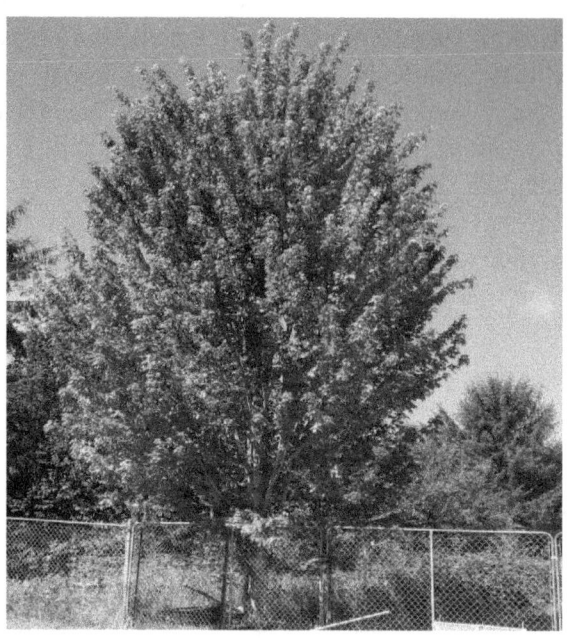

Butch's Memorial Tree 2019, Oregon

    I ask Traci and Mike about individual and societal responsibility when it comes to addiction. Mike feels that until someone is ready to get over it, we are not going to convince them. One of the biggest issues we are dealing with is acceptance. Mike talks about some of the addictions are accepted in society when it should not be; like working all the time, listening to music all the time, he feels that as a community we have to have the resources available for those people who are ready to commit. We have some resources available and they are overworked. He feels we need other options to help people get over addictions. Mike states we should stop accepting the social norm of drinking. He feels like if we work together, we can do something about addictions. It takes being able to figure out what is it that we can do, how we are going to implement it, it takes a group of people to work together, to figure this out. Mike is a pastor as well. He talks about doing stuff as an individual and wondering if we are making a difference. He has been working on a visualization to show what the collective is doing. He describes a tree with leaves on it. Each individual would be part of the tree. Working together we can accomplish a lot of stuff. The collective impact can make a big change. It is about communication, listening, letting people know they won't be judges and they have choices.

Traci recalls a conversation she had with her daughter about drinking and driving. She told her daughter that no matter what time and where if she ever drinks or one someone who she is with drinks call Traci and she will come get them. That would not make her happy, but it would be ok. Drinking and driving is never ok. Traci could not live with herself if she found out that of her daughter or someone else while she was in the car was drinking and driving and something happened to them. Traci feels like when people have to hide things it becomes more dangerous; they feel that they do not have options. A lot of people get into their addictions because they are lonely, and they are hurting. If they could just talk openly and honestly about their problems with somebody and just being accepted, not judged that would help. People are cut off each other nowadays. She tells me we used to believe it takes a village to raise a child. Now she thinks we more and more moved away from that. She tells me about multiple generations living close to each other in the same area to support each other. We can link together as a community to support one another, be less judgmental toward others as a human race. Go beyond the stereotyping Mike adds. Accepting that we are all humans and we all have faults. Just be open and supportive, prevention is be key. Now in our society we tend to deal with the aftermath of things instead of trying to prevent them. Traci recommends working with kids with ACE's (Adverse Childhood Experiences) scores early on, help the kids that are struggling in school, support the young parents who are just barely making it. If we can take a good chunk of money and put it in prevention it would save a lot in the bank end and we would be better and healthier. It will take time; we can't save everybody. ***We can't just keep chasing the end tail of things we have to get ahead and the only way is to do prevention***. Mike tells me, look at it, it took us 50 years to get to this point. It is going to take a while to get back to something reasonable. We talk about prevention and cost benefit. We all agree prevention is the way to go. Traci and Mike tell me about reenactments recreating an accident and show students what happened, then they have a conversation about it. Mike shows me pictures of previous reenactments he participated in. Kids can get an idea what an accident really looks like. We talk about different experiences people do in the community to fit in like drinking in sports events. Traci tells me about people who are fine drinking something and then driving. She does not feel comfortable with that. Mike is showing me different education slides. He tells me that every 15 minutes in our highways a teenager is killed. Traci tells me she has one more story for me. When she was working at the sheriff department for a little while she was marine deputy. She was in Seaside and observed this gentleman who was drunk driving his boat. She asked him to pull over. She gave him a ticket. Not too long after that she went to work for the state. This guy came in and looked at her: do you know who I am? I am your garbage man. (the way Traci was imitating we all busted out laughing) He was trying to get out of his ticket by saying that I am your garbage man at the office (the office where Traci works), she ruined his life he lost his job, it financially impacted him and his family. He went from being a happy garbage man to getting a ticket to losing his job and having to go on food stamps. She was telling me the different way families can be impacted. It was his choice to drink. We hear about the drinking and driving on the road, but we don't hear much about drinking and water accidents. She is telling me about oil tankers that have drunk captains. Traci feels like every single ticket she wrote hopefully saved somebody's life at some point. We finish our conversation and say goodbye to each other. Lots of hugs and well wishes. Traci and Alexi walk me to the door we talk for a few minutes and I drive off. Lots of stories swivel around my head.

7. Toni's Story

    I drive over again to Traci's house where Toni is visiting her sister for a few days. It is a nice summer morning. I know the way I was just here a week or so ago. It is fun to meet a fraternal twin. They look so much alike. I instantly like her it was the same way as with Traci. Both wonderful people. Toni invites me in, and we sit down at the dining room table. I ask her if she has any question before we begin. Traci already told her everything, so we began the recording almost immediately. Toni had an accident a major one. I cannot see visible signs now. She was asked a few years back to speak about her accident and she stood up in front of a group of people and openly shared. She tells me it was one of the scariest things she did, she was really nervous. Toni feels that it is very important to be up front about our experiences, good and bad, in order to start a conversation on issues affecting our community. Both Traci and Toni tell me that they would rather be the patient then the family member who has to deal with seeing their loved one's injured. Toni tells me her personality is if we have a problem, lets fix it. It is so funny we said it exactly the same time. Nursing brains. We laugh. She tells me Traci and she are total opposites in this regard. She feels like even that they are twins and went through the experience, have the same memories their perceptions were very different about their upbringing. There are things that Traci remembered that Toni did not. Toni felt that a bad thing happened her, attitude was let it go and move on. We discuss some of the memories Traci and Toni had that were different. They had talked about the water bottle in the fridge that was their dad's. Toni has no recollection of that. She was like what water bottle? All she remembers is the milk. When her father picked up the glass and set it down, that meant they were to fill it with milk. We are all different and how we perceive things are different. Toni has so many stories she was not sure where to start. She decided to start with early memories. She is telling me that her mom was the main person at the home, she was the one who kept the family together. Her dad was a workaholic. He did not know how to be a person outside of the Coast Guard. He was in the Coast Guard. When he was home, he was the stranger that come in and really disrupted the household. He was abusive. They even had to watch how they look at him. She gives me an example. Traci was looking up into the ketchup bottle to see if it was getting ready to pour. This angered her father, so he grabbed the bottle and proceeded to pour it all over her. He made her sit in it. That made no sense. Growing up she said when their dad was home, they were so afraid of doing anything. They were afraid to even look at him or do anything to draw his attention. Toni feels that looking back their dad only knew work, did not know how to be a husband or a father and this frustrated him. Toni feels that when her dad came home, he expected the family to be all over him and get permission from him for things to do, but the kids did not really know him, so they went to the familiar and that was mom. He was the stranger for them in the home. Toni feels that was where she thinks his aggression came from. He was frustrated and did not know how to correct it. He went back to what he was used to with his dad being physically and psychologically abusive. Toni said what she is grateful that he showed her what she did not want to be in life and her mom showed her what she wants to be in life. She is grateful for those lessons. Even as kids they asked their mom why she is staying with him. Finally, when they were sophomores in high school the parents divorced. Toni become rebellious; she wanted the separation yet after she did not know how to handle it. She started smoking and was hiding cigarettes. When her mom found them, she lied about it and said they were someone else's. She always was trying to do it in secret. That was her first addiction. It took her accident when she was 30 years old to quit. She had tried to quit many times before, but it was unsuccessful. She quit for 7 days then it would take her a ½ pack of cigarettes to feel herself again. It seemed always be on the 7th day. She also got into drinking. She was out drinking with friends and she was thinking that if she can walk a straight line then she could drive home. Now she thinking back is going:" you idiot, how you are being drunk could think that you are walking a straight line, but it does not mean that you were". Toni describes that her drinking then threw her into using marijuana. She remembers being a teenager cadet at the sheriff's department. There was one day when she went in to go to their meeting and she forgot that she had a marijuana joint on her. She went into the station bathroom and hid it so she would not be busted with it. She did not see a problem with it at that time. She felt she was just being rebellious and pushing the limits to see what she could get away with. This all affected her grades and she ended up not graduating from high school. She was behind and started to take some college classes to make up, but it was not enough. They told her during the rehearsal that she could not graduate. She did not walk. Her Mom had told her that if she did not graduate, she would need to move out. Her mother felt that would put the fear in her and cause her to walk the line. She went home, packed and moved out. She moved in with some friends who were a couple years ahead her from high school. In that apartment there was a lot of drinking, drugs and partying. One day she woke up and walked out of her room. People were passed out everywhere. It clicked in her head. She has got to stop this because if she does not something very bad is going to happen. That day she went to her best friend and told her that they need to move out. They got their own place. Her best friend was a diabetic and she wanted to be like everyone else. She was always eating sugar, drinking alcohol and smoking. Many times, Toni had to give her insulin, when she found her passed out and not breathing. She was afraid that she would lose her. Eventually, they met their partners and went separate ways. Toni admits she smoked when she was pregnant. She realized she was in a bad relationship with a man that had similar trait as her father. After her divorce Toni met another guy. He was big into cocaine and alcohol. He was running around with local friends who were big into doing cocaine and alcohol. This started Toni down a path where she felt if they were drinking, she needed to drink. If they are doing coke, or smoking marijuana she felt she needed to do the same thing to fit in. This created a long time in Toni's life doing drugs and alcohol almost every night. This was all the precursor to Toni's accident on July 28, 1997.

The accident

The day of her accident Toni and her boyfriend were meeting his cousin and his girlfriend. They went to a beach in Portland and played games, drink, had a good old time she calls it. There was barbeque, it was a nice, warm, sunny day. At the end of the day Toni remembers eating, playing, but she does not remember the rest. Her boyfriend later told Toni that she said that they could not go home, and they need to go to his cousin's house that was right down the street. He decided that he did not wanted to go there, he wanted to go home. Toni passed out in the passenger seat. He drove through Cornelius Pass on their way home. Toni does not know what made him go off the road. They ended up going off the road at Cornelius Pass, rolling down to the bottom with a railroad tie sticking out. During the roll over the top of the car ended up on the railroad tie and it come through the roof, hit Toni's seat and her neck, pinned her against her legs, shattered C6 and C7 of her neck. Piecing together the timeline she thinks that her boyfriend was knocked out for about 20 minutes. The only thing Toni remembers is waking up against her legs and feeling something warm. It was her blood. She was folded in half. Imagine sitting in a chair and pinned against your legs. The next thing she remembers is arguing with the ED doctor about Traci's phone number. Next thing she remembers is being in ICU. She was in a halo because she had a broken neck.

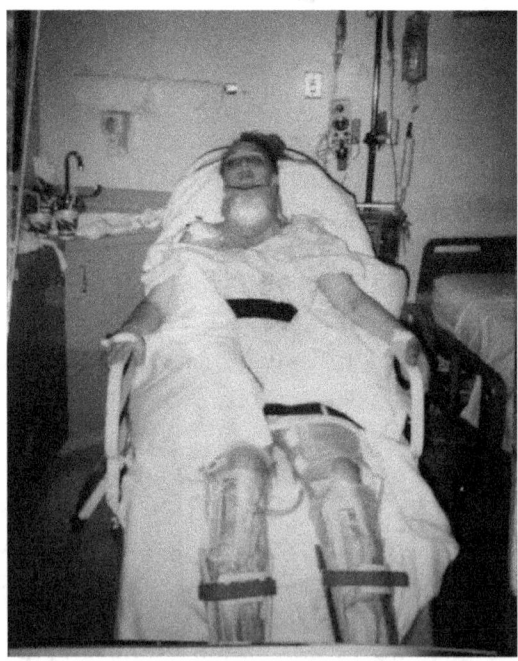

Toni few weeks after the accident

It was really weird she recalls. She woke up and she thought she had been abducted. She felt like she was tied down, she could not move. She thought she had to be abducted, because why she would be tied down. She was not. She was paralyzed. She did not realize it. She started freaking out. She remembers the male nurse coming in and talking to her, Toni kept saying it is not right. The only thing he was able to do to calm her down was rolling her bed out of her room so she could look at the nurse's station with other people and monitors. Then she was like ok, something did happen, although she did not know what. Her hands were all injured she had a lot of scars; she shows me her hands. I hold her hands and look at old scars. Trying to imagine what she went through. She almost lost a finger. Looking at her scars one looks like a cross. She laughs. What she just told me that was all she remembered from the first two weeks of the accident. She has no other recollection. Then she remembers one more thing. The doctor came in and told her that they can try and attempt a surgery with the worst-case scenario that she does not make it off the table, best case scenario she might get some movement back. She said, ok sounds good let's do it. Even today she has a hard time saying this around her sister and her mom. When she does, it takes them right back. She did not want to be paralyzed, it was just not an option for her, she wanted them to try to fix it. After the surgery if the doctor said to do something two times, Toni would do it ten times. She never wanted to play the victim and get caught up in that cycle. She saw others doing that and were having a hard time getting out of it.

    Toni recalls a horse accident as a teenager when she got thrown off the horse and the horse landed on her; it broke her pelvis. She was trying to get up and she could not move. She was paralyzed temporarily from the waist down. It was a mortifying experience for Toni. The neighbor showed up and the whole Knappa fire department showed up. They were doing training that day, so everyone was there. They all wanted to take their turn with Toni checking vitals, doing this and doing that, prepping her. She brings this up to tell me that even then she had never seen herself as a victim. She had seen some people jumping into that role and then getting into depression. Pushing people away.

Toni then starts to tell me a funny side story about her family and how in her family they like to surprise each other. She makes me laugh so hard. She tells me an example when her sister Traci was going to see her daughter in Hawaii. Toni found out and she conspired with Traci's daughter that both Toni and their mom will go and surprise Traci at the airport. They arrived a few days before. Traci had no idea. Their mom was hiding, Toni was upfront and a had a big camera and when Traci walked by with her daughter all she sees is the camera and Toni's hair. She walks right by her. She said" boy, somebody is really waiting for someone". Toni turns around and follows Traci. She just walked up to her and up put her arms around her, she was like what and looked Toni and was so excited, crying and super happy, gaining the attention of everyone at the airport terminal. When Traci comes down from her excitement their mom comes out. She taps on Traci's shoulder. Traci turns around thinking it might be Toni's husband Danny. She sees her mom and the excitement and crying starts again. I wish you could hear Toni's voice telling this story I cannot stop laughing. It is nice to have family fun. Toni tells me they love to do things like that. Wonderful. Surprise each other.

    We then get back to talk about the accident. Toni saw how it affected her family. Toni does not remember the initial time; she did see photos of the initial tubes and bandages. I ask her if she looks at the picture what she thinks. She never saw it as her, it was a problem that needed to be solved. She likes to think glass half full; she likes to find something good in everything. With her broken neck Toni describes herself as the princess and the pea. Toni was hypersensitive to pain she could feel the slightest little wrinkle, it felt like a boulder to her. She hurt from head to toe. She could not regulate her body temperature. She felt like she was in a furnace, she was hot. She tells me the ice water story Traci told me. Toni also noticed she cannot say: "sounds good". It sets off memories. She was told that her dad came and saw her in the hospital, but he could not walk through the door to her room. Her brother also had a very hard time coming into the room. She described her mom as a rock. Her mom held it together until Toni was in the ICU, then she broke down and lost it once she was safe and transferred out. Toni does not remember any of this. She tells me something weird for her. Prior to the accident she could not stand the smell of whiskey and liked rum. Right after the accident till this day she cannot stand the smell of rum and love whiskey. I don't get it she said. The accident and seeing how it affected other people around her made Toni realize the effect of her actions. She was trying to put on a good front to help her family overcome the trauma. She tells me it did not work as well as she would have liked it too. Her boyfriend at that time never got over the accident. He knew it was his fault. He knew that his actions caused Toni to die twice. He lost his license for 5 years and did one month in jail. Toni knew that the accident was equally her fault and she was so grateful that no one else was involved. I asked Toni for some clarification about feeling responsible for the accident. She explained that she was talking about her prior actions drinking at a bar and driving home. That could have taken someone's life. It could have taken someone's loved one. She is very passionate saying this and feeling a lot of regret for her actions in the past. She remembers the poor choices she made in the past drinking and driving. She did not want to drink and drive again. She decided to make her accident a good experience and stop smoking. After years of physical therapy, she was able to join a volunteer fire department. She said she wanted to help others as they had helped her. This led Toni into a wonderful career as an EMT in Oregon and California. She realized how precious life is and how it can be taken from her at any moment. She believes in heaven. She died two times, once on the way to the hospital, she received CPR (Cardiopulmonary Resuscitation) and during surgery. She tells me the story of her boyfriend's grandfather and his headstone. Grandpa took her to the headstone, and she was able to describe it exactly after the surgery. It was the most loving, peaceful moment in Toni's life. Filled with tranquility and love never experienced before in her life. Toni has a hard time finding words to describe the experience. She tells me that if heaven is anything like that, she is not afraid of death. She does not want to die, but not afraid at all.

    We skip to when she met her husband Danny 20 years after the accident. You can read his story in this book later on as well. When Danny found out about the accident it changed him. He touches her scars. He reflects on; "what would happen if she wasn't here today". Danny sees the brightness and joy Toni brings into other's lives and wonder what life would be if Toni was not there. If she did not make it. Danny wonders what he would be like. He feels Toni saved him. It is his way of looking at it. Toni's accident affected people even long after. Toni tells me a little about Danny. Both his parents were using substances drinking and drugs. Danny did not drink at all before he met Toni. They did start to drink some wine and now they are having some conversations about drinking wine and how much. Toni prefers to do something else instead of drinking wine One thing is that Toni is in the process of getting a dog and hoping that will help them focus on other things. Toni and Danny just got a new German shepherd named Ruby. They look forward to the healthier lifestyle and focusing on greater things. She is worried about the addictive traits running in the family. They make wine from their fruit trees. She started to see herself drinking one to two glasses of wine a day and realized she did not want to go there. She refuses to go there. She been there before. She is scared to go back to that place of addiction. I ask her straight up what about just not having any? Exactly, she said. She is working on that now. Danny tells her: "you say one word, and everything is out the door". I say at this point to her: Say the word. She said: exactly and she wonders why she does not say let's just get rid of the wine. She is really thinking about this and contemplating on it. She knows they don't need it. When she is sad, have a bad day or depressed she does not turn to alcohol she turns to ice cream. Toni admits that she likes her drink every once in a while. Sometimes she has too much. She admits that she goes there sometimes. She does not want to go down the same road. She has to have this conversation with Danny. She sees the same road she been down before. She feels it is exactly what it is this book is about. She has not touched anything else since the accident, but alcohol is still an issue, obviously. Toni looks at me with an honest realization. It is like a light bulb going on. I can see she does not want to continue with this trend.

    Toni then tells me about her fruit trees and her garden. She has one of each fruit tree and freezes and dries fruit as much as she can. They also give them away to homeless shelters. They eat as much wholesome food as possible from their garden. They don't like junk food and all that fattening stuff when they go out to eat. I could not stop myself I said: Just ice cream. Her voice rose up. Yes, she adds: "I don't eat as much I could". She was defending her ice cream. She did notice that she been leaning more towards sweets lately. She looks at me and another lightbulb goes on. She tells me in a way someone knows this is an addiction she is asking herself if she could throw away everything that is sweet at her house. I ask, could you? She does not know. When she was trying to lose weight, she went to Costco and got the jelly belly's. She tells me she could have 10 and it is 40 calories. She did that as her reward system. If she stayed with her diet and her calories and her exercise, she would take them. She looks at me with the realization that is where it started. Then she started to make brownies and count out the calories and cut them up how much she can have then got three musketeers chocolate bars; the fun sized ones, she keeps them in the freezer. That was her reward and since then she started to go more and more towards it. Another thing is she tells me that if she has any sweets in the house and Danny finds them, they are gone. She has to hide stuff. It is kind of funny, but it is not because she does not want it all the time, but when she wants it, she wants it now. She does not want to have to go to the store to get it. Traci's story is very similar about hiding and defending their chocolate. That is funny she tells me, and she laughs. Another addiction she sees them having is the phones. They are on the phones a lot playing games. Now when they are out eating, she asks her husband to put the phone away. She tells me that she needs to do that more. She also tells me sitting in front of the TV. She asks me why to do people have to sit in front of the TV to eat? It is another bad habit they have she tells me. She is not sure if that is an addiction or just a bad habit. I ask her why she thinks we do bad habits that we don't like to do? It is a comfort she tells me. She feels it leads back to the rebellious stage. **I can do this. I can get away with it.** This is something I can do and no one else can keep me from doing this. Toni feels that addiction has a lot to do with that. It is my choice good or bad, I have the right and I am going to do it. The more people do it, the more it becomes an addiction. She tells me a lot of people become addicted to pain meds. That was one thing that always scared to death. She was terrified of it. She had to take medications for her neck, she rather not took any. Traci is the same way. She tells me about chemical imbalance that is causing addictions. Toni tells me about caffeine. Caffeine is a huge addiction. She cannot imagine not drinking her 1-2 cups of coffee in the morning. She cut way back. She used to drink couple of pots a day. She told herself no, I cannot do this. For a while she was drinking those coke frosty things, like there is no tomorrow. Then she started to have stomach issues. She stopped. Her mind said:" no you cannot do this anymore". She needs to do that with the alcohol and the drinking and need to cut Danny back too. Yeah, she said, that is big, it is a big one and it has always been an issue. We have a reassuring conversation about roads we know and self-reflection. It is hard to recognize when somebody is in it. We discuss food addiction for a while. We talk about paths and how easy it is to fall back on what we had done previously. We discuss moderation and how that works for some people but not others. Toni knows that her sweets and her phone is the biggest problem now. Toni likes to problem solve and trying to figure things out. We discuss benefits of volunteering. Toni just started out with a new group; she loves to help people. She feels on top of the world when she can help others.

    I ask Toni what addiction means to her. There is silence for a while. Then she said, boy that is a good one. Then she comes up with one of the most amazing definitions. To her **_addiction is anything that takes a person's attention and time away from other things and becomes a greater part of their life._** She gives me an example about smoking cigarettes and how she timed everything about smoking. Her focus was only on when she is going to have the next cigarette. Anything that takes a person away from something that is truly important that is their friends, family, career. It separates people. It pulls people apart. She gives me an example at sitting at dinner and having a conversation. It is more important to be on the phone for some people, she asserts that that is not right. There is a lot of aspects to it, rebellion, being bored to anything. It can slowly work up without realizing they become focused on just that instead of other aspects of their life. Toni feels this is very scary. Toni feels paying attention to our own life is important, look at where our focus is and ask the question what is truly important in my life is it that cigarette, or is it spending time with my kids because I am not out smoking a cigarette. What is truly important. Facing up to what is it that we are really doing. Is that piece of bread being it that important she asks. Instead of having that piece of bread. Let's go for a walk. That candy, she continues. Do I really need that candy? Or should I just drink a glass of water.

> *Toni suggests if you have a craving wait 15 minutes. Are you still craving it? What is going on? Paying attention to your family and friends. Speaking up.*

    Toni feels this is hard to do. It is hard to do a difficult conversation. Trying to have a discussion without saying it is wrong what the other person is doing. She feels that is the worst thing someone can do. It is difficult to have these conversations and not to ruin the relationship. Toni tells me that when it comes up to the difficult conversations, she went through with that with her daughter. She was rebellious and got together with a guy who was using substances. He was addicted to pain killers and meth. She kept calling Toni for money. She kept sending money and enabling her. Toni was hearing from her son about all the issues his sister had. To try to get drugs they would drive 3.5hr to another doctor just to get drugs. It come to a point that they were living out of a house that had no electricity, no water, no nothing, going down to the local gas station to try to bathe in the sink. Toni's daughter kept calling and asking for money. Toni was wondering if this money was going for food or for drugs. She did not know. The hardest thing she ever said was no. Toni told her daughter that she will not help her out anymore. It was hard, she threw everything at Toni. After a while her daughter got into a better relationship.
    Toni then starts to tell me about social media, gun violence, school shootings. She feels like kids do this sometimes to gain notoriety, so people will know their names. Whenever someone shoots someone their name is mentioned over and over again in the media. Toni feels that when something like this happen that person and their family name never mentioned. She does not want to hear about who caused the issue. She wants to hear about the victims and their family. She feels this have a lot to do with social media. She brings up cyber

bullying. She feels like cyber bullying and social media turns people against each other. Toni feels families should talk to one another and discuss what is being said on social media and together decide what children should see. Then they need to discuss how to process and deal with all the negative media.

Toni tells me she has a Facebook account, but she never goes on it. Danny is on it every single day. Toni brings up news and how all they talk about are bad things. She suggests talking about the good things in life. We talk about brain oversaturation with news. She asserts that people need to see the good in other people. Then she tells me about cursing and how we don't need it. Take away from Toni: If you can't say something good don't say anything at all. Take the negatives in people's life and use them for good by using previous knowledge to help others in similar situations. Focus on the good and get away from all the negativity. Be family oriented. Pay attention to your kids. Get back to the roots. Bring families closer to each other would bring us away from the addictive elements.

8. Causes of Addiction

What causes addiction in our society? Rory believes it is trauma. Beth believes it is Marijuana shops in every corner. Peer Pressure, a lot of peer pressure is out there, competition where people are comparing themselves to others. Stress, including financial stress, especially in rural areas with seasonal jobs, people might want to cope in a bad way like drink or use. Genetics, family history of addiction, environment can be some causes that were described to me by many people whom I talked to during the creation of this book. Dr. Tedd Levin describes causes related to genetic predisposition, family history of substance abuse disorder. Not everybody has a family history of socioeconomical factors, broken families where children and youth are raised by one parent, foster care system, no housing, lack of close relationships with people who can look out for them, nobody to lend a helping hand. Additionally, the peer group young people hang out with, so many factors, it is pretty complicated and there can be multiple causes why someone ends up in the addiction trap.

When I was talking to Angel, the small-town influence came up, where she felt that excuses are made up, that kids are just kids and if they are at my house, I at least know what they are doing. Then, she said all of the sudden parents have these "monsters" that they did not know existed, and don't know what to do with anymore. She feels this is very sad and unfortunate. She describes that the kids that were lost locally to addiction were kids she did not think that would end up that way. They were athletes, intelligent, well liked.

Fun fact: At this point we were both amazed because a hummingbird just came up to us, very close as we were sitting outside and talking. Angel started laughing, she said she loves them. Neither of us ever seen a hummingbird this close. Angel then burst out laughing more and said, "why are you not at my feeder, I've been trying to feed you".

These kids Angel describes seem to have everything going well in life. When these kids get close to graduation and don't know what they want to do, where to go and who they are supposed to be. The identity they had in their community as an athlete or a good scholar or something else is now up in the air. Angel feels that we (schools, parents, doctors, everybody she said) don't do a good job saying it is ok not to know at age 18 who you are going to be at age 30. It is normal, it is ok to be scared. It is ok not to know where you want to be. It is ok to go out and fail and come home and go and try again. She feels that a lot of the kids she had seen who lost their lives either permanently or lost who they are because of drugs or alcohol they don't know what to hang on to so they start self-medicating trying to cope with the feelings they have and it just never works. The loss of potential, she thinks is the most awful thing, when she sees what a kid could be. What is lost. This is probably the most difficult part of the job, seeing this happen. (She works in a school system). She mentioned to me that there are a lot more ways to self-medicate now than before and it is not just drugs and alcohol, but food, sex, shopping, all things youth trying to use to make them feel better. We discussed smoking and vaping in the schools and how many times it is a first step to addiction and addictive behaviors. Angel describes a youth who lost his mom, he was caught vaping, the first thing he said: "I just miss my mom. I just miss my mom". Not the best coping skill, but probably he had nothing else or no one else to comfort him. He was trying to cope by picking up a habit that is not necessarily healthy. It takes his mind off of it Angel thinks so he does not have to feel the hurt.

    We also had a discussion with Angel about life in general and the misconceptions of expectations of this great life for all. She said this is not how this works. Life throws curve balls. It is ok to fall, and we have to teach our kids that it is ok to fall then they need to get up and keep moving forward, work through it, whatever it is.

    Paige asserts that sometimes there is just a kid who is in the wrong place and at the wrong time and gets caught up in addiction. The majority of time there are root causes before the addiction begins. Paige had met people from both ends. People who got caught up in addiction very quickly, they were not prepared what it will do to them and others who had been able to try meth for example once or twice and decide it is not for them and stop. She feels combination of lifestyle, brain make up, impulsivity and society as a whole play a part in addiction. Chief Jason feels that there are a lot of broken homes and kids do not get the attention they need growing up. Then kids start to hang out with friends that are more involved in addictive behaviors. Jason gives an example from his daughter's class in middle school where just before spring break there were 13 kids disciplined because of vaping in class. He was wondering how this can go on and teachers not paying attention to this? This is not easy. What could a teacher do? I talked to teachers and they are not sure how to handle this situation. They take the devices away and more comes. With all the broken homes and poverty how would people deal with this? We also discussed how alcohol and smoking looks better in advertisement. It looks good on TV, posters, it shows something that people might want to do. Having models and famous people who look good doing it might give the suggestion to other people that they can get healthier by using those products. He talks about how advertising still shows that people are having more fun when they are drinking. He also talks about marijuana and heath and natural advertisement and the chemicals and additives that come with it and how harmful that can be. It is a continuous battle.

    Kayla describes learning about addictions in the classroom while attending classes in psychology. The brain can change and made her realize that there is a lot more to addiction than what it first seems. The problems are more deeply rooted. She describes from personal experience a time when her dad had a "low" in his life because of issues with his job and marriage and he started drinking. Kayla was unsure if she wanted to share this, sounded like this is still a painful reminder of what had been going on. She describes that there hasn't been alcoholism in her family before that and they did not know how to recognize the signs until it become a "massive problem". Kayla describes that different people have different weaknesses and strengths and no matter how strong someone is addiction can touch anyone just the same way it touched her father. Rory feels that people will always seek out drugs for different reasons like having an altered consciousness. He describes mammals seeking out trees with fruits that are fallen and fermented, and elephants and baboons go and seek that tree out. Then they get staggering drunk. He said that the videos are hysterical. He is wondering if there would be a way to offer people a different kind, a healthier way to do an altered experience. He describes meditation, yoga, chanting, humming, sweat lodging, dance for example. Rory feels that there could be a lot of ways we could help people do that and we don't. We don't teach them. We tell people there is no reason to be out of that experience. Rory said he disagrees with this mentality. Could we prevent addictions by teaching youth about these alternative experiences? Rory describes addiction as a youth disorder. A pediatric condition. He said that research shows that if a person is not addicted by age 25, by the time their brain is fully developed, it is highly unlikely that they will develop an addiction after that. Rory mentioned that the last thing a treatment facility personnel at one place he worked would tell people when they left is if you relapse be sure to come back to us. It is thought in treatment that relapse is expected to get the next client. It is outrageous Rory felt.

Diana talks about her daughter Lana who got addicted to drugs after drugs were introduced to her by her boyfriend. Looking back Diana thinks she should have not brought her Lana into a small town from living in a big city in her sophomore year. The drugs took over so much that Lana wanted nothing to do with her family. She was battered by the boyfriend but would not leave him and cut ties with family. Lana finally got out of the bad relationship but could not get away from the drug abuse. She had 3 beautiful boys by then Diana recalls. Lana had good jobs, hid the addiction well, but started to get into trouble with her employers. She still had the boys at that time, Diana would go with her husband on weekends and asked if the boys could stay with them, she was getting more and more concerned about her grandchildren's safety. Lana was getting more and more verbally abusive with her. Lana eventually got into trouble with the law by driving the car with the kids in it while on cocaine and smashing into other cars. Luckily nobody was hurt badly, but she was arrested and taken into jail. DHS (Department of human services)/CPS (Child protective services) proceedings started to look into the case. Diana and her husband ended up adopting the boys. Lana did not fight for them at that time. Lana has now been clean for 11 years. Before she got clean there was a lot of up and down and when she was using Diana did not let her see the boys, when she was sober, they allowed visitations. This was very hard on the boys as well. When all this happened the kids were 10, 6 and 1 years old. Lana was also abusing oxycodone (opiate) and possibly meth she was not sure, and alcohol.

Lana was mandated by the court and went to treatment twice. Only for 30 days, Diana felt this was not enough. Lana ended up going to prison in Tillamook and that is what "cured" her. After prison Lana turned a corner and jumped in, doing everything she was supposed to do, she found help. Lana started to attend counseling, she felt this saved her life. Diana sent me a picture that represent new beginning in her life.

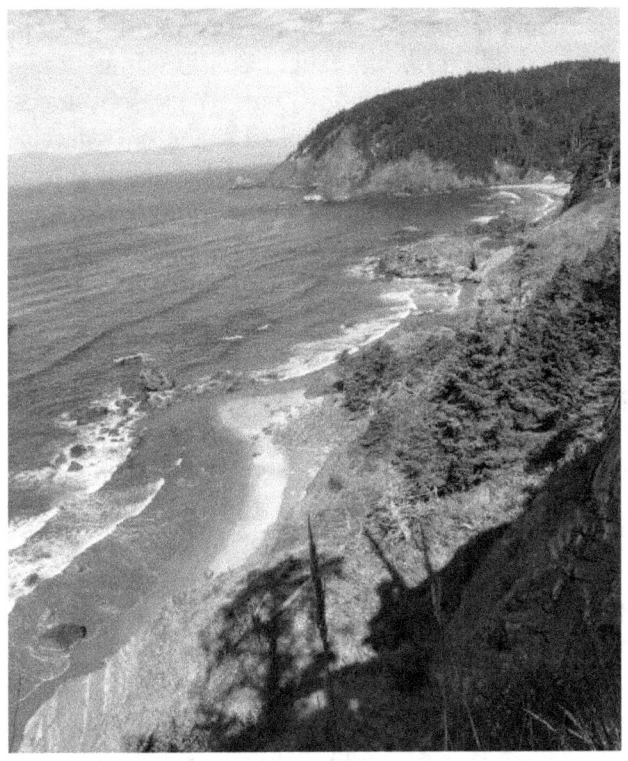

New Beginning, Cannon Beach, OR 2018

Chloe describes peer pressure as a cause for addiction. Especially if someone is in the popular crowd in high school or college. Ron adds that the causes of meth addiction from his experience with his friend as coming from non-acceptance in family, community as a gay man. That group become a chemical community, created a sense of belonging, become a social activity that sucked people in. Ron felt that people got really wrapped up in the party drugs and sex. Sex was a big focus too. People were dying. Once it got out to the literature and to the CDC (Centers for Disease Control) and the negative effects came to light then people had support to get out from the cycle, some did not. The ones who were too far gone and they lost everything, cars, homes, jobs. Ron describes that for many people it was easier to stay in the addiction then to try to get out. Ron describes a luring evil drug scene.

    Joel wonders if domestic violence is a part of why people might turn toward addiction. She feels like it is a huge topic. Bernadette senses that a lot of people start to use substances including alcohol to cover up trauma that happened to them. It starts as a coping skill and then becomes an addiction she said. Trauma examples she gave me included being raped repeatedly, seeing her mom being beaten by her boyfriend. She describes a lot of kids in homes where there is a lot of trauma going on. How can we stop all this trauma? She had seen a lot of people with addiction abuse or neglect their children. It is difficult because on one hand nobody wants to take the child away from home. We also would not want the child to be neglected and abused. Better parenting. Can we make parents be better parents? Quality education, good jobs, schools, teachers, social worker. What happens to the kid when they go home from school and they get neglected at home or abused at home. She describes that all the power is with the parents a little with the schools. How about watching out for each other's children? She sees parents not caring for their kids in grocery stores, on the street, kids crying, she feels like just picking them up. Now we can't. It is illegal to care for other people's kids. She feels that is what many kids just need to be held, touched, create attachment. Kids are not attached to their parents; parents are not available. Could we live in a society that allows us to help others care for their children? She wishes we lived in places where everyone could take care each other's kids. She had dealt with so many adults who had bad parents. Lack of good education and good parenting is a big issue when it comes to our society and addictions, mental health issues. Kids grow up and become bad parents. They use addictions to cover up the pain that was caused by their parents. Very bad cycle to continue. She sees this over and over again. She feels like even if a person does not have a lot of money, and they have good parents they are going to be ok. Because they would have good emotional stability. Also have a good mentor at school. How can we make better parents? She describes having cooking classes for parents she might have 15 people sign up and one or two show up. Hard to make a change that way. She feels like people don't show up unless things are mandatory. Teaching emotional intelligence in school helps.

Albert feels like a lot of addiction comes out of depression, anxiety or hopelessness. People fall back on using alcohol or drugs to kind of try to cover it up, bury it. He struggles when people say it is not a mental health issue it is a drug issue he feels like no, why are we separating the two, there is a core here where we are getting it. This person is not drinking themselves to death because they are happy. A person is not using meth because things are going great in their life. It is usually because there is something else going on that they are trying to bury, it might be feelings, trauma, or something similar. Albert feels that there is a lot of overlap with mental health and addictions. He gets a lot of throwback when he is trying to get help for some people for mental health and the jail or the district attorney's office would say no it is a methamphetamine induced psychosis or problem. People do not get the same treatment if someone is bipolar or schizophrenic. Albert feels like why not, their brain is broken, he does not care how it happened that is not like they did it in purpose, why can't we give them the same help we give other people? The distinction there does not make much sense to Albert. People have the misconception that using drugs is a choice. He said" yes of course maybe the first time when they took a Vicodin it was a choice but not now, not when they are on the street shooting up heroin and they can't stop. Even if it was a choice, they are in trouble" Albert said, "I don't give a s*** how they get there, but they need help now". Flower feels like there are many reasons that can cause addictions to happen, it could be past trauma, an element of escape, then it becomes a necessity and a dependence. It can happen at a high school party, it could be an advertisement that looks cool, it could all start just for fun, and benign in the beginning or presented as benign. Flower believes that when people use at the first time, their intention and goal is not to be addicted, but it happens anyways. People fall into it, she explains. Nobody at age 7 for example sets the goal to be addicted to anything.

Nobody sets the intention to become addicted to anything with the first use and for some people they might be able to use one time and never again, but others are not so lucky. Flower believes that we as humans are built a certain way to respond to chemicals in our brain. She brings the examples of nicotine and how strong the response is in our body. She personally knows she is wired to nicotine so she does not even want to try she knows what the response will be. She feels that when people start there is an assumption that the use will be benign. Then many years later people recall, oh yeah first I tried this when I was 13 or so and so gave me this at a party and it went all downhill from there. Another issue is when the whole family is using a substance and it is a normalized behavior in the family. Family can be a great influence to use or not use a substance.

9. MY GRANDFATHER

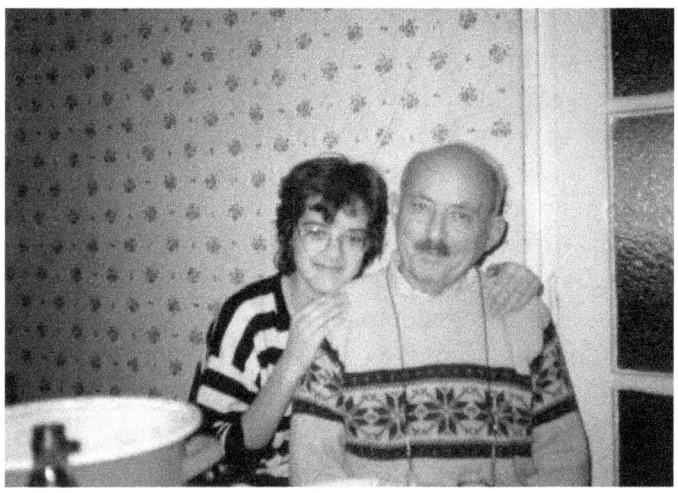

Budapest, Hungary around 1987.

He was a wonderful person. He was super smart, humble and lived simply. Never saw him cocky or showing off. I was afraid I lost this picture in a house fire. It brought tears into my eyes when I found it. I just woke up this morning knowing exactly where it was. I opened the album, and this was the first picture, him smiling at me. I don't have a lot of pictures with my grandpa, but I sure love this one. I can see the calm and kindness on his face. I just cannot look at this picture without smiling back at him. I am now kind of feeling silly sitting here just keep smiling back at his picture. I was talking to my dad (Zoltán Kőrösi) the other day about my grandfather (András Kőrösi, born Kauffman). After the war there was still a lot of hatred toward people with Jewish heritage and it was recommended for my grandfather to change his name from Kauffman. He was a great man. He has an amazing story. I will describe a little of his life history for some context. My grandfather went through a lot in his life. He was in Siberia as a prisoner of war, part of his foot froze off there. He was there because of his Jewish heritage; he was part of the working section that got executed by Germans. Well, most of them. It would have been too much for them to bring people back, so they just shot them. They shot my grandfather too. He got shot in two places but survived. The bullets went through in his right shoulder and left leg luckily. I remember him showing me those spots. I was too young then to understand why he was shot. I was just glad he was ok. The family at that time did not know he was alive. There was a notification that his mother, my great grandmother received that he disappeared. He was declared dead. From the 100 people in that specific work section 2 people made it home to Hungary. Luckily for our family he was one of the two. Life experiences took a toll on him for sure. I am very happy that he made it. He created a beautiful family after surviving all this. Three wonderful children. My father and two aunts. Many grandchildren and great grandchildren.

    I loved my grandfather very much. He was a wonderful man. I remembered some stories when my father gave him some money when I was young and asked him why he needed money. My dad told me it was so he can buy a drink that he needs. I just acknowledged the story at that time like ok, grandpa needs it ok. Thinking back, I never saw my grandfather drinking much; an occasional half Deci of vodka, but never saw the effects, he was always very quiet, super friendly and loving. Loved when he made food. I am not sure what he did with salads, but it was always amazing. Potato with parsley was one of his specialty. My dad tells me a story when my grandfather got his engineering diploma, there was a celebration. At that time, he was not used to drinking he had a half Deci (dl) pálinka (Hungarian fruit brandy) and he was staggering on his way home. He had to walk 200m. People who told the story after told my dad that my grandfather walked like someone was pulling him on a rope. Once he got home, in the hallway he was walking from one wall to the other staggering. Later he started to drink but only half a Deci pálinka a day he did not even had money to drink more. My dad told me that my grandfather started drinking when he was sent to Moscow, Russia in 1969, for an assignment for two years by himself and his family could not go. Dad recalls that he was sent because there was an opportunity that he could have been the CEO at the cable company he worked at, instead they sent him to Moscow and while he was gone someone else took the seat. Dad says that grandpa really learned how to drink there. People in Moscow, Russia know how to drink and know how to drink well he learned how to drink vodka with sour pickles. Eating the sour pickle allowed people to drink more. I talked to my aunt Kati (Funk Sándorné) today, she said the same thing about grandpa a drinking in Russia.

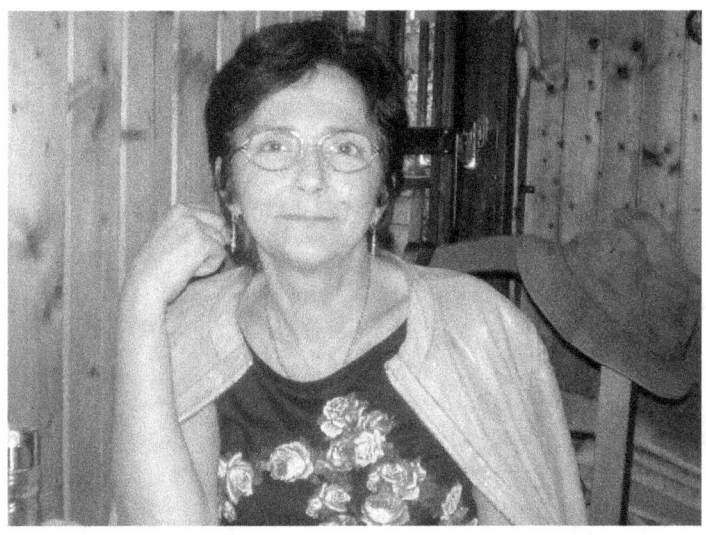

My aunt Kati, 2011 Slovakia, Zsolyom region

Kati was remembering how wonderful he was, and she started sharing some funny stories about him. She recalls a story that happened. There was a phone call that got to my aunt that my grandfather took some medications and he was not responsive. They sent an ambulance out. My aunt called my grandmother (Szarvas Magdolna) to find out what had happened. She thought her father was a happy, well rounded person, so what happened? She was telling me how nothing was wrong with him, he had his little pálinka, then everything was ok. My grandfather always used to say that he had a beautiful life. My aunt feels that all that he suffered through in his life he just looked everything in the past and had fun on it now. It is like looking at our fears in the eye and laughing. My grandmother told my aunt, why what would be wrong with your dad, he is snoring on the couch he had some drinks. My aunt thought that she was just trying not to tell her what is going on because my aunt was pregnant at that time. She insisted on talking to him. She was panicking and told him what she heard. My grandpa said: Well, bum, then they can come and pump my stomach if they want to that is not something I had done before, anyway. They were laughing so hard. It was a mistake; it was the wrong person. It was somebody else in the family. My grandmother ended up redirecting the ambulance to the place they needed to go. My aunt Kati describes a bar that grandpa used to go to (Dagály utca 7, söröző in Budapest Hungary). The bar is nonexistent now, but I found a picture of the location of it, see below. I guess grandpa stopped there every morning before work and a half deci pálinka was already there for him to get every morning. It was a custom apparently that it was on the table waiting for the regulars.

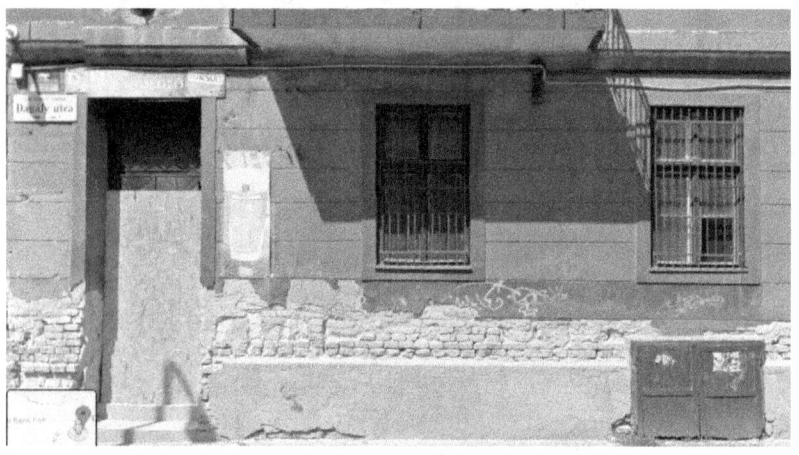

Dagály utca 7., Budapest, Hungary

Kati was also telling me that my grandpa had a license to drive a tank. Never heard about it before. Kati asked him why he don't buy a car, life would be easier to get around. He told her, oh no, I like alcohol better. (We had a good laugh on this) Kati recalls that my grandpa was hungry many times in his life and the only time she saw him upset when my father was young and he did not eat the food that was front of him, it was potato with parsley (it is so good, especially from fresh young potatoes in the spring). This was my grandpa. Most wonderful man someone can imagine. My grandfather died of a heart problem when he was 75 years old. Was it from years of drinking alcohol? Was it his time? We will ever know. My dad was telling me that when my grandfather came home from Russia, he was sick from the alcohol. He was an alcoholic by that time. He was around 48 years old. Dad recalls that before my grandpa was an engineer, he was a roofer. He worked on the Basilica in Hungary and a museum. There was no way he could have had a drink then dad recalls, since roofers did not drink because they would had fallen down from the roof. My dad said this so funny I was bursting out laughing. He also said: "if you drink as a roofer you just die". I try, but sometimes the translation to English from Hungarian just does not sound the same. Grandpa sometimes talked a lot if he had a little too much to drink, then dad would tell him, ok, that is enough, and he would just say, ok son, and go to bed. I wish I had more time to spend with him. He was a teacher in college, he was teaching Math. Alcohol maybe was not the direct cause of his death, it contributed to it some. Alcohol is not good for the body. Once my grandfather invited Dad and Erika (his wife Erika Kőrösiné Budás) to dinner. When they got there in the afternoon the door was closed. They ring the bell, nobody came out. They smelled smoke. Dad tried to call; he did not pick up the phone. At that time the phones were down the street. Dad broke the door. It took 3 tries then my dad fallen through the door. He tried twice then he put his hands together and said God let me through this door. It worked; he fell through the door. My grandpa was sleeping, snoring, like there is nothing going on. My dad woke him up, asked him what he was cooking. He was making pacal a Hungarian specialty, well dad said, lets then repaint the kitchen. Everything was black in the kitchen. He put up the food in a pressure cooker. The kitchen was painted 2-3 weeks before. It was a lot of work to get the kitchen back to normal. Dad recalls the bean soup that my grandpa used to make; it was wonderful with smoked ham. Dad said he loved all his grandchildren very much. He was ready to help any time. I remember him watching my sisters when they were young. I stayed at my mom's and just saw dad on the weekends, so I did not have a lot of time to spend with grandpa. My maternal grandmother (Nagy Borbála) lived not too far from grandpa so when I visited her, I tried to see my grandpa too. Many times, I would find him sitting at a bench in front of the condominium with the neighbor, smoking or just talking. Cannot really turn time back, he could be still alive today, maybe. I know he is here in spirits and I am forever thankful that I met him and was able to spend some time with him here and there. I was very sad when he died but did not fully realize what I had lost until much later. Spend some time with loved ones, because we just never know how long we have. Sit by them, listen to the stories they have to say. Just be there. Dad said the drinking got worse when my grandmother died. While she was alive his drinking was more under control. My dad said my grandfather's view on making money was that it is difficult to earn it but anyone stupid can spend it. All the money he made he would give to my grandmother. If he would ask money for a drink, she would give him money for one. Only one. She knew this, he knew this. There was never a problem. Not until she died. When he was alone, he would drink to forget things.

    My grandfather and father had a little cabin on a lake where he liked to go and fish. I have been there many times. My dad recalls that about each Thursday grandpa always really wanted to go fishing. He did not drive but we had a family friend Zsiga who did. Zsiga usually drove my grandfather fishing. It was more than about fishing of course. They left this particular Thursday just like any other Thursday. My dad and his family were going to go that Friday as well. It was a regular weekend activity to get out of the city and hang around with friends; it was a great place for kids too. My grandfather and Zsiga took wine with them for the whole weekend, by the time my father got there next day with his wife and my sisters all the wine was gone and some palinka as well, then they started to drink beer that my father was going to have that weekend. In these cases, my dad might get a little upset. My grandfather was a "good drunk" dad describes, never got violent, or aggressive. Zsiga however did, dad recalls he would keep saying he is not drunk then actually fall down from the roof which actually happened then he would call my dad for help. I am not sure what he was doing on the roof drunk. He stepped wrong and broke a bone. My grandfather never even thought about treatment.

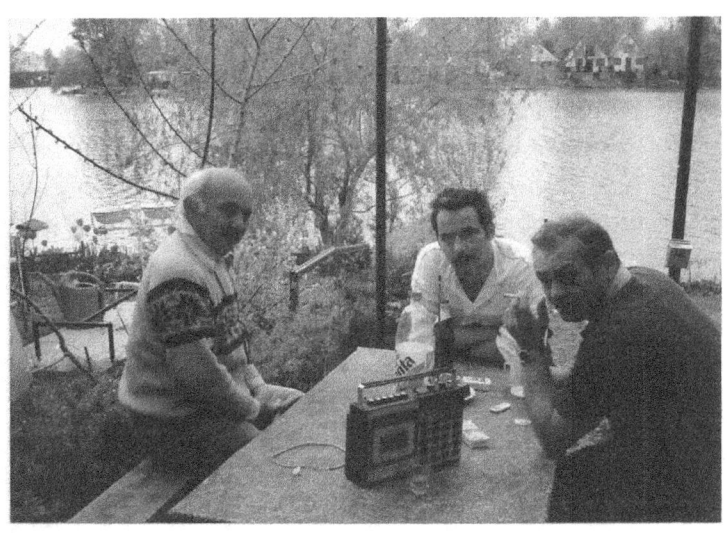

My dad, grandfather and Zsiga at the fishing cabins, Hungary 1994

The last time my grandfather went out to fish he went to a party that was at a friend's fishing cabin. He went back to my dad's fishing house after the party which was about 50 meters away. Everything was really close; small little cabins around a little fishing lake. He did not go back to the party and next morning friends asked their grandkids, two teenage boys, to go check on my grandfather. He was not out fishing in the morning which was unusual. This was 1995 August 2nd. The boys went in, the door was unlocked. He was dead. He was sitting on the edge of a bed. Dad thinks it was a breathing or heart problem. He died alone which was very sad. All his family remembers him with great love. My dad would love if he would be still around, he would not mind taking care of him. He misses him, so do I.

10. Alcohol - Drinking

    Beth did not realize that her husband was drinking heavily after her brother died. He was drinking a lot, not just on the weekends, but he was drinking every day, missing out on family events, spending a lot of money creating financial difficulties for the family. When he started drinking her gorgeous, beautiful husband lost himself and the ugly come out. He lost control over spending money. His behavior changed. Sometimes we all miss things. Beth was in deep sadness about her brother's death from opiates and trying to cope herself, she cried a lot. It is hard to stay behind. Beth ended up going to an Al-Anon meeting, she found an all-girl one, went to the meeting where they told her she cannot change the person they got to go and figure out themselves and they cannot come back until they figure things out. This is exactly what she did, it was hard, but it worked. Alcohol was affecting everything, the family's finances, his job, their marriage, he did go into treatment when he was offered the choice and he is been sober for 5 years now. Even after treatment getting their life back on track together was no easy, finances had to be sorted out, family issues had to be resolved. It was hard for them. They did make it through. Treatment can help. It can work. It worked for Beth's husband and for her, it created a deeper understanding for her what addiction is. Beth remembered her mom saying that alcohol runs in her family. She did not realize it then but realizes it now that deep down she knew it was a disease.

    Mary described her father as an alcoholic who stopped drinking when she was 10 years old. He started drinking again later in life before he died. Even though her father was drinking Mary does not recall her father being drunk or having any discussion about alcohol in the house. She remembers bottles with interesting labels in the cabinet, thinking back she thought it might had been whiskey. Once when she was about 10 years old when she heard some noise, walked out and all family was gathered around her father. His head was bleeding, and he had been in a car accident because he was drunk. Her brother in law was a police officer who brought him home and did not take him to jail. Her father ended up going to treatment for about a month and everything was back to normal after that she did not notice any major change. Mary describes 3 of her siblings who are also alcoholics, one of her sisters had died. Her older brother also used methamphetamine with the alcohol. Mary's sister did not start to drink until she was 60 years old. She started drinking so heavily every day that her kids had to set limits of her being around grandkids. She was able to stop after about 4-5 years. Her other sister Evelyn, who died 10 years ago started drinking at age 13 and was drinking very heavily. Mary remembers Evelyn always was gone, always at parties, skipping school. Mary felt like Evelyn seemed to have something better to do than to be home. Evelyn had a very active social life that was evolved around drinking. The drinking did not stop even when she had kids. Mary remembers watching Evelyn and knowing that is not the type of life she wanted. Evelyn never looked good, never looked healthy or felt good. Evelyn was smart, but her intelligence was kind of blocked by the alcohol. Mary also felt very sad to see Evelyn's kids grew up around alcohol, be around it all the time. Evelyn was diagnosed with breast cancer, was drinking through treatment until she died.

    Mary grew up people around her drinking at all time, yet she was never a drinker, nor she was ever interested in alcohol. It is interesting what makes someone more susceptible then others. Mary felt that people don't drink because they are happy, she felt like her sister was medicating some kind of pain she had. Mary had heard stories from her older brother who is also an alcoholic and used drugs that he was molested as a child by a family friend. Mary knows what this does to the child's brain and was wondering if the same thing happened to her sister, maybe that was the pain she was hiding. Childhood trauma can cause serious mental health and substance abuse in life. Breaks my heart that this happened to Mary's brother and maybe to her sister as well. Evelyn never asked her own daughter about her feelings and never talked about her own feelings. Mary feels that something happened to her sister when she was a kid that she never disclosed and just covered it up. Mary has 7 siblings and feels very sad that a few of them took the route of using alcohol, while others never even smoked or had a drink, yet they all come from the same household. Mary felt that is very confusing. She was wondering if the time between youngest and oldest kids have to do something with this, as the age difference between the oldest child to the youngest is 17 years.

      Dr. Tedd Levin tells me a story about his wife's father who was a brightly functioning alcoholic, who was an engineer. He took care of him as a doctor, his father in law just did not trust anyone else. He insisted to see him as a doctor. He died of liver cancer. This condition was related to the cirrhosis of the liver that was caused by drinking. He stopped drinking when he was in his mid-50's, even though it was too late, he developed cirrhosis, he died at age 73. His cirrhosis was treated, but it was a set up for liver cancer. Liver cancer usually develops in a cirrhotic liver. The pre-existing cirrhosis can be caused by alcohol, or infection by Hepatitis B or C, explained Dr. Levin. It was challenging at times to take care of him since he was a family member. He died by his choice with assisted suicide, which had only recently become legal in the state of Oregon. Currently the preferred term is physician aid in dying. His whole family was there. Once he could not get out of bed without assistance and become incontinent, he just called up the family and told them this is it. Today is the day. He could hardly walk by that time; he was wasting away recalls Dr. Levin. He was in pain by that time and had no quality of life. All his children decided not to drink alcohol. They learned from their dad's mistake. He discussed how some people just cannot control drinking alcohol and the use escalates while others are able to control their drinking. It is complicated he continues it is genetics as well as personal decisions. We discussed difficulties about alcohol that it is everywhere. He said yeah it is a pervasive part of our culture.

      Paige shares that there is a lot of addiction issues in her family, her stepfather has been a "big time alcoholic". This created a lot of difficulties in the family especially for her mom. Her stepdad was close to Paige's husband they were doing things together, they both liked the outdoors. Her husband could not figure out that he had been drinking he was a "closet alcoholic" and they moved in with them to save money and that is when they realized what has been going on. He got himself into a hit and run, Paige went home from work to have lunch and there was an officer on her doorsteps looking for him. Paige had a talk with him about the unsafe environment for her children. Her stepfather went to treatment. The problem was then that after treatment all the issues come up that originally started the drinking. Her stepfather was abused very bad as a child by his dad. Both him and his sister as well, Paige believes that there was molestation happened to both of them when they were kids. His sister talked about it, but her stepdad did not, he could not go there it was too painful. Things were good for a while, but then he slipped back to his addiction. In a way Paige felt that her mom preferred when her stepfather was dinking, because then she did not have to deal with all the other issues, and she know what he needed. Once stopped he become depressed and her mom did not know how to deal with it. Paige describes an occasion when her stepfather got very sick from alcohol, and they needed help from the neighbor to get him back to the house. This was very embarrassing for her family. He was not responding well, and they did not have medical coverage. Her mom was not sure if she should call an ambulance. Paige told her: "if you don't, he will die". He made it through. Paige is still amazed how long has he lived with the amount of Alcohol he has consumed. His behavior does get very embarrassing for the family.

    Chief Jason describes alcoholism as very strong in his community, he feels that this is very sad. He describes a personal experience when a field training officer told him that alcohol is a way to deal with stress. He was laughing and thought that this idea was ridiculous. He found this comment very amusing because it was thought in the academy and growing up that alcohol is not good for anxiety and stress. We talked about the misconceptions of alcohol that people think that going out and having fun and relaxing is connected to alcohol somehow. In my conversation with Tracy who work as a counselor helping families, she recalls that addiction was a big part of her family when she was growing up. Lot of her family was addicted to alcohol. Three out of 4 of her grandparents, both sides of her family owned bars and she was raised around the alcohol industry. She learned how to poor a beer and top a beer at age 4. She had worked in the bar after hours to serve her family. She played bartender. Addiction was a big part of her life. She did not realize until she become a young adult how unhealthy and dysfunctional that was. She feels her experience in her family is what drove her into her current occupation working with families. She is working with families that are having issues with addiction, addiction had touched their lives.

    Diana describes her mother's side of the family where all the boys were alcoholics. There were 6 boys, and all had alcohol issues. I asked Diana how this affected the family. She said her grandmother just did what she had to get from morning to night. Diana describes being a young child and spending time on the family farm not knowing what was going on. She said they had a great time everyone was happy all the time (at this point we both laughed). When she got older her mother talked to her about the problems with her brothers. Grandpa loved the family but was not a nice person and he was not nice to the boys nor to her grandmother. She discussed the personality changes in people who drink alcohol how it can change from day to day. We never know from day to day if they are going to be good or bad and this is hard to live with. Chloe describes a lot of drinking, but she feels it is hard to know who is an alcoholic and who is not. People can hide alcoholism very well. I was just talking to Thomas today who was deep into alcoholism for about 15 years and he hid it very well from his family. Ron describes his experience with Circuit parties and his relationship with a boyfriend where they would travel from one party to another. In these huge parties were drugs and alcohol present it was part of the party scene. Traveling, party culture, big names, big venues. Ron got out of it in 2004, he got out of the craziness. There was a publication on just circuit parties. It was huge. He describes going to Spain for a 5-day Circuit thing called mad bear. It was all over the world. Part of it was the party drugs and alcohol. Ron ended up getting out of the relationship.

    Joel talks about her mom's drinking and also her struggles with weight. Her mom would take diet pills and not lose weight at the same time sitting with her Joel describes her mom drinking 4000 calories worth of rum and coke while they sit and have a conversation. Not recognizing that this is a problem. She feels that her mom has been going back and forth throughout the years, now she moderates her drinking. Alcohol used to be the main focus and it was a daily and everyday activity, now her mom drinks on the weekends and on occasion. She has been successful on moderating her drinking. Joel was wondering if her mom was really addicted or was just drinking to feel the time and space with something. Can someone be addicted and do something in moderation? Maybe the prediabetes scared them Joel asserts. She is very happy that her mom is doing so well now, she looks much healthier and she can go over there and have a cocktail with dinner but that would be the only thing they would not drink anything else after.

Janett describes her mom's side of the family struggling with addictions. Janett's family has Irish heritage, grew up outside San Francisco. Janett describes all her mom's family having issues either having addiction themselves or marrying someone who had addiction. One of her uncle's died on the streets using alcohol or drugs, she was not sure. Another uncle lives under a bridge at the next town over where Janett grew up. Her mom was struggling with drinking when she was growing up. Her mom had 7 siblings. She was not abusive, but for a little while she was neglectful, and for a long time, she was just very angry. Janett forgot for a while that her mom had a personality; she was just this angry cloud. She was able to stop drinking and now she has been sober for 20 years. Janett now laughing said then she started to realize that her mom is a human being with a personality. She describes growing up in a chaotic situation and feeling more comfortable with people who had similar problems even though it made her feel crazy, she was dating people who had addiction problems. It made Janett feel like when she was a kid again and had to deal with whatever was going on. Janett went to Al-Anon for a few months and she describes that this had changed her life when she had heard other people's stories. She feels Al-Anon changed the trajectory of her life, she was originally going to work on the fears of her mom relapsing and hoping to resolve childhood issues. Then she realized more is going on and she broke up with her boyfriend who was addicted to cocaine. In her mom's family Janett's grandmother died of alcohol poisoning when she was 51 years old. Her grandmother was a binge drinker in her mom's entire life and one night she had too much to drink. She died.

Janett's aunt was married to someone who was alcoholic, had two children, he was abusive, he ended up getting worse. Ultimately, they divorced. Unfortunately, and ironically one of the kids, Janett's cousin was walking on the side of the road one day when **_he was 17_**

and got killed by a drunk driver. There was more tragedy to come. Janett's grew up with her other cousin. They went everywhere together from kindergarten through high school. He went to a party one night where he hot drunk, he was messing around with his friend and hit his head on the floor. ***He got a traumatic brain injury; he was 21 years old*** and died 2 years ago. He was disabled, unable to speak or care for himself. He lived in a care home and two of Janett's aunts dedicated all their time to care for him for 3-4 years before he passed away. He died from pneumonia. All his systems were compromised by his time and he could not fight it off. This was very hard for Janett. He partied a lot, he drank a lot and smoked a lot of pot. It was difficult to tell she said if he was just going through a phase or had an actual problem with substances. He went through a lot before with the abusive father and her brother being killed so young. He was 15 years old when his brother was killed. Janett feels he did go kind of reckless and drink more he should have. By that time even though they knew all the same people because they went to high school together, they did not hang out with the same people. Janett is scared of using any alcohol of drugs because of her family history or doing anything habitual. She would drive a different way if she come one way, do things differently when she can, eat different things just to make sure nothing becomes a habit for her. Janett wonders where is the line between young people experimenting and addiction. She recalls when all this happened to her cousin a lot of people were doing the same thing who made it through that phase, but he did not.

    Tragedy seems not to stop for this family. The boys' father drank so much that he was having alcoholic seizures and become unable to care for his finances, people were taking advantage of him. He had money. One time a taxi driver talked him into buying him a $100,000 car. At this point Janett's aunt took over the finances even though they were divorced and made sure things were paid for him. He was mentally disabled. Within the year after the traumatic brain injury accident he died. Janett's aunt literally lost everyone in her immediate family related to alcohol. She made it through somehow. She is still doing well, has great coping skills, she is healthy, exercises, spend times with friends, she is in a very stable relationship. We had a discussion on how many people in Janett's family were touched by addiction. So much tragedy and loss in one family. Janett does have a brother who also went through a phase of drinking and smoking pot, but he hardly drinks now. Janett's mom was lost for a long time, but now her life is back in order, their relationship is good now.

Janett also describes an aunt on her father's side of the family who is very active in her addiction to alcohol now. She describes this aunt living out in the mountains, farther away from society in the woods. She has a boyfriend who also lives in the mountains about 45 minutes away from her. She drinks a lot. Every time she goes to see Janett and her family she drinks so much that after 7 or 8pm at the evening she cannot even have a conversation with her. She also smokes pot. She becomes very loud, ridiculous. She starts earlier in the day than she used to and drinks more. Her aunt would say she is trying to drink less for her health, but the next time she sees her she drinks more again and finds excuses to drink. She would ask Janett's husband if he wants to drink another martini. He would say, no I am ok. Then she would be like: "well why don't I make you another one?" He would say, ok, but not sure if I want to drink one. She would say it is fine. Then she would proceed to make another blend and would make a double or quadruple shot of something in a name of sharing. This way she can have another one justifying it.

Janett really loves her aunt, she is like a second mother for her. The alcohol does affect their interactions. Janett used to spend a lot of time with her aunt, she is a very independent and capable person, she built her own house, she is so awesome, but now she drinks so much that her assertive personality comes out. There is just no planning with her Janett said. Examples she gave me were planning a dinner and not getting there until 10-11pm. Additionally, if there is a plan to get somewhere, they always arrive at least one hour late. Janett decided that she will never drive with her in San Francisco again. (She laughs here) Then she gets serious and tells me that especially her daughter can never go anywhere with her aunt. She just drinks way too much and she smokes pot while driving. It is very sad Janett adds. She knows it is her life, she respects that she can live her life any way she wants but it is still sad that Janett can't spend the quality time with her that she used too before she was drinking and smoking pot. She still tries to spend time with her but in the back of her mind it is there, hoping it will be ok, it will not be too overwhelming. Janett really has to prepare herself before spending time with her aunt. There is a fight about everything. It is exhausting. No, we can't do that, no we have to do this, no we have to leave now. She has to be very hyper assertive. Janett now sometimes just gives up on having good conversations with her aunt. Sometimes she calls her, and her aunt just talks her then said I have to go and hung up and Janet was not able to have the conversation she called for. They used to have wonderful conversations together. It is upsetting to Janett that she cannot be as close to her aunt as she would like to be. She is also sad because her daughter will not be able to see the strong amazing aunt she grew up with. She is just trying to accept it for what it is. Then the difficult part for family comes. Janett is not sure what she could do for her aunt. They had some conversations. Her aunt at least about pot felt like that it is better than using other stuff that can kill her faster. Janett does enjoy spending time with her aunt, after a certain time at night she needs to go to bed. (she is laughing here and saying she just does not want to deal with her past a certain point). Janett never told her aunt this. Probably same thing I hear over and over from others. People are afraid of confrontation and losing the relationship with loved ones.

  Chelsea describes growing up with addiction in her family, her mom struggled with alcoholism. Her mom went to rehabilitation, they have done family counseling. Her mom is doing better now. Chelsea feels like this was a reason she was attracted as a provider to work at a FQHC (Federally Qualified Health Center) where she dealt with addictions, mostly opiate crisis she adds. Growing up with a mom who was addicted to alcohol was a heavy experience. It changed her world view; she did not fully realize the effects until she was older. She has a hard time finding words to describe the experience. She wanted to help people because of what her mom went through. She became a provider. It was a shameful and isolating experience for her, she did not talk to her friends about it. She did not have any resource and when she went to her high school counselor to talk about it, they did not have anything helpful for her. She describes the counselors as fish out of water. Now as a provider she knows that there are resources like Al-Anon, but she felt it was very taboo for some reason when she grew up. She felt like growing up with an alcoholic parent was a huge effect on her, she had to grow up faster, worried about her parent, if they went to counseling for example. She kind of had to take on a partial parenting role for her own mother. Her mom has been sober and doing good, but she has slip ups every once and a while and then she has to re-focus. Chelsea thinks her mother turned for drinking to cope with stress, she was not in a good relationship. She got divorced and got with a better support system, put positive influences in her life. This helped her to stay sober.

Era tells me a story coming home one night from work around 1230 and seeing a commotion in her basement. Two kids were there who were drunk. The boys were about 15-16 years old. Her son was playing nurse, he was trying to give them water. Era was trying to get the parent's number because what if something happens to the kids, she would be responsible. She checked vitals on the kids it was normal. She was thinking to call 911 but her son did not want her to do so. They pushed water for them. They were ok next morning but it was very scary for her. Era was drinking some wine back then to help her go to sleep after she come home from work but had no other alcohol at the house. She thinks the boys brought alcohol from somewhere else. She experienced feelings from alcohol like walking on clouds. She was using wine as a sleep aid for 2-3 years. She stopped drinking wine for sleep when her schedule changed, and she got home earlier. She drinks wine now with meals sometimes, she describes as a culture thing in Europe. She feels that people might be drinking wine to go to sleep then wake up and drink more to fall back asleep and become addicted. One-time Era and a few friends went to a place after work and had some wine and chips with cheese, it was nice. She was joking with the others what would happen if police would stop her on her way home. That night it actually happened. The police did stop her. She spent maybe 2 hours with friends. Then she headed home. She likes the back roads. She describes seeing the sewer tops in the middle of the road, she does not like to go on top of them, so she went around it. Police thought that she was drunk and swirling on the road. She was in uniform from work working on an addiction unit. The police officer told her: "ma'am, where you have been?" she told him, he asked if she had a drink she said yes, he asked how much she told him 2 glasses of wine. He did the breathalyzer on her, but it showed a low alcohol content. The police officer still did not feel comfortable with Era driving so decided to take her home. Era never explained to the officer what happened. Why she was driving the way she did. She had to wake up her son said sorry son we have to go get my car. It was funny, but not at the same time. She always just tried not to damage the sewer tops for the city. She was ashamed regardless. The police officer was a very nice young men, and he took time to make sure Era was safe.

Era tells me another story. It was a Halloween celebration. On a party bus. One of her co-workers had a little too much to drink. She had a little too much fun, dancing around the pool, on the bus, flirting, singing, and just acting way more loose than usual. It was very funny. Thank goodness she was amongst friends. Once they got back Era told the co-worker she should not drive. She wanted too, Era said no, she insisted. She took her home. Every minute she would ask Era where she lives. She did a lot of repeating; she would not digest the answers. She never talked to the co-worker about this. Era just made sure she got home safe and watched her walk in the door before she left. Era feels very glad she did this for the co-worker and feels everybody should do this to avoid loss of life.

Bonnie tells me a story about her first husband who was an alcoholic. She mentions that people did not used to talk about his kind of things back in the day. Bonnie is in her 80's. Both of her daughters drink more than they should. She does not say anything to her daughters, she does not want to jeopardize their relationship. She tells me it is very hard to deal with addiction unless the person wants to deal with it. Her great grandson's father has been addicted to things, she was not sure what, he is going to AA and uses pot. In her personal relationships she never experienced anyone wanting to get help to get out of addiction. She had to make a choice for change, she divorced her husband. That was the only way she could fix it. Her ex-husband was never violent, he would stop on his way to home and drink a lot, then come home so drunk that he would barely make it through dinner then fall asleep on the couch. This is how Bonnie lived during her 20's. Watching her husband sleep on the couch. He always smelled she recalls. It is difficult she explains to have romantic feeling about somebody who is like this kind of problem, she felt she was better off without him.

Bonnie's second husband was a binge drinker, he was violent, he would go out once in a while he might do nothing for months then he would go out, drink all of a sudden, then come home, turn the furniture upside down, rip the phone out of the wall, acted like he was going to hit Bonnie, she left before that ever happened. She never married again; she tells me: I am sure you can understand why. She tells me that she did not pick very good men, they picked her. This situation made her feel terrible. She had to go through two divorces. She had two children, two girls, she did not want them to grow up in a home where this sort of things are going on. She could not deal with it anymore, went out on her own and feels she done ok. Bonnie feels that the addiction is handed down in generations and it is a weakness, she talks about both of her girls who did not live with their father only when they were very young, and she is wondering why they are drinking too much. They don't drink or work under the influence but drink way too many glasses of wine once they are home Bonnie thinks, too many for her anyway as she does not drink. She will not talk to them about it because they just get defensive. It can damage their relationship. It is the best for her to stay out of it, this way when she gets old-old, she will have children. She does not think saying anything will help any way if they want to stop drinking, they can do that on their own they don't need her telling them what to do.

    Brenda tells me about Pamela who was really close to her, she was a nurse and she was addicted to alcohol. She was the first person in Brenda's life who had any type of addiction. Her friend was very resistant to get any type of help. Pamela was lonely and alone, she lived in Chicago and her family lived in Las Vegas. Pamela had run a car into a house. Brenda and her fellow co-workers were trying to help Pamela get into treatment and get help, she was resistant. She eventually ended up falling after getting out of the bathtub and died. Brenda describes Pamela as a brilliant nurse, but even though she knew all she knew about medicine and everything she could not assess herself and ended up dying as a result. Pamela was in her early 50's when she died. She was still young to die. I asked Brenda how it makes her feel what happened to her friend and dealing with her addiction. Brenda asserts that dealing with addiction is very difficult because she might have an idea what is right for the person or what would be the best thing to do but the person themselves might not want to do what is best for them. In the end we cannot make the choice for them they have to make it for themselves, they have to be in the right place and make the move themselves, just be there to support them. It is a difficult and frustrating process.

    Susan tells me about her older brother who had been an alcoholic and now he is sober for about 4 years. He could not handle his life really well. She had seen him drunk, provided transportation for him sometimes. He is married now. Susan was surprised his wife stayed with him; they went through a lot. Susan's maternal grandfather died of liver cancer because of drinking. He had a heart attack when he was 36, developed bad anxiety from that and decided to self-medicate with alcohol. Susan's dad used to drink but stopped when she was around 4 years old. One day she brought him a beer when he got home, and it seemed like he did not like that image of his little girl is waiting for him with a beer. He worked in a very alcohol-soaked environment. They had martinis at lunch. Susan's parents talked to her about addictions. She was not sure if they talked to her brothers about it. Her parents were so afraid that she might end up like her brothers that they sent Susan to a private school. She used to be a bartender. She tells me that in a service industry when someone work at a bar there is a lot of drinking. She is not sure why, but a lot of people she worked with would get pretty hammered sometimes. Sometimes even at work or right after work. She saw some regulars at the bar.

    Dolores feels like there is a very alcohol infected culture that we live in. It seems like nobody does anything without having a drink. She feels that the kids see that and think that it is being adult to drink and the only time the adults have fun when they are dinking. It seems that every single entertainment after age of 16 that is available has alcohol. She feels this is a societal issue. Around where she lives the culture is very much involved in drinking. She brings up a very good example. At her work they have been wanting to do a team building exercise. There is a place in town that she heard of and recommended where they have people come in and create a piece of art, and they also serve wine. So, she tells me:" we create art while we are drunk". Interesting concept. We had a discussion about why you even need wine to go paint? Why can't the activity be just to go paint? Dolores said, yeah that is a very good question. She is not much of a drinker; she might have a glass that is it. She feels though others might have a lot. Things could get uncomfortable. Dolores tells me she does not understand why people drink it just makes her tired and she want to sleep. She chuckles. She does not want to drink she can barely stay awake as it is. She said this with such a funny tone that we just both burst out laughing. I listened back to this like 3 times I admit I just wanted to laugh more. Got my daily dose of laughter.

    Fuchsia and I talk on our porch in a nice afternoon. She does not have any addiction in her nuclear family. She tells me that her story begins with her great grandparents on mom's side. They were both alcoholics. They lived on a ranch in Idaho and her great grandfather was selling dynamite for railroad people. He died from liver cancer. Family have not heard much of the dark side of their life only the glorified stories. Fuchsia felt that because she grew up without knowing much about addiction, she was pretty naïve about it. She feels that she had difficulty in the past picking up on when people are using substances.

11. Kevin's story

Dr. Frazier Beatty was telling me about Kevin during our phone conversation. Kevin lost his job with a 6-figure income and over time he has changed. He tells me that Kevin has an incredible story. Dr. Beatty told me that his friend works for the VA, he has been in prison twice, he works now to help veterans and other people. Later I had a chance to connect with Kevin and he told me more about his life. Kevin sent me this picture:

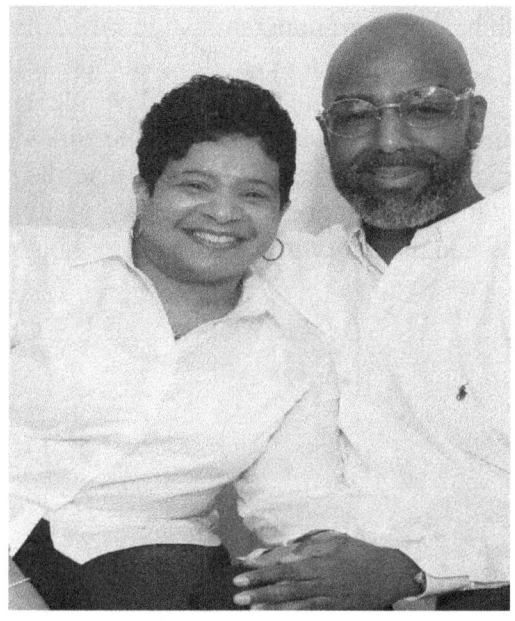

Kevin and his beautiful wife Sheila

Kevin describes his beautiful wife Shelia as an instrumental person that kept him in the quintessential epitome "tough love"! I was talking to Kevin on the phone. Kevin does have an incredible story to tell. He went through a lot in his life and was able to turn it all around and do good. Kevin has been having issues with addictions in the past 30 years. He told me he wants to be as transparent as possible telling his story and chose to fully disclose his identity. He is very kind and humble throughout our conversation. He calls me Dr. Gabriella. He is the first person who called me that since I just received my PhD recently. He first engaged using illicit substances when he was 16 years old. He used alcohol and marijuana before, then he started to use crack cocaine. Cocaine led to this 30 year of addiction with intermittent sobriety. Addiction brought Kevin legal issues, unemployment, it cost him a marriage, loss of home, jobs, incarceration. Kevin is a Marine and also has a good level of education and this made things even more difficult for him. Being a military veteran, he had a lot of pride and humility to reach out for help. Kevin started to use cocaine because he was drawn to the subculture that comes with it. The cocaine took a tremendous hold on him. Once he crossed a threshold from intermittent addiction, there is no way to go back through the door he adds. Have to accept it to face the demon. He remembers that he had a motor vehicle accident in his senior year in college, he was an athlete, playing basketball and was getting a scholarship. He was 22 years old. Because of the accident a young lady lost her life and lost her child. After the accident Kevin went through clinical depression and self-sabotage related to lack of self-esteem and lack of value. Whenever Kevin would get to a good spot he would go and revert back to a bad behavior. It took him 25 years and a lot of clinical hours of therapy to overcome this problem. The irony of this is he tells me that now he is a peer support specialist in the state of Michigan, and he is helping military veterans doing the same thing that he had to work through. This work has been a wonderful experience. Nobody wants to be addicted. It is a difficult process.

  His first sobriety happened in 1990. Kevin had a spiritual awakening at that time, that lasted for 8 years before he relapsed again. At that time, he got a promotion he worked at IBM. He worked for corporate security in a high position. He was doing very well. His youngest son was born at that time. He thought he was invincible. His words. He thought he had this all under control and started to go back out again and actively using cocaine. It took 15 months for him to lose everything. Kevin thought that he can just have a little bit and he is going to be ok. It did not work. He tells me that to this day that is a greatest lie he told himself. He told himself: "look at you, look how good you are doing, you can have a little". It was a loophole for him, and he relapsed. He knows the signs now very well; it helps him when he works with others. Kevin just attended a community event last night and telling me that people are dying of addiction. Not in small numbers he tells me. I asked Kevin how many times he relapsed. He told me too many to count. He would sober up for 3 months or 4 months or 6 months and relapse again. Now he is been sober for 3 years. Kevin's addiction took him to prison twice. He has a felony record. He feels it is remarkable that he was able to get a federal job and able to help others. Kevin tells me that for him there was a point he knew that he can never go back, it's been a long battle, he knows if he would go back again, he would die. He heard this voice just as clear as he is talking to me know. He knew that either the drugs or the lifestyle would kill him. He felt the seriousness of this, he put himself in harm's way before. This time he knew it is his last chance to get sober.

      The first time Kevin went to prison it was for 20 months he got out in a year and a half. He violated a personal protective order and the judge told him he is not getting it and sent him to prison. He got home, he did well for 2 months then got back to his addictive behavior. Not even in a year he was back in prison. The second time he was accompanying someone who was breaking into a home and he got 2.5-3 years in prison. I asked Kevin how his prison experience was, because by this time I talked to many people who told me that they were happy when their loved one was in prison at least they know that they were safe and not using drugs. Kevin was laughing when I asked him. Once he stopped laughing Kevin told me that the first time, he went to prison he was angry and blaming his mother who called the cops on him. He tells me he would be crying in prison and did not wanted to feel like this about his own mother. It did not happen for a while. It took months. Then he tells me one day he was sitting in his cell. Kevin's voice changed here he was excited, like making a discovery. I knew something good was coming. He heard a voice telling him: "listen if you were going to a stranger's home at night at any hour of a night beg them to give you money wouldn't that be stalking?" He realized that the answer is yes, then he asked himself, so then why isn't it stalking when it comes to his mother? Kevin realized that he put his mother in a situation where she thought the only option, she had was to call the police. Kevin accepted what had happened. He tells me that first when people go to prison, they blame their family, they blame someone, they feel betrayed, there is a lot of anger. He feels that people are so disconnected from feelings at that time that they do not want to take ownership of what had happened to them. He changes his tone and he sounds like a teacher now. He tells me that **addiction is a selfish disease. People don't understand while in it how much they hurt others**.

He tells me people have to be selfish to be addicted. He now looks back and knows that his family never turned their backs, they were enablers and he believe they were ecstatic when he went to prison, they knew that he was safe, and they were safe. Looking back, he feels it was absolutely a good thing that he ended up in prison. He met a pastor in prison who was his polar opposite, he talks about him with a lot of compassion and love. Kevin was a young black man; the pastor was an older white man. He made a great impression on Kevin, how he cared about others, how he carried himself, the humility he had. Kevin keeps in touch with him still today. Now he works with people in prison and act as a mentor, providing support for them. Kevin received much help to be able to be where he is today. He feels that it is important for him to turn around and provide as much help to others as possible. Sometimes people don't know that they need help. I asked Kevin how he stopped using. He tells me that he put himself in a situation where he was robbed and beaten. He speaks a little slower now remembering what happened. It was people who he knew, it was all a set up. It was his sub circle of people; he had a large amount of money on him. He was furious, he was telling himself things like he is going to go kill them, and he talked himself out of things. He did not want to go back to prison. He slept on it, woke up the next morning, and realized he needs to quit to be ok. It was not immediate. In about 2 months he needed surgery, but the surgeon told him he cannot do the operation with cocaine in his system. There was a risk of him dying on the operating table. He was living on the streets at this time, by choice. He heard the voice inside his head asking him again: "Do you want to die? You will die if you keep continuing with this addiction". He decided he did not want to die. The way he tells me this both he and I burst out in laughing. Death is not supposed to be funny, the topic is certainly not funny, but the way he said it, I wish you could hear his voice. We laughed for a while. It gave a moment of pause and release of energy while we were talking. That was the last time he used cocaine. He had his operation and started over. He stopped smoking cigarettes, he changed his life around from his diet to exercise, he did a complete shift. He runs a mile every day.

  I asked Kevin how did he make the change, who he called for help? He had relatives and he was staying with his sister through this time. He had a long road ahead of him. The biggest thing he had to re learn was how to handle money. He did not want to have more than 20 dollars on him even 20-dollar bill as a previous addict can be the worst thing to have. Addiction can get started again. He needed to learn how to go to the store and buy things that he needed like deodorant, razors, pay a cell phone bill, just to do small things. He put up a stop sign, created an accountability team around him, call him out on his "BS". This is what he did. He started working, got back to his fraternity and went back to church. He is now involved with his community doing at least 2 community events a month, he is mentoring a 7th grader, he believes in giving back the gifts and tools that God gave. I ask him about cravings. He has not had any. Kevin tells me about his job, he used to work for the VA before he lost his job. About 3 years ago he tried to get a job back, but he was denied because of his background. He was upset, but he understood. Another job came up 6 months later. He talked to them and told them he just went through this process he wanted to make sure he was eligible before applying. He got the call that he was. 2 months later he found out that the job offer was rescinded. Kevin got back to a real dark place then. He was contemplating suicide. Before he opened the denial letter, he went to pick up some Chinese food and went to his sister's house. After reading the letter, he knew he wanted to go use cocaine. He talked himself out of it by eating first. Then Kevin tells me he was sitting there contemplating, he heard his voice again: "if you go out on that door, you will never come back again". He decided to pick up the phone and call a peer support specialist who he was in training with. He used every tool he had learned to make sure he does not do something he would regret later. Kevin tells me just think about that I almost went out and used and tried to kill myself because I did not get a job offer.

Kevin just lost his friend of 50 years recently and he is very grateful that he was able to be at the funeral, support his friends' family thought he process. Kevin has been very successful and has been able to provide housing and other supports for veterans and people coming out of jail. I asked Kevin what addiction for him is. He paused. He told me people have been trying to define addiction so long. Kevin defines addiction: to engage in a daily lifestyle that prevent him from enjoying life. Making a choice to give up being a father, son, brother, husband, and to be the most anti-law obeying social person he could be. Every day he made this choice. His job was to get high. That is the only thing existed. We took a pause for a moment. I was not sure what to say, it was just kind of soaking in for a second. Then I told him I would sure love that if everyone would have the little voice in their head that he had. He laughed. Kevin kept laughing, then he told me that the funny part is that we do we just don't listen to it. He tells me he heard the voice so many times before, but he did not listen to it. So many times. He describes his experiences while using as insane. He just made a choice to stop. He laughs again. Kevin had a great laughter. He just made a decision that if he can stop the drugs he can stop smoking too. He was able to make good choices. Kevin feels that society drives on addiction. He tells me that people in America want instantly what pleases us. He is in Detroit; Michigan and he recalls a big thing about bringing casinos there. Everybody was against it because people knew what is coming with a casino. America has the strongest consumers Kevin asserts. He is upset by this. Kevin describes addiction as a 100-billion-dollar enterprise in America. He feels this will never go away; it is too much money people make on addiction. Again, it is all about money. It is sad especially when so many lives are lost, and families torn apart.

    Kevin feels like society has a moral responsibility. If there is no moral responsibility, then we can never have a humanitarian responsibility. He tells me about policies and legislations and that people can never execute a legislation to eradicate moral injustice; and brings up addiction treatment. Kevin recalls that addiction treatment used to be 18 months now you ae lucky if you get 30 days. You know he tells me that even 60 or 90 days does nothing. The brains need much longer time to recover at least a year. That is a minimum Kevin tells me. He sounds upset. People need a chance to get better. We are sending people to rehab to 30 or 60 days he tells me when we know it does not work. The data is overwhelming in both qualitative and quantitative studies that that is a flawed policy. Now, unfortunately it all depends on what the individual and the family can do. This is very hard because those who have low socio-economic status, don't have the resources to get help. The more money someone has the more resources they can get. The inner cities, the major metropolitan areas like the Detroit's, New York, New Orleans, Chicago people don't have the resources. It impacts the whole family. He starts to tell me about the opiate epidemic as an example. There is policy to combat this because it reached places where it was never thought that it could go. It is everywhere. It is not just the stereotypical anymore, we are talking about moms, surgeons, pilots, young high school kids. Increased use in 16-25-year-old white population male and female. We agree it is all about money. Some people are making money while destroying other people and their families. Kevin describes the United States other than the Roman empire as a greedy capitalistic society that is the worse in the history of mankind. He tells me nobody wants to stop the drugs it is money. We have to step up as individuals and support others in wellness, by providing education and support throughout the communities. He tells me that there used to be a time when we knew our neighbors. Now people are afraid of people and we have to eliminate that fear. Kevin feels that we need to get back into being a more social society. Now we are a violent anti-social society.

  Kevin tells me about his family. He had 3 children and 4 grandchildren. He makes effort to keep connected with them. He tells me that it is very rewarding to be an active part of society. He tries to be connected and do his part. He tells me we all just need to do our part. He is making sure he does his part. What else we could do he asks? Is there anything else we could do? How else we could make things better? Kevin is being very open with his family sharing his experiences about addiction. He talked to his kids about having an addictive gene as a possibility. He talked to his kids telling them not to even try anything, asking them to trust him. He feels like there is a lack of common courtesy in our society today, lack of saying things like excuse me, please and thank you. I made Kevin chuckle again by bringing up my magic wand question. Kevin, if he would have a magic wand, he would make addiction awareness education mandatory in our school system. Continuous education in each grade. He tells me it needs to be upfront, the data, the reality, it needs to be ugly, it needs to be real. Kevin had watched individuals drink themselves to death. He feels kids to know how long a physiological recovery can take if a person is even able to recover. No one is removed from it anymore. It has touched every household in America in some shape or form. Very true. Kevin tells me face it, in this country people will always have the option to use illicit drugs because the demand for it is so high.

12. OPIATES

Many people I talked to said opiates are a big problem. I had many informal conversations during my career with patients and providers about opiates. One thing is clear, they can be very useful for acute pain, but can be very addictive using long term. During our discussion Dr. Tedd Levin had mentioned that more people died of prescribed opioids then car accidents in the United States. We talked about that many people were prescribed opiate pills like Vicodin or Oxycontin first ten become addicted to other non-prescribed drugs. Prescription opiates can be very expensive Dr. Levin said, so people could not afford it and ended up buying heroin on the street. He gives an example of Oxycontin 80 mg twice a day costing over $1000.00 per month. Compared to that, heroin is a fraction of the cost.

Chief Jason describes doctors who are willing to give out prescriptions very easily. He feels there is a lack of standards to determine if a person really needs the pain medications or not. He feels it has gotten better over the years. He remembers when he grew up his mom would just call and get a prescription. Now people have to go in in person to see the doctor to get pain medications. Kayla describes opiates as a whole another problem. Especially when people had known that they can be addictive. She asserts that before a medication is distributed to the public there are more research that needs to be done around it. Additionally, more education for the people who are distributing it. Rory talks about opiate problems this country had before in the 1800's. He said it was outrageous. San Francisco looked like people were just draped over stuff. It was very common. Now the pill poppers are closing, they got shut down.

Tracy describes her sister who is 8 years younger from her and addicted to opiates. She lost her first child because of opiates and Tracy ended up adopting her sister's baby. Now her sister just gave birth again and the baby was born very ill with multiple problems. The baby was born 3.5 months early, had hydrocephalus, possible brain damage from that, cerebral palsy. Tracy feels like the cause of all this was the drug treatment her sister was receiving while she was pregnant. The doctors are saying not, but Tracy looked at the CDC website and the side effects are listed there. She is very frustrated about this. No matter what the baby will have the consequences for the rest of her life as well as the family raising this child. Her mother is helping her raise the baby. She is able to take care of the baby when she is sober otherwise mom helps said Tracy. Tracy describes her sister as a "pill popper" she has had periods of being clean and sober, been in treatment several times. Tracy's sister used to have a great job in the medical field then she lost it after stealing prescription pads from work and was writing out prescriptions pretending it was for her significant other and his family.

Most of the families Tracy works with people who are in trouble because of heroin. It is the biggest problem she sees out there now. We talk about difficulties to break the cycle of heroin addiction. It is very difficult. She calls it a tug of war how the drug gets hold of people. I asked Tracy if she had seen success stories when it comes to heroin addiction. Tracy describes success stories with heroin as little successes to celebrate the small things. She describes moms who go through treatment, get sober, follow support that was provided for them and even it is just for 6 months, it is a success Tracy feel a small one, but a success. She sees families coming back. Families that were doing great for 6 months, one year or two years, then there is a relapse and the families come back again. She feels like long term support would be helpful, all the resources she is aware are short term. Most things she describes are intensive and short term while addiction is a lifelong disease, need lifelong support.

I talk to Susan on the phone. She tells me about her older brother Emanuel who was a heroin addict for about 10 years. It was pretty bad. Luckily, he was able to get clean for 7 or 8 years now. Susan was 10 years old at that time. It was a lot for the family. I ask her for more details, it is still a painful memory. It was hard for her to understand at that young age what is going on. Once Susan was in high school, she started to understand more. Emanuel was homeless for a while; she would go and look for him on the streets of downtown Portland. He was missing for a while. After rehab, he was sober, the family was so happy that everything else from the past was brushed under the rug. It is very complicated she asserts. Susan never really talked more about this with Emanuel.

He is still very defensive about his addiction. Susan feels he did not work through it mentally what was going on with him. He is not doing any recovery work now. Emanuel went to rehab about 9 times. He was on methadone for a while, attended groups as part of that, but nothing else. He uses cannabis now. I asked Susan how their relationship is affected by Emanuel's heroin use and recovery. She was telling me that it is funny that I asked this they just got into a fight. She tells me about enabling. It is difficult for her to draw boundaries. Emanuel gets upset if she draws boundaries. Now he is been trying to move in with Susan and her boyfriend. She does not want to do this. Emanuel takes advantages of things. Susan describes her brother trying to make her happy, butter her up to try to get what he wants. He is manipulative. He has a job; he grows medical cannabis. Susan saw him high. Emanuel was on Suboxone for a while, he was out of his mind and talking to the wall. Suboxone had a funny effect on him. Susan's mom became a drug and alcohol counselor to be able to do something about it. Susan's brother still has difficulty today to take responsibility for his actions and would blame family for things that happened to him. He can't see that he did anything wrong. He stole things from his parents and took things to the pawn shop.

  I been talking for Dolores for a while, when she recalls that she does have a cousin whose son died of an opiate overdose. She thinks it was accidental, not intentional. He was admitted to treatment, he had been in treatment for about 6 or 9 weeks, Dolores was not sure. He came out of treatment and he was living with his parents. Dolores saw him after his sister's wedding. The treatment program did not let him out for the wedding, he arrived later and met the people who were still there. He was doing very well at that time. He had a friend with him from the program. He was getting ready to have a job. Two weeks later they found him dead. He was 25 years old. Dolores feels that he failed to realize that once he was sober, he cannot use as much heroin as he used before. She feels people can be arrogant about this and use the same amount. This was a big tragedy in Dolores's family. Dolores was far away when it happened, she was removed from the tragedy, her cousins were just devastated. One of their children get married and the other died just a few weeks after. Very sad situation. He had been using a long time. He seemed to have other problems too and previous trauma was present for a sexual abuse.

Fuchsia tells me about her experience dating someone who had been dealing with heroin addiction. When they were dating, Paul was clean and sober. He spent a lot of time focusing on staying sober, which makes sense she asserts, that is what was keeping him alive, and it did take priority over everything else in their lives. Every decision thy made carefully had to be weigh if it would be a good decision for Paul, and his sobriety for example where they live. Paul was big in the AA community as well. He got sober when he was 22 years old, he is 29 years old now. Paul lost family and friends as he was growing up, he lost more than a dozen people around him related to overdose. This was his world. That is what he knew. Fuchsia tells me Paul lost so many people during the years they were dating. Paul's friends were into addiction, some of them were people relapsing. Paul had a friend who relapsed one night, overdosed and died. Very sad stories of people who are really struggling. Fuchsia describes this: "***huge dark world of pain that they are living in***". Knowing the people and hearing their stories gave her a lot of empathy for them and what they are going through. Paul had hepatitis C, did not tell his stories to other people besides AA. He was ashamed. Fuchsia does not like to lie and keeping his secret was very hard for her. It became complicated when they would go out and do outside activities, she was concerned about not telling her parents because if something happens, they need to protect themselves from his blood.

Paul did not even want to share that he has Hepatitis C. He had a lot happen in his childhood, divorce, family deaths to deal with. He had been through a lot. Fuchsia was wondering where all the shame come from, he was very private about his story. Paul had an overbearing personality. Fuchsia felt maybe he thought he would not be accepted if people knew. Paul's story is very difficult, he was homeless for a long time, for Fuchsia, for months after she heard his story and see a homeless person she would cry. It was him; it could be him. He was living in a big city, with nothing. She saw pictures before he went to rehab and how he looked. It took Fuchsia about a year just to process all this. It was hard for Fuchsia to understand addiction, the process of rehabilitation, AA. She wanted to understand and talked to him about it, but on the other hand it was traumatizing for her to hear all these stories. Then he told her about Al-Anon meetings. She did not know what that was. She went to him with one AA meeting Saturday night. The regular meetings she could not go to with him they were closed. There was a meeting for men and one for people who been sober a long time. They were both closed meetings. This was a whole world Fuchsia was never going to be a part of. Fuchsia had this problem with AA with he is thinking that others don't understand what is going on with someone who went through addiction and in recovery. Paul told her that too, that she does not understand. She felt Paul would minimize other people's problems or what they went through because they did not use substance as a band aid.

Another issue she had with AA that her boyfriend was so service oriented that he ended up volunteering for people all the time whom he just met and things that needed to be done in their life for example mowing the lawn would not happen. He helped a lot of people; this effort was not carried through at home. **All his energy went to other people and he did not put much energy on the people who were actually around him.** Paul would be quick to tell Fuchsia if she expressed a feeling about something that this is not her story and don't be co-dependent. She tells me that it was her story too because everything they did impacted her. It was amazing to witness what Paul had done with his life. Turned it around, graduated from school. Paul has a good job now. I asked her if she knows what made him start and stop his addiction. She tells me he started at age 14, he grew up in a place where everyone used. Paul had a pretty sad childhood. He used for 8 years and he been in different phases of using alcohol then heroin. He tried to get sober 3 times. He 3rd time worked, he got himself into school, he had good community and sponsors. He got away from his hometown. He still has friends that are dying today. Fuchsia wanted to leave him for a while, but she was scared, she did not want to trigger something, she had a lot of struggle with this, she did not want to be a cause a relapse.

I ask Fuchsia, how this experience impacted her. She tells me that is really opened her eyes and she was more judgmental before she knew his story and other people's story. She also feels that **she put her own needs on a hold for a long time to take care of him**. While

Fuchsia was with him it was always about him and anything she wanted to do had to put on hold or really think about if it is safe or ok for him. Is it going to be a trigger for him? Not being open to other people was challenging. After she left, all this trauma came up that she had not processed while they were in it. She feels freed not have to think about issues she had to think about while she was with him. It is kind of freeing, she adds. I ask Fuchsia that based on her experience what addiction means to her. She thinks for a moment. She tells me she thinks it is a manifestation of trauma and repetitive behavior that is damaging to oneself and others. She does not believe that addiction is a choice. She also believes that people either have an addictive personality or they don't. She does not have one.

13. Bonnie's Story

This is a very sad story. My friend Era told me about Bonnie and the story about her granddaughter, Ella. Bonnie was kind enough to talk to me on the phone. It is a fresh wound and I truly appreciate her taking the time to share her granddaughter's story. The events and the loss is still very upsetting to Bonnie. She knew she will get a phone call one day, she thought that phone call will be about her kids not Ella. She never suspected Ella taking anything. It was a complete shock for the family. I ask Bonnie if she could tell me about her granddaughter. It was 8 days before her 31st birthday. Ella had a 6-year-old son. She died on April 11th from a cardiac arrest. The family was trying to figure out how did that happen at her age. Then the tox screen come back and they found out what Ella had drugs in her system. It was a shock and felt that she just died all over again. Bonnie thinks Ella had been taking drugs since she had a c-section. It made her feel good, it does not take much time to get addicted to Oxycontin. Maybe a week. Nobody knew what Ella was doing, there is a lot of guessing in the family. They think she bought pills on the street and she happened to get one of those pills that had Fentanyl in it. She died instantly of a Fentanyl and Oxycontin overdose. Ella was home alone with her son, she took the pill and she fell on the floor, he did not know what to do what was wrong with her, he started screaming and the man who lived on the other side of their duplex came over. He tried to revive her and called 911, they took her to the hospital, it did not work. We all left with this mess Bonnie adds and a child who has no mother. It's been a terrible, terrible time.

The child has been living with Bonnie since the death of his mother. He will be going to live with his father when school starts. Bonnie is not really happy about this, but not much she can do. She is concerned because the father had his own drug issues. The family is watching him very closely. He knows it, they had this conversation with him. She will go to court if there is any sign of use. They are both keeping a diary every day the child is with them; this was recommended by the lawyer they have. In case they ever have to go to court to try to get custody of him. He has been cooperative and thankful for Bonnie. She feels they did everything imaginable for Ella to get through life. When she had he baby and she was not married, she lived with Bonnie's daughter for 3 years, did not have to pay rent.

Now looking back Bonnie thinks Ella used that money for drugs. At the time they just thought she was not making enough money. Bonnie is mostly doing ok, but there are many days when she cries a lot. She is ok when her great grandson is there, but when she is alone it is difficult, and she will be seeing a therapist soon. It is been about 5 months now, it had been so overwhelming for the family, that they could barely function. Bonnie calls Ella the master of disguise and lies. When the child's father was going through drug stuff Ella would not even let him see their son, she was so upset for him using. Ella would not let him see his son until he went to rehab, he did go. She told Bonnie how upsetting it was when her child's father was using drugs and she did not want her child to see that. Now they find out Ella was using pills during that time too. Nobody knew, none of her friends knew, family had been hacking into her accounts of social media and e-mail and found no reference for use. Ella was living this secret life and Bonnie thinks a lot of other people might be doing that. Ella was working two jobs, she had her own little business, and worked at a store as a salesperson. Her workplace loved her. She was a great salesperson. Ella was a functioning drug addict. She was going to be in trouble financially very soon. She was not paying her bills, not renewing her car tabs, not buying car insurance, not taking care of her business insurance and about to lose health insurance through the state both for herself and her son. All these things were going to come down on top of her. Family had no idea about all the money she owned on visa cards and lines of credit. They had been trying to reconstruct her life and they feel very bad that they did not picked up on it that something wrong. There is a lot of guilt of failing her. She was her only grandchild. Bonnie thinks Ella would be still alive if she had not met the father of her child. Bonnie suspects that he did not treat her well, went through with him using drugs, she got no financial support from him. Bonnie's daughter has no child and her great grandson has no mother. Bonnie's mother died when she was 8 in childbirth and she knows what it is to grow up without a mother.

Bonnie feels that we need to get rid of the Fentanyl, the bad Fentanyl she calls it that is coming from China through the post office.

The government needs to work on what is coming into this country. Bonnie asserts that we need to find a way to examine packages that come through the post office. Maybe dogs to check the packages. As long as there is a demand there will be a supply. They will figure out where to get it as long as people are on drugs. If we stop the supply people will eventually have to get clean and have to get off of the drugs. She feels it has gone too far. Bonnie had a recent experience after surgery. She was getting ready to go home and the physician assistant (PA) came in and gave her a prescription to hydrocodone, she told her she can't take it because it makes her throw up. She told her just take it anyway, the PA told her just take it, she told her I don't want it, she told her just take it. She took it, she brought it home, immediately ground it up because she did not want it to have it in her house. She told another PA about this incident after her granddaughter died. She feels this is why we have a drug problem. She asked the PA to talk about this in the office. The PA exactly knew which provider she was talking about. Bonnie didn't want a prescription like that automatically. She took it because she did not want to argue with the PA. She feels like the doctors have a great responsibility when prescribing to do this appropriately. She is wondering what we did before all this drug for pain in the 50's and 60's? This pushing medication was nonexistent.

Bonnie feels like people need to be highly educated when it comes to addictions, effects, be responsible, a lot of information is needed. The general population is weak and just want a pill to fix something. There is a need to change the mentality of people through education in the schools, at the doctor's office. Don't even manufacture Oxycontin. Morphine in the hospital if needed. People need to learn to live with a little pain. Start when kids are young in a health class or set aside time to talk to kids and offer the opportunity for them to talk to people who went through addictions. Bonnie things people can manage through things without taking strong medications like Oxycontin. She just had a mouth surgery before she talked to me, she is using ice and non-opiate over the counter pain relievers for pain. She feels strongly about people needing to be stronger and not use oils for a solution that can be addictive. She tells me: "people just need to buck up and be stronger". Bonnie believes that it is individual responsibility as well as societal and that the pharmaceutical companies caused a lot of the problems as well when it comes to opiates. They were telling doctors it was not addictive and they were prescribing them like crazy. Then, people started taking them and realized how great they feel on it. Bonnie sometimes took prednisone, she took it for one week to help her back, she knows the euphoric feeling. Others find ways to carry it on. We all like to think that life is a bowl of cherries. No pain, full of possibilities. Wouldn't that be great she said, well life isn't like that. We have to learn to deal with it. Prevent doctor shopping. People keep secrets for different reasons, she feels Ella was afraid of losing her son and that is why she did not seek help. There is a lot of stigma around addiction, it is not treated as an illness.

    The government has a big role to step in and help. The high doses Fentanyl comes from China she asserts, and the government needs to stop it. In Ella's apartment 2 pills were found on the counter and a rolled-up dollar bill which they assumed she used to snort the medication. The father of the child called a sponsor from AA, went to the apartment and took care of the pills, they got rid of them. They also found an empty bottle of Suboxone from 2016. They were wondering why she was taking Suboxone in 2016. Bonnie thinks she was already addicted to Oxycontin at that time. She was probably trying to get off. This is very hard for Bonnie's daughter, because Ella lived with her during that time and did not know any of this. She is also seeing a therapist to help deal with all this stuff. Bonnie had a hard time finding a therapist for herself who takes Medicare, she just found one. She is hoping that the therapist will help her get through he transitions of her great grandson going to his father. Trusting him to take care of him. She still will be involved in his life, but just can't trust the father because of the history. Grief will take time she tells me, but she needs help with this transition. She needs guidance.

14. Marijuana

Era tells me a story about her husband Will and marijuana. Will had difficulty sleeping. They went to a sleeping center in 2017 to try to figure out the problem in Edmonds, WA. He did a sleep study with all the wires and everything. They found that he does not go into the stage of deep sleep. It made him tired all the time. It was difficult to concentrate for Will on anything Era would tell him. Will was complaining again that he could not sleep. Their son told him; he will find a little marijuana to help him sleep better, more deeply. Will said ok, smoked some marijuana then he went unconscious. He dropped to the floor. They called 911. Will was rushed to the emergency room where did all kinds of test, nothing was wrong. The doctor told them this is the side effect of marijuana in some people. Maybe the marijuana was not clean. Will was not responsive for 24 hours; they were very scared. He was receiving fluids, his vitals were ok, but he was not responding he looked like he was asleep.

Will's breathing was very slow. Before the ambulance come Era did CPR on him, pushing his chest with her hands and giving breaths. She was shaking him, slapping him, trying everything to get a response, he did throw up. It was a very bad experience with marijuana, and everyone was blaming her son for it which was also hard. Will described the experience as feeling very weak and darkness. If he would have been alone, he would have died. Era wanted to try marijuana once, so she knows what her patients are talking about. She got some tea drink it and she had no effect. Then she chewed some of the leaves. Little later she saw fireworks, the beautiful colors of purple, blue, red, it was beautiful. She thought this is what actors and painters must see in Hollywood. She was laughing. Her husband was laughing because she was laughing. She said it was completely stupid. Then she was hungry remembering opening the fridge eating something and going to sleep. That is, it she said, never had it again. She is just not interested. Era said she is hyper as it is.

I asked Susan about marijuana. I was wondering if she has any conflict about her brother growing it. A little bit she said. She is trying to find the right words. She had some problems with it, but she also knows that cannabis can help people too. She was giving me an example of her boyfriend's mother who had brain cancer and was using marijuana as a vape. It helped her improve her quality of life. It was the only thing that stopped some of her seizures and nausea. Still she argues with him about it. She knows that there are good things about it, but she also feels it needs to be more regulated. There are a lot of chemicals used to grow marijuana and then people are inhaling it, not much better like cigarettes. There needs to be more research about it. In California there were more medical dispensaries and it was more under control than in Oregon. She had discussions with her brother. His view is who is anybody to tell anybody else how to live their lives. He felt that people should be able to do what they want. She talks about the controversy if people make something illegal people want to do it more. She was not sure if she believes in that. We discussed benefits and damage for a while especially when youth are using marijuana. She definitely feels like more collaboration and research needs to be done. When comparing to heroin marijuana addiction does not seem as big of a deal.

15. Joe's story

I talked to Joe on the phone. He first tells me that he has no experience in addiction. Then he starts to tell me about his best friend and his brother who did have trouble with addictions. Joe grew up as a youngest child and he did not do things that involved substances, he was afraid of everything. As he got older, he become very outgoing in his community, he liked to help people. He did not realize his brother had an addiction until he become an adult. His friend relapsed and went wild and crazy he describes. Joe had not had any issues with any types of addiction, neither his children. Joe describes his brother trying everything including pills, different types of drugs, but Joe is not sure of the full story. Joe's brother Tim always looked at Joe as his little brother and when he talked to him it was just for encouragement and support. Tim would come Joe to talk to someone, to share things he was going through. Joe does not know specifics; his brother would just tell him he used everything. I asked Joe if he knows why Tim started to use drugs. He tells me yes, he thinks mostly from humiliation, having low self-esteem about his own sexuality.

Tim is gay, he had grown up with a lot of self-doubt, feeling of not being worthy. Joe feels that sometimes people respond and act out because of the societal pressure. I asked Joe what made Tim stop. He did not know, and he was not sure if he had stopped. He is functional, he has a job, but he always done that he always had a job and used drugs before. He had problems with drugs and reckless behavior. Joe never asked, he does not want to be that person. He does not want to be judgmental. Joe perceives that his brother seems to be well, not seem to be having problems. Although he did not seem to be having problems even when he told Joe about it before. Joe he tells me:" you don't know what you don't know". Not getting involved, not getting too personal. It would be problematic for him. He would be concerned, keep thinking about it and try to fix it.

He tries not to get too invasive even in his children's lives. Joe feels that his brother told him what is going on to tell someone and for Joe to listen no to do something about it. Tim does things that Joe would not. Next month Tim is going skydiving. Joe does not feel this is something he would do. He tells me: "It is a perfectly good plane, why jump out of it? "This makes me laugh. Joe describes himself as very frugal and very conservative. He does not like to do things that are not logical. He drinks alcohol but never to a level of not being able to function. He wants to know what is going on around him. He was always that guy even in the military, he was the guy who made sure everyone got home safely. Joe does not like to do anything risky. He does not judge but it is hard for him to even process why would somebody do stuff to themselves. He knows people have their reasons, still he does not understand addiction, he does not understand why someone would do something to hurt themselves, why would they drink in access or why would they do drugs in access. Joe would be still there to help out. Another friend was on heroin, he would help him with money, food, clothes, needed a place to sleep he would help and let his friend sleep at his place.

    He does not know what happened to him. He is wondering now if his friend still alive or where he is. Now that Joe thinks about, he realizes he used to have a lot of friends who did drugs. He used to own a coin laundromat in the early 2000's and he met a lot of people there who did drugs and alcohol. So many people would come around and they would be the "town's drunk or the town's druggy". He met a lot of people, they accepted him; he was not sure why he was always trying to do nice things for them without getting into their business. He never asked anybody why they are drinking or why they are doing drugs.

16. Smoking – Nicotine

Talking to Chloe she describes a lot of smokers in her workplace. Many had tried to quit smoking multiple times but could not. They had tried to switch products to quit. Chloe describes chewing tobacco to smoking to vaping, then start the cycle again. It is very hard for them to quit. Her grandfather had bowel cancer which she feels was related to smoking in all his life. He still smokes today. Michelle describes family members who are smoking and heard the warnings for years yet have the attitude that people can die from anything. There is a certain truth to this she said. Her family can hear the problems with smoking, but the addiction already took hold, they choose not to do anything about it.

I just talked to my mom about smoking. She used to smoke. She was never a strong smoker; she did not have time to smoke. She knew people who used to make pasta and smoke at the same time. She would only smoke if she had free time. She did not have a lot of free time, so she never smoked a lot. She did not smoke just to smoke. When she was pregnant with me, she stopped smoking completely. When I was born, everyone went to smoke, mom had the cigarette with her too, she went out to the hallway to smoke, took two smokes then she did not want any more. Later like 17 years later she went back to cigarettes when her new partner was smoking. Also, at that time my uncle Attila and his partner were smoking. Everyone was smoking around her. Still then she was only occasionally smoking. She was the same way with alcohol as well. She knew her limit and too much just did not feel good. Then she got pregnant with my sister, stopped smoking and never started again.

Growing up I remember seeing her smoking occasionally. She would smoke sometimes these minty, thin elegant looking cigarettes. I had no concept then that smoking is bad for people except that I did not like a very smoky room. Mom feels that if someone really wants to quit smoking they can. She was able to stop as well as my uncle and his partner. It is probably different for every person. Mom did smoke a lot when Józsika died, she was smoking one cigarette after another then like a chain. Probably because of the stress. A lot of things had fallen on her shoulder. After a while smoking so much decreased.

Mom tells me for some people smoking is difficult also to stop because people are bored and don't know what else to do. It just becomes a trend, something to do during a break at work. I am glad that my mom was able to stop smoking.

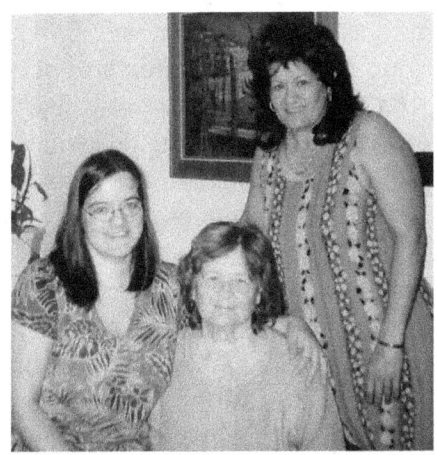

Me, Grandma and Mom, Budapest, Hungary, 2011

It is a nice summer afternoon when I go and visit Bill. We go to a conference room area with a big dining room table and chairs around. We have a conversation about the book project then I start my recording. I ask Bill about his experiences with addiction. Sitting in a church with Bill and we have a conversation about his mother. His mother passed away about 5 years ago related to smoking. Bill feels like that as a society we pay attention to drugs and alcohol but not as much to other addictions like smoking. He talks about how smoking was even elevated into a fashionable level and become accepted in society.

Throughout his life he been witnessing his mother enjoying cigarettes at times and breaking from the habit at times. Then go back to smoking again, then stopping, then going back to it again over and over again. Bill felt that watching his mother confirmed for him how he wanted to live his life. He did not want anything to dictate how his day began, how his day progressed, the way the day ended. Bill talked about public advertising and how acceptable the behavior become. It seemed acceptable at least. He observed his mother's struggle, she really did not want to do the smoking. In the beginning it was comforting and had emotional soothing effect, but other times she was at odds with it. When she got to be a point when she was not able to be without it, she spent time sneaking around thinking that she is disappointing herself and her family. She was trying to hide it, so family does not know she was smoking again. For a while Bill told himself that an on again off again addiction was better than a full-on addiction from age 16 to 80 day in and day out. It bought her some time, but ultimately it was doing the damage inside that ended her life. She had lung cancer that metastasized to her brain. Now, Bill understands the complexity of our lungs and lungs carrying oxygen in our body when there are other elements from cigarettes those are carried as well. Ultimately, the lungs communicated the cancer along with the oxygen to her brain. This was devastating for him to recognize. It makes sense now. He did not realize that this could happen. His sister is a nurse practitioner, he felt she always knew what was going on, she told him what happened physiologically when he was ready. Bill describes himself as a professional hearer, listener and his sister as the clinical person with the knowledge and expertise to provide information what was happening to their mother. We talked some about loss and grief and he felt that because of his sister's clinical brain she did not allow herself to grieve the same way he did. He tries to check in and support his sister in this process. Loss and grief are very important when it comes to addictions.

  Bill's story about his mother reminded me of my stepfather Zoli who used to smoke a lot. He died many years ago around 2010. I did not even know until after the fact. I found out from my father who heard it from people in town. I just thought he want to be with his new family and lost touch. He loved cars. One thing he did was to get a car, fix it up then sell it. We used it a little sometimes. He just loved to hang out in the garage and work on his cars. Spent a lot of time with the cars. He was very proud of them. He loved his cigarettes and smoked a lot. It was a trend, everybody seemed to smoke then. We did not know about secondhand smoking and its effects. Both my mom and I would sit in the same room when he was smoking. The company he worked for was a very stressful place. So stressful we were receiving letters to go to funerals, people seemed to die of a heart attack very frequently. I was young but it scared me. He just told me that his job was very stressful and there was a lot of pressure. He also would have some beer or wine every night a few, or more. I remember bringing him the beers when he wanted one. He switched from beer to wine because he did not like the stomachache the beer started to give him. He would drink the wine with sparkling water in a tall glass. I learned how to make them. I was young, I did not know any better so when he would ask for a drink, I bring him one, he smoked, I sat in the same living room. We did not know then what we know now about secondhand smoking. I certainly had no idea that I will lose him to smoking. He lost vision in his eye for a while I believe that was to be smoking too, then developed lung cancer, then developed brain cancer, then he died. He originally recovered from the eye problem. He was still so very young. Way too young to die. He could have lived another 40 years or more. He has 2 older sisters; he was the little brother. His sisters are still alive today. He never had children on his own. He and my mom separated after about 10 years or so. I wish I would have known he was sick; I wish I was more educated to warn him, maybe I could have talked to him. I wish he would have known what smoking will cost him. He was the godfather of my son. A very sad loss. Here is a picture of him on his 40th birthday:

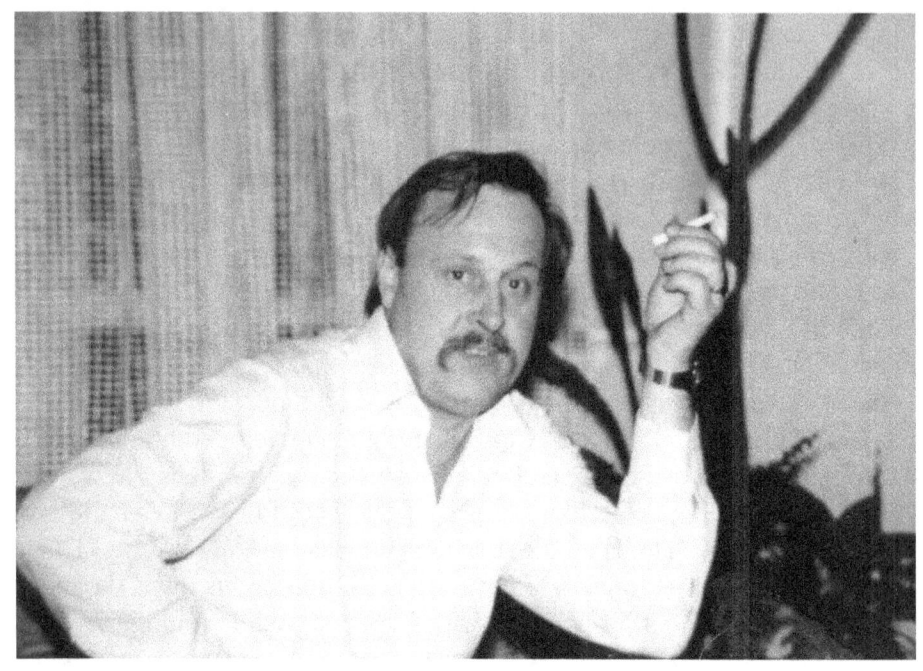

Kiss Zoltán, 1988. March 11, Dunakeszi, Hungary

My father also smokes. He knows the risks, but still smokes. It is scary. He also had cancer, survived it so far. It was super scary. Was it related to smoking? I don't know. I don't like that he smokes, but it is his decision. I am just hoping he is going to be ok. He told me recently that he has no intention of stopping. For a while I was very upset and angry about him smoking, I learned not to be. It was hard for me to accept that it is his choice to hurt himself. I am here if he needs help with it, but I don't think he will ever ask. My dad tells me he grew up in Angyalföld in Hungary. I just talked to my dad and he told me he started to steal cigarettes and smoke when he was 7 years old. He used to steal the cigarettes from his mom. She did not know about it for a while then my dad got caught.

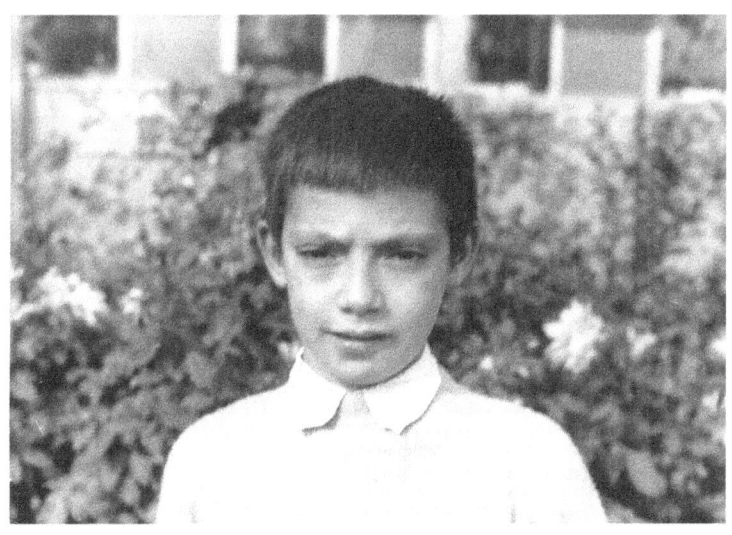

My dad around age 8, around 1961, Budapest, Hungary

It was a proletarian era. There were two types of people lived in the area, either people who worked in the factories or police officers. Both of these groups smoked like a machine. So much so he tells me that my grandmother got part of her paycheck in cigarettes. This was the end in the 1950's and beginning of the 1960's. The police officers instead of getting more money than people who worked in the factories got cigarettes.

Everyone was smoking back then it was the trend. One pack of cigarettes then was 4 forint and for 5 forints. With the equivalent amount of money people could have a nice lunch. This would include a soup and a main entree and a drink. Dad grew up in this environment. He tells me to become a full citizen in this era people had to be smoking. This was in 1960's. He could go and buy one cigarette or just a few depending on how much money he had, many people did not have enough money to buy a whole pack. They lived in the Dagály utca. There was a small market. Right next to the bar. The owner of the market would open the packages and make little bundles of 5 cigarettes a time, people did not have enough money to buy the whole pack. When he was attending elementary school on the way to school if he had 20 fillér he would go into a small market and buy a cigarette. There were two types Sport and Mátra that were half a size of other cigarettes. My dad tells me they were big boys from smoking in the bathroom in the breaks. This was still going on even in high school. Kids smoke in the bathrooms. Sometimes a teacher would come in and say 2-3 kids need to go out because the smoke is so bad, they could not breathe in there anymore. Then there was a trend started that the end of the cigarettes that had the filter on them were licked and thrown up to the ceiling. The butts were hanging of the ceiling. The school did not like this. After that the school sent a teacher to the bathroom in each break. The school forbade the smoking but if kids went into the stall like they had to go to number two and smoke would come out the teacher did not care unless there was a butt flew up to the ceiling.

Now my dad had been smoking for almost 60 years. He stopped once for few months and pretended to stop some other times but did not really stop. He would go to the basement where the wood is to heat the house and smoke there. Erika would get suspicious why he keeps going to the basement in springtime, then she found the pack of cigarettes in his pocket. He was denying it at first, he thought he would get into less trouble. Dad is so used to smoking that he does not even think about stopping. He could stay maybe 2-3 hours away from a cigarette but not much longer. I could watch a movie he tells me without smoking. Then Erika asks him what about 5-6 hours, he said he did not know never had to go that long without a cigarette.

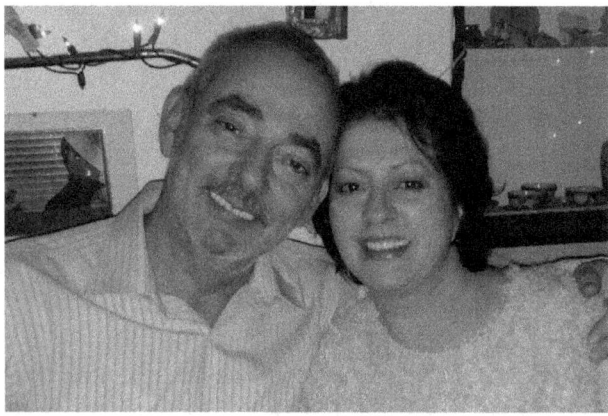

My dad and his wife Erika, Hungary, 2017 Christmas

Erika also smokes and she tells me her story how she got started. She was a teenager in the 1970's. She had a friend/neighbor her name was Gréti. At that time, she explains everybody was smoking in the whole country. People could smoke everywhere even at the birthing center, movie theater, playhouse. It was normal then that 90% of the country was smoking. People knew it could cause problems, but nobody talked about it. Erika was around 13-14 when it started by Gréti asking her to light her cigarette for her. It was a big deal. Next was that Erika could light the cigarette by putting it in her own mouth, it was a very cool thing then. Gréti smoked a lot Erika describes her smoking as a factory chimney. In about six months they were smoking together. Thinking back Erika is horrified what was done to her. Gréti made her start smoking and become addicted to it probably she adds without knowing what she had done. Same with "konyak" which is cognac.

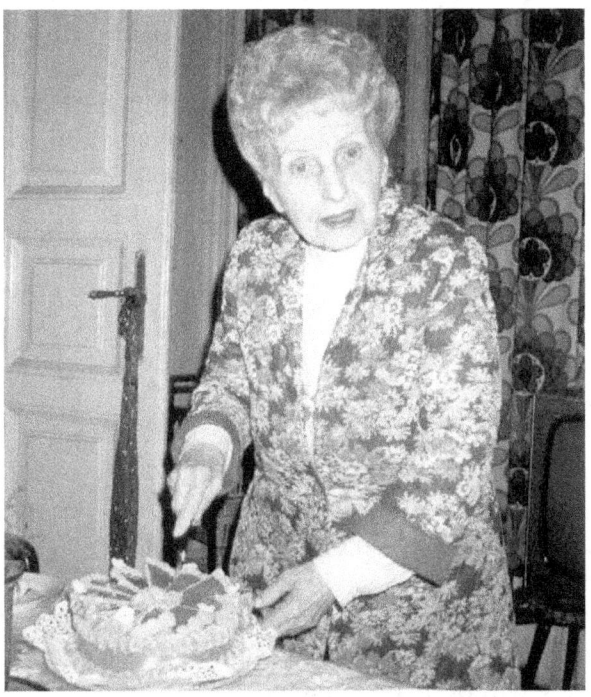

Gréti (Ditti) around age 80, Hungary

During pregnancies Erika did not smoke but after she went back to it. With my sister Hédi, who is my youngest sister Erika did not smoke for 3-4 years. It was hard because both my dad and Zsiga was smoking at the house. There was a conflict in the family that created a lot of stress for Erika and she had one cigarette. She thought she could have one after not smoking for so long. She did not smoke again for a few months then she had another one. In about 3-4 months she got back to smoking. She likes it. She laughs. My dad laughs too. They both like to smoke that is the problem. She would like to stop too.

She remembers that when she did not smoke for years it was a very freeing experience. She gives me an example of going to a play and it was nice that she could enjoy it without feeling after 1.5-2 hours that she does not care what they play she just wants to smoke. She also gives me an example going shopping where in the end she would not care what they sell just go so she can smoke again. It is an addiction she tells me, and she feels sorry that she robbed herself from the freedom she had. She is still dreaming that she will stop one day. Right now, she tells me that the addiction is stronger than her willingness to stop smoking. Gréti did stop smoking when she was 70 years old. From that time, she was upset with Erika why she was smoking. Erika had observed that people who stop have a hard time when others smoke around them. They give comments and saying bad words. Even more than others who never smoked before. She thinks this might be related to being unconsciously scared that they might start smoking again since they were addicted before. Could be also she adds that they are so proud that they stopped, and they want to keep preaching it to others.

We have a conversation about people who smoke and do not die from smoking and others who don't and still die from lung or mouth cancer. Gréti started smoking as an adult which was unusual at that time, usually smoking started at the teenage years. Erika brings it up that even in all the movies in the 70's everyone is smoking. I said at this point that now everyone drinks in the movies. Erika laughs. Yes, she said, they will probably stop that at some point too. Erika also remembers that when she was very young the schoolteacher would send the kids to get cigarettes for her from across the store.

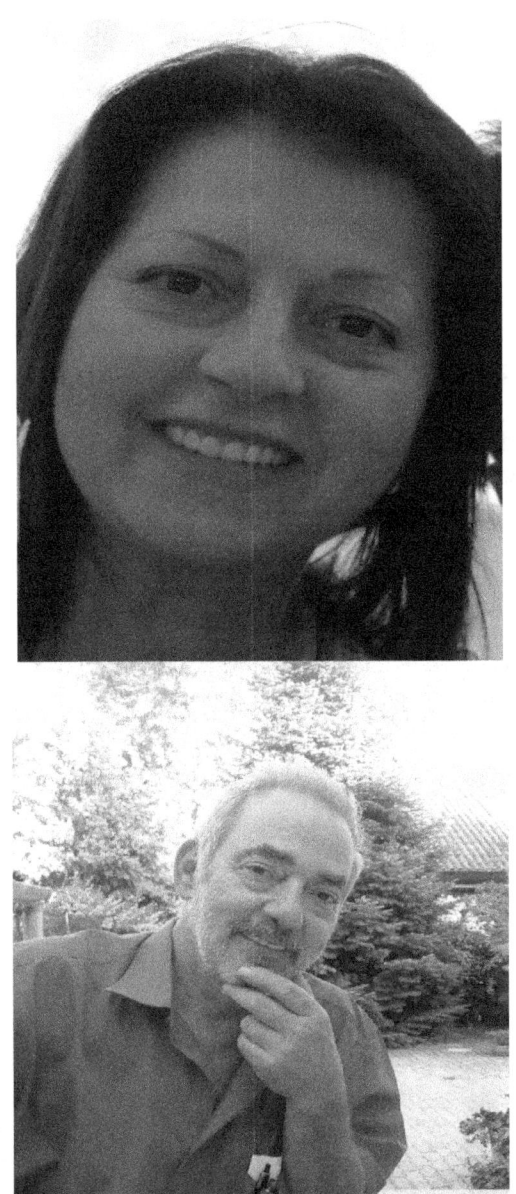

Erika and dad Hungary 2017

My grandfather liked cigars. My dad just told me he used cigarettes too, I had never seen that. Apparently, grandpa stopped smoking when he was in Moscow. This was around 1968-1970. He did not smoke for about 5-10 years. Then he started using cigars and a pipe once he come back. I remember buying him some. Because he liked them, I bought him cigars as a present. I had no idea that they were harmful to him. He died. Probably smoking did not help prolong his life. I bought him something that caused him harm. I was young I did not know, but still. My father told me grandpa would be happy if I get him a cigar for a present, so I did. My dad just told me that yes it was very true, grandpa loved his cigars. Later in his life if he had a cigar that is what he used, he loved them dad tells me if not then he used cigarettes. Erika found a picture of grandpa with his pipe, see below.

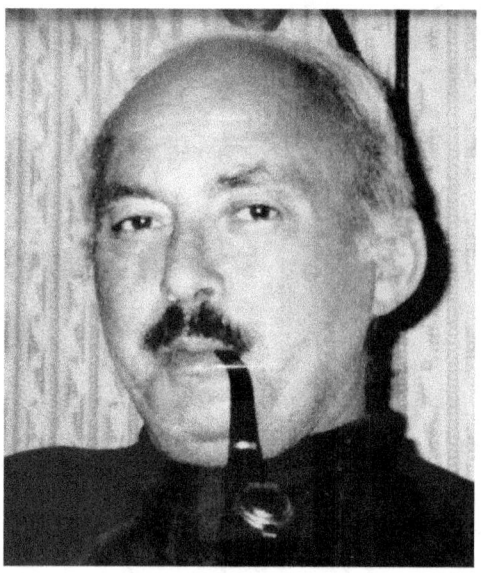

My grandpa with his pipe

I talked to Bob about smoking and vaping. He tells me that in his experience a lot of people are still doing this, and vaping is popular now. He feels like most people who smoke it has to do with stress or something that happened int heir life and not sure how to deal with it. Nicotine is very addictive. We talk about cool advertisements. He tells me that he feels like something bad has to happen a lot and then slowly change happens. It is democracy and people want what they want. People still smoke. People still start smoking or vaping.

17. Thomas's and Nicole's Story

    I was talking originally to Thomas's sister for an interview for this book. Her story was under Susan in the book. While we were talking, she thought her brother and his wife might like to talk to me. I received their number and got in contact. They both decided to talk to me. I was delighted. I love when I can talk to more than one family member it gives a nice picture and different points of view within the family. I talked to Thomas first, he lives farther away from me, we arranged a phone call. We talked for about an hour and 20 minutes. Thomas has now been sober for 4 years. He had been struggling with addiction from age 15-30. He had used multiple substances. He drank a lot of alcohol and also used "hard drugs". He mostly used alcohol and marijuana in the first 13 years and the last 2 years of his use he describes ramping up and using cocaine and methamphetamine as well.

    His condition was getting worse quickly. He describes waking up every morning thinking he just had a hangover, now he knows that they were bad withdrawals from the alcohol and drugs. He describes cold sweats, racing hearts, light headedness, he had trouble standing. He was drinking a lot of caffeine to try to counter act how he was feeling. He would then just go about his day to drink and use drugs. It sounds like a very painful experience. I tell him that. He said yes it was, he become very isolated and withdrawn, he was trying to hide all his usage from friends, family and his partner. He would keep alcohol hidden around in his bedroom; in his hamper he would have 2-3 bottles of hard alcohol that he could use. He did not just want to drink he wanted to black out, he tells me just being drunk was not enough, he was looking for oblivion. He wanted to stop thinking, that was the goal. This was the reason why he started to use other drugs as well. When alcohol was not enough anymore, he started to touch the drugs he swore before he would never use to forget things. To be honest he tells me just before he got sober most nights he went out and used and hoped he would die. He calls this passively suicidal. He would start drinking and using and hope that he will not wake up the next day. He did not want to live this way anymore. He was able to turn his life around. I ask him why? Why did you not want to wake up Thomas?

He tells me he had previous trauma and underlying mental health issues. He was diagnosed with Bipolar 1, severe obsessive-compulsive disorder (OCD), he is dealing with a lot of anxiety, he was trying to self-medicate to manage his mood. He would either be incredibly depressed or uncomfortably manic. His drugs and alcohol helped to balance his mood out, it helped to prevent the experience of a very uncomfortable high and low from the disease. He had a lot of depression because of the way he was living and the notion of living in a way that went against his values. He wanted to be numb and not to deal with his feelings. After he got sober, he realized his low tolerance for distress and his uncomfortableness for emotional pain and discomfort. Thomas went through a lot of therapy to be able to sit with emotions that are uncomfortable and feel them.

He was diagnosed with OCD at age 7, it shaped his youth and young adulthood because it was difficult to manage, and it impacted everything in his life. He had problems with socializing with other people because of his OCD, performance in school, diet and health. It impacted every aspect of his life. It made him miserable. He found out about his Bipolar diagnosis after he got sober. He had some suspicions, but he was not formally diagnosed. After he got sober, he had intense manic episodes where he would not sleep for a week then he went to a psychiatrist and got his formal diagnosis. Not being able to sleep for a whole week was terrible. It made him incredibly anxious, and the anxiety would not stop, very uncomfortable and unsettling. He would hallucinate because of the lack of sleep. Hallucinations were unsettling even though he knew he was seeing stuff because he had not been asleep, still it was very uncomfortable. I ask Thomas if he would feel comfortable sharing the cause of his emotional pain that he was going through. He is willing to share some aspect of it. He felt isolated because of his mental health issues, he was different than others, he still struggles with this, not as much as before, he also felt pain from the stigma he felt because of his mental health issues. He was secretive about having a mental health issue. There were two people outside of the family who were aware he had mental health problems. When he went out with new people, he just tried to pretend to be as normal as possible. Now he is open about his mental health struggles. He has support from people in his life now. He is in a good therapy program.

He feels in America we view mental health issues as a moral failing. The more he used to drink and use drugs the worse his mental health problems got. It was just taking him further from people. He had this secret life nobody knew about. He felt shame because of the illegal things, it was counter to his value system he had done during his addiction, it made him feel demoralized, isolated and monstrous. Once he become sober and started to address the shame regarding his addiction, he became less isolated and more connected to the people around him. This experience now is amazing he tells me.

    He has open and loving relationships with friends and family. It is a huge change from the way he was living before. Many people I talked too brought up the connections to others as an important part of recovery. Thomas was able to find support and loving relationships with friends and family. Asked him what the turning point for him was to get out of addiction. Thomas tells me it was fear, he knew this life he was living was not sustainable, he tried multiple times over the 15 years to get sober. He been in and out of AA starting at age 19. He had periods of sobriety but kept relapsing. When he was having severe withdrawal symptoms, he realized he will die unless he changes something. He knew enough about alcohol withdrawal that it was dangerous; it was a kind of a wake-up call for him. He realized that even though he been suicidal he did not want to die. He researched what could happen during alcohol withdrawal and it scared him. He stopped using cold turkey. In hindsight he tells me he should have used a medication assisted withdrawal. He did end up being ok. He been doing DBT (Dialectical Behavior Therapy) and working with a private counselor. This really helped Thomas to get through the first year of sobriety. He is now to a point where he could be around alcohol and it does not bother him anymore if he is in a bar or if others drink around him. There can be alcohol in the house, he won't touch it. He wakes up grateful that he is not hung over and he remembers what happened last night. He feels gratitude and this really helps him staying sober.

    Thomas started to go to an AA meeting with a group of people who are agnostic or not sure there is a God and wanted to talk about other aspects of AA but not the religious part. Thomas feels that AA is a valuable tool, but it also has a lot of issues it was hard for Thomas to go to regular AA meetings because they can be so dogmatic. He felt that there is a stigma in AA about relapsing and it is hard to come clean about a relapse in an AA meeting. AA does not take a harm reeducation approach only an abstinence approach. Thomas feels that in a lot of cases that is not what a lot of people need, people need a method where there is support and a harm reduction model. The group he is attending in the past year does have a harm reduction approach, someone might be sober from alcohol but still smoking marijuana. Thomas feels this is really helpful for people to keep them from problem behaviors. Build connections and help people feel less isolated. People can relate to each other. I ask Thomas what addiction is meaning to him. He tells me it is a good question. Then he said:" ***Addiction is a hell of your own making***". I felt this is a very powerful statement. It was his own personal hell, he got trapped in and had to crawl out of. Thomas feels nobody sets out to become addicted to something. When he was in the thrills of addiction, he had no idea how to get out of it. He could not fight his impulses enough, could not figure out the best way to get sober, could not stay sober more than a day here and there, felt stuck in a cycle. He knew he was causing damage to his life, and people he loves, and he could not stop it. He felt powerless, but also knew he is responsible for everything that is going on. He describes this cycle being very lonely and awful. I ask him if anything could have helped to prevent him starting to use substances or help him crawl out of his cycle. He describes a good feeling free of anxiety that was like an out of body experience. He tells me maybe more education when he was young about drug addiction, something effective that would have told him that what he was doing could lead to addiction, he might have at least given it a second thought. More information could have helped. Access to better mental health care, tools and coping skills could have helped to prevent trying to self-smooth with alcohol. Tools would have helped a lot. He also has a family history of severe addiction issues. He could be genetically predisposed. His father and grandfather were alcoholics and his brother were a heroin addict.

    He feels early intervention could have really helped. Once he was in it then it was too late, he lost jobs, it become his first step to quit. The impulse to use was so strong. It overrides our sense of self control, self-preservation. The most someone can do once they are in addiction is to offer support and be there when they are ready to quit. His dad got sober when he was 6 or 7 years old. He did not see a lot of bad behaviors from him. He would just see him sometimes passed out on the couch. Thomas remembers his father losing a job because of alcohol and getting a DUI once. His parents did not really talk about it. He remembers him used to drink beer and one day that just stopped, and he was not drinking beer anymore. His grandfather on the father's side, the family would get reports on his behavior like locking himself into the room for weeks and only leave to go get more alcohol. He died soon after Thomas was born so he never knew him. His maternal grandfather died from liver cancer caused by alcoholism. He used to have a coke can and Altoids (candy) with him to mask the sense of alcohol. His brother was using marijuana at age 12. He also had mental health issues going on. At some point in high school he started over the counter medications, later started using heroin. Thomas describes growing up in an upper middle-class environment in the suburbs and he feels that both he and his parents were really naïve to think that addiction is not something that could be an issue for them. They did not find out about his brother's heroin use until he was well into his addiction. He was 17 years old. When Thomas found out about his brother's heroin use, this was hugely devastating for him. His brother was one of his best friends. Sometimes the only friend he had. It also allowed Thomas to compare his use and justify it by saying well, I am not using heroin. With his brother into heroin his parents focus was on that and Thomas and his addiction and mental health issues flew under the radar. Family did not know until much later about Thomas's use.

    Thomas got good using and hiding it, he would go work high, going places drunk. His parents did not really know the extent of his addiction until he got sober and started to talk about it more openly. He tells me about his brother. He is clean of heroin but still high on marijuana continuously. They have a hard time connecting. He has not addressed his underlying problems of addictions. It is frustrating for Thomas; he wants to be close to his brother. Thomas used to think that the world is against him and not take responsibility for his actions and that is where his brother is now with his addiction, it is difficult for Thomas to see that. His brother still has the view of him against the world and if anything goes wrong it is never his fault, it is everyone else's. This is hard to see and creates a lot of damage to their relationship. Thomas has been working on setting very healthy boundaries with him. Family is doing the same thing. It makes him mad. They are firm on not giving money and not crashing on anyone's place long term without a plan. Thomas describes their relationship as arm's length. Thomas is happy to support him emotionally, but not financially. When Thomas first set this boundary, his brother did not talk to him for a few years. We discuss the fine line between supporting someone and enabling their habit for addiction. It is very difficult to draw the line especially for family. Thomas talks about this when it comes to their parents. Their parents did not want to kick his brother out, but they knew he was bringing heroin to the house and shooting up at the house, in the end regardless of parents' efforts, his brother ended up choosing to be homeless. Their parents put some boundaries around behavior and where he can use drugs in the house. He was homeless for a few years on and off until he got some stable housing again. Thomas then talked about his mom and his partner finding support to deal with the loved one to set healthy boundaries in Al-Anon meetings. There is not an easy solution, it all comes down making hard choices Thomas asserts. It is hard to set boundaries because then people can feel responsible what happens to them next.

Thomas feels that we as individuals have a responsibility to reduce the stigma around addiction issues and this could save lives. If people don't feel stigmatized, they can reach out for help, reducing isolation. We are all humans worth dignity and respect. He brings up some examples he heard people saying about addicts. He heard people say shouldn't provide Narcan (medication to reverse opiate overdose) because if someone is a junkie they are choosing to die. He had heard people say addicts are choosing to become addicts. He feels that this shows a fundamental misunderstanding on what addiction is. Doing our part to educate others is our individual responsibility. On a larger level we need more funding for recovery and harm reduction services to provide more support. Expanding education programs, MAT (Medication Assisted Treatment) programs, training for primary care providers in addiction issues and how to treat them. On a federal level Thomas feels he is radical in his views and asserts that we should use

Portugal's model to decriminalize all drugs and put the money that was used to incarcerate people to create recovery centers, recovery programs, stable housing, caseworkers. He tells me we need to change views on how we look at addiction. He has no hope that this will actually happen because people's view on drug use and drugs. He feels like if we would follow Portugal's model, we would see a huge change in drug use and an overall decrease of people suffering from addictions because they would not be exposed to the criminal system. Not be punished for addiction, they would get the help from mental health providers, case workers, social workers. It would be a more humane way to deal with addictions. It would be the ideal situation to help people with addiction by decriminalization. More realistically he tells me that he would like to see relaxing some of our drug laws. More emphasis on the federal level of trying to treat the roots of addiction and improve mental health and addiction services, research.

    Our conversation circles back to stigma and working on reducing stigma in mental health as many people with mental health issues have addiction issues and for them to access mental health services in the first place to make the decision to go to a mental health provider, mental health stigma would also need to be decreased the same way as stigma around addictions. He feels that stigma about mental health is getting a little better he feels people don't view mental health problems as a personal or moral failing anymore. He feels like health care providers are in the front line to treat addiction like EMT (Emergency Medical Technicians), primary providers, emergency physicians. The providers and people who interact with patients could be trained in addictions and how to have a conversation about them to increase competency, as well as be knowledgeable about resources available. We have a discussion about training doctors about options for patients who need to get off of drugs or alcohol. We discussed benefits of using different drugs to get off opiates and pill popping Suboxone clinics that want cash for pills and don't provide other support for patients. I have a tendency to kind of get worked up about this issue. We had an intense conversation with Thomas. It was good. He was telling me about some county efforts for training providers to be able to provide Suboxone for patients who need it. We talk about full-service treatment not just a replacement like methadone without additional support. This is what happened to his brother he was on methadone for 5-6 years, he tapered off his dose himself he did not wanted to be on it forever. Just replacing heroin to methadone is not enough people need additional support minimum counseling Thomas asserts with the ultimate goal to get people off of opiates.

    A few days later I talk to Nicole on the phone. We have about an hour of conversation. She starts out by saying that she does not believe people just wake up and decide they want to be addicted to a substance. Nobody wants that. She was excited to talk to me. Nicole has experience in addictions and dealing with addictions as a health care provider and she also a has a family member, a loved one, Thomas who you just read about who has been dealing with addiction issues. I ask her about her experiences. Nicole tells me that addiction has permeated her life. She grows up in a family where nobody would identify themselves as an alcoholic and everyone in her family uses alcohol for coping. Interactions had been difficult growing up especially with explosive emotions. I can tell she said this with a heavy heart and there is a big sigh after she finishes the sentence. As she got older, she told herself she will not fall for someone who had a problem with addiction, it impacted her youth so much. Then she tells me: "I ended up marrying an alcoholic" – she laughs. I push for a little more detail; I ask her how it affected her growing up in a family of alcoholics. Nicole is willing to share. She tells me that her family cannot really be around each other without drinking. They get together for holidays, for dinners, her aunt and uncle from the moment they wake up to the moment they go to bed they are finding excuses to drink. Her mom would have multiple ales every night. ***As a small child she could tell if it is going to be a good night or a bad night based on how many ale bottles were besides the kitchen sink.*** Nicole tells me that if it was just one or two bottles it was a standard just wanting to unwind after a hard day of work, if she saw 4-5 bottles, she would know her mom would end up crying sometimes during the night or getting mad and yelling at her over something. She tells me even as a kid she started problem solving around caretaker's relationship with alcohol. As an adolescent she would put her mom's ales in the fridge for her during the daytime because she put them in the freezer the night before and if they exploded, she would get even angrier.

Nicole tells me it was better for her to put them in the fridge for her mother before she got home, so it could be one less thing that she could get upset over. When your loved one has an addiction people kind of learn how to cater to the addiction to make life easier. ***One of the proudest moments she had when she started to set healthy boundaries with a loved one***. Many people I talked with have difficulties setting boundaries, they don't want to lose their loved one. It took Nicole a year going to Al-Anon to be able to set the boundaries. Hearing other people's stories with similar situations give Nicole the strength and the courage to set boundaries out of love, not punishment. Out of the need for self-preservation she adds. She tells me about a first time. Her partner, Thomas come home drunk, he could not remember things Nicole told him, he was falling all over himself. Nicole politely told him: "hey I love you and I don't want to talk to you when you are like this, please drink some water I am going to bed". He had to sleep on the couch that night, she did not let him back in the bedroom. Next morning, they had a conversation about how he acts when he drinks like that, Nicole told him she does not want to be around that. It was a wake-up call for her setting boundaries and for Thomas to realize how annoying he is when he is intoxicated. She laughs. Her mom stopping drinking as much and the two of them now been having conversations about her mom's drinking and the effects on that for Nicole when she was growing up. Nicole does not touch alcohol much, occasionally she might have a drink, but she is not interested in alcohol. She feels like because she does not have anything positive with alcohol. I asked Nicole how this is working for her with our society being so alcohol friendly everywhere. She tells me it has been so hard, and people get so weirded out if somebody does not drink. People get really nervous. She has to come up with some sort of excuse why she does not drink. It is so common in our culture. She feels it is odd to her that just saying she is not into it is not a satisfactory answer. She works in mental health and addictions field in about 8 years now. It is surprising to her that more of her co-workers are not more thoughtful about their use.

A lot of holiday parties are at bars. It seems very hypocritical to her that while they are trying to help people and show them how substances effect their lives, yet, then go and have a work party at a bar. Nicole tells me that she thinks this speaks to a larger societal issue about comfort and socializing. She calls alcohol a "social lubricant" that people need to feel comfortable being themselves around other people. It is an interesting phenomenon. Being married to Thomas who is a recovering alcoholic Nicole has been watching people's reactions to him if he discloses why he does not drink. It makes people uncomfortable. I ask Nicole why she thinks that is. Deep down people know and have some feelings about the need to drink and social interactions. She feels that there is a fear of judgement and stigma. Nicole feels that people in recovery are the least judgmental people she had ever meet. They went through so much judgement and stigma themselves.

Based on what Nicole witnessed, she feels that **_addiction is filling a void_**. Feeling an unmet need. She saw this with her loved ones, loneliness, inability to cope, something missing. She sees it with her patients too, either because of a persistent mental illness they are trying to self-medicate for or PTSD. Their substance of choice is trying to minimize whatever they are experiencing so they don't feel so intense. Sometimes nothing feels like a lot. We talk then a little more about society. Nicole tells me that she feels our society breathes addiction and it has a responsibility to help and support people with addiction issues. Our society normalizes a lot of addictive behaviors. Class plays a huge role and how we treat addiction because a soccer mom with a drinking problem is laughed about while a homeless person with a bottle in a brown bag is looked at with judgement. It is a same problem, but it is treated differently. She feels like we need more access to help with addictions and a different mindset.

We discuss society and acceptance of who we are without alcohol. Nicole feels like that there is not enough focus on emotional intelligence. She feels we need to talk to our kids about mindfulness, acceptance, compassion, boundaries, with those skills she feels people would feel more comfortable being who they are. This is very difficult now with social media and unrealistic expectations on how someone should look like. For sure she said, she tells me it is getting harder and harder. She works with adolescents and the kids are connected to their phones they live on it 24/7. They are addicted to social interaction that is so surface level. It is like there is a need for connection, yet there is no deep connection forming. It is very superficial, lacking deep friendship. Nicole feels we need more sober spaces for people to hang out in. Making more places that are not bars to meet others. She tells me as individuals if someone suggest meeting at a bar, suggest meeting at a coffee house instead. To help with addictions we need people to have access to things, to light up their reward pathway, that are not harmful to their bodies. Create a society that makes coping skills acceptable. Self-care will look different for everybody. Knowing our community and coming up with realistic alternatives can be a first step Nicole asserts. She talked about coming up with ideas how to make affordable spa days, make body scrubs, make it out of sugar and essential oils that people can get the experience for $3. I tell her about the coffee scrub that I make. She talks about diet a lot with her clients. Nicole tells me about food addictions. Studies show neurotransmitter receptors in our gut, it is a very strong brain gut reaction. Sugar and carbs have a dopamine rush in our brain, and she tells me this makes us feel better by eating these things. The problem is when people are eating that much sugar, they end up getting a crash then maybe not feeling as well, it is not healthy for their body in the long term, it does damage over time. She encourages replacing them with healthy alternatives. A little bit in moderation it might ease the craving she feels, that when it comes to food, she gives me an example with ice cream. Nicole tells me a lot of people love ice cream; it makes them feel great. The nutritionist Nicole spoke with suggested eating frozen bananas instead. See her recommendation below.

Frozen bananas to replace ice cream Recipe: blend bananas up in a blender add a little milk, maybe a little vanilla, it tastes just like vanilla ice cream she said. Put it in a freezer. An alternative to milk can be used like almond or coconut milk. Nicole uses almond milk herself, she said it tastes great with it. Enjoy.

She suggests eating a lot of food for vitamin and fiber. Eating less processed carbs. We are talking about pastries, pasta, bread eat much less of these items. Eating rainbow, as many different colors as possible can when it comes to fruits and vegetables. Be open to a variety of things to eat. It gets us exposed to more nutrients. Moderate food intake. Eat on a smaller plate. Use a salad plate for a meal instead using a huge plate. Nicole tells me the importance in alcohol use and the lack of vitamin B and iron. When someone is recovering it is very important to eat things high in iron and Vitamin B. With methamphetamine and heroin, people don't eat as much because they don't feel it, too sedated or too ramped up to eat. Suppressing hunger with drugs and alcohol is also a problem Nicole had run into. People with eating disorders sometimes use substances to make themselves not feel hungry anymore. Ask Nicole my magic wand question. I ask her what she would do. She tells me she would completely change our society structure, make it more available for people to have free time for their interest and hobbies outside of needing to work for survival. Give people more opportunities to find pleasure in day to day life. More opportunities for people to grow their own food and support their local agriculture. She feels like this is missing from modern day culture.

People now have no idea where their food comes from and how it needed to be grown and raised. This might seem weird, but she would like if we could use the knowledge, we have now but go back to a simpler time with less technology. Interestingly when I was talking to Chloe, she told me the same thing, she wanted to go back 100 years and live on a farm. Have less mobility, Nicole adds, create communities again, foster connection to the earth and to us. Let's just revamp society. She laughs. She said: We can always try. There are a lot of problems with our health care system, it is not that people who work there are not trying, so many try their best, and there are more problems than resources. Mental health and addiction get the least funding. Less money with more issues. Many people utilizing the ED (Emergency Department) for overdoses, mental health, liver failure. Nicole feels that there is still a lot of misunderstanding and stigma about addictions. She hears phrases like medication seeking as a label. Sometimes people and their pain get brushed off because of their history. Nicole feels awareness could help. In Portland, Oregon there is more of a shift now to MAT. She tells me about Suboxone and how it can help some people. We discuss benefits and problems with Suboxone. Patients also need support and mental health work. I tell her about my experience with Suboxone and detoxing with Suboxone, then switching to other options. Just prescribing a pill is not enough to achieve sobriety.

The government could allocate more funding for social services. She feels this would not happen, but it is her dream. We discuss legalization of drugs and jail time for using or possessing substances. She tells me a lot of people died in Jail from withdrawal. We discuss prevention and coping skills and how we could help youth and kids to prevent addictions. Nicole feels that we could have conversations about boundary setting, for peer pressure, teaching boundaries at a young age. Teaching how to handle disappointment, overwhelming feelings, teaching that feelings are ok. How someone handle their feelings is what important. There are a lot of people who are afraid of their feelings, feel like they are not allowed to have feelings. People might have also never learned how to sit with discomfort she adds. It is hard to sit with discomfort and people need skills to learn and accept discomfort. When someone cannot sit with discomfort then they are starting to look for ways for the discomfort to go away. **_We really need to teach our kids healthy coping skills_**. Life will not always go the way they wanted it to go. I ask her what those heathy coping skills could be. See Nicole's tip below.

Heathy coping skills:

Breathing – take a deep breath – take a moment taking yourself carefully out of the situation

---

I ask Nicole about happiness and joy. Nicole lets out a big sigh. She is learning to find happiness and joy in the little things in life. Looking at her cat rolling over. Taking a moment to stop and smell the flowers. She was diagnosed with persistent depressive disorder and it is hard for her to find joy. She likes to share meals with others and cooking. Trying new things. When somebody deals with addiction, it is harder for them to find joy in small things in their life. Closing out our conversation Nicole tells me that addiction need to be addressed with a well-rounded approach. Get enough education and information and get support as needed. I ask her if she had trouble accessing the mental health system, she feels that we need more beds, more support and there is a lot of band aids currently in the system. I ask her about treatment, she feels it is very short and people are cycled through to get beds for others. There is a lot of burn out. She feels that the system could be restructured to support more people. Take away message from Nicole: **Compassion.** She thanks me for doing this book. I thank her for participating. It has been wonderful to be able to talk to 3 members of the same family and hear their experiences.

18. Food and Sugar Addiction

    I was talking to Sheila about sugar addition. She describes difficulties stopping eating sugar once she starts. She wants more sugar when she eats some. This is hard around the Holidays. Is this a true addiction does the mind or the body craving it? She asks. It does not really matter it sure feels like and addiction she adds. Sheila thinks people need to wean off themselves slowly. Paige describes that at her work she sees food addiction more than anything else. Working with her clients who were previously addicted to drugs and alcohol and now they are addicted to food. She sees depression and lack of money bringing out the food addiction. Creating a habitual spoiling each other with food. Paige recalls when she did this herself. Her kids were little, and she went to the store and spoiled them with junk food, and it can very easily be done. They had no money so she would get them treats and played cards. It is so easy to turn to food especially in the wet and gloomy area where we live in, there are not a lot of things in the winter months that kids want to do outside. Paige is grateful that it did not cause problems in her family and her kids are healthy.
    Talking to Kayla when I asked her what foods she thinks we should avoid she said sugar of course, it lights up the same place in the brain as other addictions like cocaine for example. She said it is interesting to think about this in a molecular level and how many other things we have in our food today that we don't even know what they are. Kayla recommends staying away from sugar if someone are recovering from addiction to prevent changing the brain chemistry. It can basically trade one addiction to another. I saw people who try to quit smoking and trading for a candy bar, then they gain weight which makes them unhappy and start smoking again to lose the weight. Kayla recommends trying to stay away from sugar, a little here and there it is ok but not every day and not with every meal. Eating whole grains, fruits, vegetables, seeds, protein, is very important. Try to stay away from things that have ingredients. Diana said: "no sugar" when recovering from addictions. Carbs don't help. Educate people what good foods are and what make people better. Chloe describes friends who are eating fast food every day and never learned how to cook. She was wondering if that is an addiction. People can be addicted to fast

food to the sugar, carbs and fried things for sure. This is even more difficult for service men and women at the dorms with crazy schedules she describes.

Joel describes how much of the food addiction we self-create, watching advertisements of unhealthy products, candy for example. Advertisements that encourages us to be skinny or to get a certain type of food, the need to satisfy something for someone else or self. Joel brings self-image and social media into this and how it is expected a 15-year-old girl to look today. Janett and had a conversation about food, and it became about potatoes and all the different way people can make potatoes. Janett tells me a story she heard about someone who decided to eat only baked potato for a year. Plus, they added a supplement. Their perception and taste for food changed after this. They ate to live, not lived to eat. Our society, food stores, wineries, bakeries, cake shops offer so many goodies for people. Is this good? If someone eats pizza occasionally will it hurt, them? How about if someone eats it once a week or every other day?

I visited Traci and her family yesterday and we talked for hours. She shared her struggles with chocolate addiction that became overbearing on her life. It all started at childhood with trauma she went through. She had struggles in her life feeling accepted in society. She threw herself into work to feel that she is worthy. She is working on those issues now. She had a car accident in February. After the accident she lost control of many things, her movement, ability to fully care for self, to drive, to work. It was a very difficult time. Chocolate helped. She would have some chocolate and feel better. She was hiding it from family and co-workers. It went out of control. She would put chocolate by her nightstand and eat them after her husband fall asleep, just eat one after another with no control at all. She wanted to stop; she did not know how. Same thing happened once she got back to work. She would buy big bags of chocolate and put it in a file cabinet. When her co-workers did not see she would go to the cabinet take the chocolate out and out it in her desk drawer by the handfuls. She would eat them at work when she thought nobody is seeing it. She felt she would be judged because she feels that she is already heavier set then other people. She has been working with a doctor and therapist to stop this addiction. She is doing much better, she still has chocolate at her nightstand and had not touched it for a while. It is a blanket security for her. She needs to have it in case she needs it. If she would not have it there and feel the need to have some she would sneak out after her husband fell asleep to the mini mart to get some chocolate. She said: "I would do it if I think I can get away with it without waking him up". At this point she looks up at her husband and tells him don't look at her like that. She has tears in her eyes. She tells me had two small chocolate covered cookies yesterday. It is a hard road for her to admit that she has a problem. It is very difficult because her family struggled with addictions so much. She knows she is vulnerable and could have the tendency to go down the wrong road and it is scary. She made a conscious decision not to drink alcohol or maybe just have a few sips here and there. Chocolate and food is everywhere. It is hard to resist. Dark chocolate can be very good for people in moderation or cocoa beans. For Traci chocolate is not a good thing it become a coping mechanism, to get a small release of "happiness" when she was not ok. Traci described the feeling of being forced to eat chocolate even when she did not want to eat it. It became a constant need. Bill describes people coming to him and telling him they have problems with food addiction. Many Hungarian foods that I grew up on have a lot of carbs and grains and sugar in it.

    Era talks about carbohydrates as an addiction. She feels she has a problem with that. Then she tells me, face it, years ago we did not know that this could be a problem. She talks about pasta, rice. She tells me about the feeling of emptiness and craving for carbs even when we are not hungry. She feels the best is to walk, exercise, hike, touch and hug mother nature. She would like to see more rehab centers in nature and food grown without chemicals. Era would get up at night to make dessert. She describes this dessert to me how to make it and she said she could even eat it now nonstop. She does feel better when she does not have sugar. She met a friend recently who had no sugar for a year, and she looks so much better. More tuned. Lost some weight. Era feels now people are more aware of problems with sugar then before. Era does describe sugar as a bad guy. She feels that the fogginess is gone when she does not eat sugar.

19. Kristen's Story

I have a phone conversation with Kristen on a nice summer early afternoon. We talk about 45 minutes. Before we began our recording, we have a conversation about this book the reasons I am writing it, she had some questions for me. I ask her about her experiences about addictions. Kristen considers herself very fortunate with not having close family members or friends who have drug addiction problems. She shares an interesting experience regarding some people who she had been close too. John was the head of the organization where she had worked before, he was struggling with alcoholism. She found out about his struggles with alcoholism a few years after he started working at the organization. She describes it as an interesting experience to go through. John shared his struggles with everyone and become very open about it. He started to come out and make amends.

Kristen tells me it was interesting to observe how people's opinions and actions toward him either changed or did not change after he shared his struggles about alcohol use. I ask Kristen how it made her feel when he shared his story. She laughs a little. Her first reaction was betrayal. John was a mentor for her, and someone invested in her career and she felt like one of her hero's let her down a little bit in the beginning. She did some self-reflection with time. She realized how much courage it takes to recognize that someone has a problem and be open about it with others. She came to admire him for bringing the people at the company into his confidence, and for the level of honesty he shared with others. She is happy to tell me that her initial reaction was changed. She sounds happy about it too. Kristen tells me it's been interesting for her to observe the different kind of addictions that people have. She feels like that alcohol is a problem for a lot of people. ***She feels that people are reluctant to consider themselves problem drinkers.*** It is legal she said. People don't want to hear about it and that causes a problem. Alcohol is responsible for one of the leading causes of preventable deaths in the country she adds. Kristen feels that people drink for a variety of reasons.

Kristen switches to talk about social media. Addiction to our phones, people cannot put their phones down. She finds herself in that same pattern sometimes. She tells me it is the same thing kind of with food or with sugar. Caffeine. In her experience it all comes down to telling ourselves a story. She used a lot of I statements: "when I am drinking too much coffee, when I am eating too much sugar and when I cannot put my phone down". She knows that she probably should not, she knows that it would be better for her to make a different choice, but she gives herself a pass. She makes an excuse. It would be something like this: "I had a really hard day and I need something to relax and this will help me relax". She feels like this is a way of avoiding doing something that is better for us, but also more difficult. Just the ways our brains are wired she adds, we get into patterns and it is hard to break out of them. She feels it is **addition to the behavior, but also to the story we tell ourselves as well why we are engaging in that behavior**. It makes perfect sense. Addiction to the story I tell myself, addiction to the justification of why it is ok to do this. Whatever it is. I like it. Do people justify why can they continue a behavior and why is it ok to do it? Kristen gives me an example. I am a very busy person and I am stressed out and if I want to look at Instagram for an hour, I deserve that. She continues, it is some kind of an escape for me and I deserve it, so and she is addicted to that vision of herself, where this particular behavior fits into that vision.

I ask Kristen if she feels like it is part of our cultural and societal norms that we tall ourselves these stories? She thinks so. She feels like that our cultural norm is that there should be a reason behind behaviors and if we decide to choose to do something that is bad for us. We better have a good reason behind it. She feels like on the societal level there are so many people are doing the same thing. She tells me that if we start noticing that other people have a problem then we also have to recognize that we have a problem as well. If I say that, of that person drinks too much, what is that mean about me – she asks. Do I drink as much as them? Do I drink too much? Or like that person is on their phone always, that is bad. How much am I on my phone? Kristen then brings up a great point. She feels **people are reluctant to point at others for their problem behaviors because then they have to look at themselves and realize they might have the same problems**. Kristen said it all comes back to a public health background she has. We have to look at the environment where people are, the environment they operate in. What are the systems and structures we have in place that help people make healthier choices? She states: ***If we have systems and structures around us that enable us to continue in problem behaviors without consequences or without being challenged, then there is little incentive to examine our behavior***.

    She thinks it is so culturally acceptable in this country to be addicted to something that she was uncertain how we can change that. She feels like most people engage in some type of addictive behavior. She sees people who are borderline problem drinkers, people who spend a lot of time on their phones, people who are definitely addicted to work, or to the idea that they are indispensable. She feels then people play that out by working nonstop. I ask Kristen what addiction means to her. The first time she tells me that addiction is the inability not to engage in a behavior that we know is bad for us. She thinks about this for a second then she decided to change this a little bit: Addiction would be a compulsion to behave in a way that we know it is not in our best interest and the interest of the people around us and keep coming back and repeatedly trying to get that feeling whatever the feeling is that we are trying to achieve. She talks about the feeling of shutting the world out and escape, maybe getting that from social media, using drugs, relationships, chasing after a feeling and using the behaviors to get there. I ask Kristen if she thinks people know what is going on with them if they have these addictive behaviors. She feels some of them know like if they went through trauma, this is a coping mechanism and they know why. Others might not, if they just try to cope with their daily life and have not recognized what some of their problems are. It might be harder for them to recognize that they have developed unhealthy coping mechanisms. We have a discussion about people growing up in an environment filled with addiction they might not recognize addiction as a problem. Kristen asserts that there is definitely intergenerational addiction. Patterns can definitely pass from one generation to the next. If that is all someone knows growing up, that is what they know. It can go both ways.

    Someone in an alcoholic household is deeply scarring for children. Kirsten knows many friends who grew up in an alcoholic household and many of them decided not to drink at all. They see how damaging it can be, but others just continue the same as their parents.

We have discussion about families. I ask Kristen about her thoughts on our individual and societal responsibilities when it comes to addictions. She felt that our individual responsibility is doing the work, each person doing deep reflection and psychological work for motivation, challenges and where are points of concern. Tell ourselves the truth of our life not a made-up story. She asserts that everybody has a responsibility to know themselves very well. To understand our motivations and challenges that we face. She tells me that there is a societal responsibility to make addiction unacceptable. ***Right now, everybody is so addicted that we are all telling ourselves that its fine.*** She gives me some examples: being addicted to opioids is bad, being addicted to cocaine is bad, doing unprotected sex is bad, but my addictions are fine. Recognizing the entire spectrum of addiction and being able to say, this is not acceptable. I summarize what we come up with the issues in addiction and asked her how she thinks we can help people who are dealing with addictions. She tells me this is a great question. She asks if I am thinking of individual or societal level. She feels more comfortable talking about what she can do as an individual to support others who deal with addictions. Be attuned to the people in her life and what is going on with them. Be aware where there might be problem behaviors. Make conscious choices when she is together with another person to do everything, she can to create a space where it is easier to the other person not to engage in a problem behavior. If she is with someone who is struggling with alcohol addiction she will not say let's meet up for happy hour, maybe instead making a conscious choice to go for coffee or a long walk instead. Choose a different activity. She now remembers and example she forgot about her uncle. He was addicted to drugs and alcohol for a long time. He struggled a long time, now he has been sober for 20-25 years, his wife is also in recovery.

    A few years back the family was going out to dinner and most people wanted to go to a microbrewery, she was all on board, then she pulled her mom aside and asked her mom if this is ok with her uncle. She knows some people are not be around alcohol. Her uncle was ok. Just tune into people. Support them so they don't even have to make that choice. We talk about that it can be difficult if we do not know that someone is struggling. Very true she said. When we do not know that someone is struggling it is much harder to support them. We have a discussion about open conversations without judgment and stigma. I wonder how we can be a more open in our society so that people can talk about what their problems are. We talk about our society and Kristen said that it is so alcohol centric that if we want to socialize with somebody alcohol is just assumed to be involved. In the past two years she is been more aware of a sober living movement she thinks the millennials are driving this trend. Not centering alcohol in social situations as much. I have to say that is great. I felt so awkward many times where there is a work gathering and people drink. It is uncomfortable. Kristen tells me about bars and nightclubs that don't serve any alcohol. She tells me about an article in the New York Times a few months back on the sober living movement. The article mentions a book Sober Curious. We had a little side conversation about frustrations on alcohol being just everywhere. I ask Kristen if she could wave that wand and make a change in society to help addictive behaviors or lessen the impact what she would do. She tells me oh, boy. Big sigh here. She takes a second then comes up with a great idea.

> *Make it part of the curriculum in schools at every grade to teach healthy coping skills. To teach kids about emotions and teach kids what to do if they feel an emotion that they don't like.*

She laughs. She tells me start young, start with healthy emotional habits. Emotions can be a trigger for unhealthy behaviors.

We turn the conversation to healthcare and healthcare systems role when it comes to addictions. Big sigh from Kristen. She tells me that the first thing we can do is have addiction recovery treatments fully covered by every heath plan. Screen for addiction as a pat of routine heath care visit. Making sure that everybody is getting access to this sort of screening. She tells me that often times the people who are underserved would be the ones to benefit from these types of services and might be the least likely to benefit from them. She feels we need a more equitable funding for healthcare and health care access. Additionally, consistency of services provided to people across income and geography. There is so much variation from state to state and urban and rural. I really appreciate Kristen's perspective and her public health mind. She tells me it is really upsetting to see how unevenly distributed healthcare resources are. I ask her what she thinks about providing healthcare for all. She is definitely in favor of it. She takes a moment to find the thoughts then she asserts a careful, complex and wonderfully worded idea: ***"It is really a national tragedy that people in this country die because they don't have access to healthcare".*** We should be able to do something about that she asserts. Everybody should be able to see a doctor regardless of ability to pay. Where that is Medicare for all or public option or completely reconfiguring our healthcare delivery system in this country which she thinks it would be a great idea. She laughs and tells me we just need to figure out a new way to do this all together. We have got to do better to make sure everybody has access to healthcare providers. We have a conversation about the cost of healthcare. It isn't pretty. It is not right. I ask her about the government's role. Big sigh again. She tells me we tried to criminalize addiction and it does not work. She feels to move away from criminalizing addiction and move toward viewing it as a public health problem and treating it as such. Putting funding and resources, incentives in place for states and local jurisdictions to change how we police addiction.

   She sees governments power deriving from where they choose to spend money. It all just ties back to money. The government can choose to pay for things that work better than putting people in jail. Allocate resources differently and putting more money into healthcare and public health. Thinking about changing the way healthcare is delivered in this country. Be more equitable. More funding for prevention, less reactionary spending on crises. It is much harder to fix the problem then preventing it. I saw so many times in hospitals and the communities how hard is it to try to fix something once it is a full-blown disease. Kristen brings up the opioid crisis and feels that the government needs to be very serious about regulations. Regulating the producers of controlled substances, doing so with an eye for the public good. Yes, public good not power and money in somebody's pocket.

Kristen thinks that in this country as a capitalistic society there is still a tendency to embrace business, entrepreneurship and the right of the company to make money and it is prioritized over the health and safety of the people who live here. She feels if the government could make this more balanced toward public good, we would see different types of regulations.

We talk about stigma a little more. Kristen feels that stigma plays a huge role because of this country's value on individual and their strength to make their own destiny. If we admit having an addiction it can been seen as a sign of weakness. Being seen as someone who is weak and not in control of their own destiny is not great, in the United States. She feels like there is a lot of stigma and that is why a lot of people stay in the shadows. More and more people in the past few years are able to be more open with struggles they have particularly with drugs and alcohol. People who are in recovery and able to share that without shame, I am 6 months sober for 6 months or 2 years and celebrate their accomplishment of being sober without the same.

20. Gambling

Paige describes that she has not seen much gambling issues with her clients at work. She does have a co-worker who has major issues with gambling. She had been in treatment a couple times. It was very sad for Paige to watch. She describes her co-worker as very smart, intelligent person. Paige would know where her co-worker is at lunch time or if she is late why she is late. She was gambling to a point that she could not make her mortgage payments. It was very sad to watch. I know of someone who had a good business, sold it and then gambled all the money away. He was tricking his family into giving him more money to live, he would tell them that he has nothing to eat, then he would use the money for gambling. This was hard for the family to find out especially when they had many expenses of their own and were raising two kids and worked hard to earn money.

Era tells me about a friend who she thinks has a gambling problem. She told Era she has credit cards to play the games. Era was wondering why this person needed credit cards when they have good pension and social security. Era is retired as well as her friend, so she was wondering at her age why she needed a credit card, no need for big items to buy. It did not make sense to her, so she is thinking there is some addiction going on. She thinks it might be affecting her friend's life financially. She asked her why she is doing it, her friend told her because she feels alone. She thinks that there are other people she knows who are dealing with the same thing. It is very private Era asserts. I might have played in a casino few times in my life but always used a limit of let's say 20 dollars and if I spent the $20 then I left. Looking at machines that are designed with pretty colors and flashing lights to get attention it makes me think of candy and sweets with all the colors that designed to get attention too. It is kind of like hiding something bad in a pretty cover. Tracy describes a lot of gambling in her family. Her grandparents had a lot of gambling debt as well as her mother. This was all coupled with the drinking in her family. She feels she did not develop any addictions; she went the opposite way because of what she grew up in. She wanted nothing to do with that lifestyle.

Dolores tells me about some patients she has who gamble. She had noticed that those patients have an associative disorder from PTSD. She explains it segue ways with the gambling addiction so that they kind of get lost in the process. She tells me they become different people when they are gambling, it is very interesting. This is just her experience and observation. She was surprised to find that there was a trauma-based issue that caused the gambling. When she figured it out with the patients it really helped them. She talks about gambling, getting a thrill and people can't stop.

21. Dr. M's Story

    I have a phone conversation with Dr. M, he works in the addiction field. He tells me that based on his personal as well as his work experience the roots of addiction come from some type of fear. Fear of a situation, fear of life, fear of not being adequate, not fitting in. Whatever the fear is for the individual. Through fear the response is to numb or take away the fear by using substances. The substance can be almost anything from alcohol to methamphetamine to heroin. All what Dr. M had seen is that the underlying cause is fear and people want to numb up this fear and become fearless by taking substances. Initially, he asserts it starts to reduce the fear, then the physiological needs take over. I ask him what he had seen people are fearful of. He tells me it is very individual; he had seen fear of being inadequate or fear from the future. Fear of what had happened in the past, how to deal with it and the shame and guilt, fear of death, injury, loss. Dr. M shares his own journey into addiction to alcohol and drug abuse. It initially started with fear of the future, fear of loss, fear of inadequacy, fear of the health problems of his spouse. He started to cover up with alcohol, then it became an obsession and compulsion. The addiction got worse and worse and he started to have more and more fears.

    The addiction was ruining his life, his relationship, his career. There was a point when his wife came to him and told him that he has to stop, or she will leave him. One of his fear was loss of spouse and friends and at that point he turned to get help. Personally, he found that acceptance of life and what is going on was a key for him. Putting his faith in a higher power and accepting things how they go was helpful for him. Accepting that there will be losses in life, there will be challenging issues. He believes that the higher power is there to help guide things and give him the grace to deal with things. Dr. M defines addiction as a compulsive searching out and using substances even though the damage the substance is causing. Dr. M asserts that the individual is responsible for the behavior before the addiction kicks in. Once the addiction took hold it is a compulsion; the individual has to do it. There is help out there he tells me, and it is the person who is addicted who has the responsibility to seek out help. Once they get help then it is their responsibility to continue in a recovery lifestyle without continuing a behavior that can put them back into addiction. Including being in recovery lifestyle and avoiding mind altering substances. Accepting life on life's terms. Dr. M describes through his own addiction that he had brief moments of sanity where he recognized that what he was doing is not working and he needed help. Most of the time it was not in his mind at all it was just about getting the next dose. In a larger scale Dr. M thinks that there should be help available for people with addiction across the board. The cost for society is losing a societal member and the cost of addiction is too high. It is the individual's responsibility to accept the help and accept the recovery lifestyle. It cannot be mandated he said, it is an individual choice. He feels that there is not enough help out there for people now, there is a mix match of available resources. Part of the problem is lack of funding and another part of is the overuse of resources of a small subset of people.

    The societal biases against with people who deal with addictions cause people with these problems to hide and not get help. Dr. M explains that a number of people in society think that addictive behavior is a choice, a moral deficit, something is wrong with this person, they are weak, they are bad or evil and it is not driven by a disease process. Then, the person is blamed not the disease. There is a fine line between the addiction disease and the responsibility of the individual to get help. The individual does have the responsibility to get help. Dr. M feels education could help change the blaming and stigmatizing mentality. He is not sure how it would look like. People who go through addiction, they have this perception of judgement erased, he adds. At that point they had seen both sides. We start to discuss the medical side of things. Dr. M asserts that addiction is a disease just like diabetes and heart disease, yet medical insurance only recently started to cover it. The medical insurances however started to dictate the duration and type of treatment, which might not be the best interest of the client. Dr. M feels that everyone has a basic right to some level of healthcare. He feels that the U.S. government had not been particularly successful in providing healthcare to U.S. veterans int the VA hospital system. His concern would be if the government totally took over, then healthcare would be run like in the VA hospital system; which is sometimes good and sometimes very bad. He does not trust the government or insurance companies to run it. He tells me that Medicaid pays under market value for all the services, and people only can get services at a small select number of settings. He feels that these services because of the financial constraint are cursory and incomplete. People on Medicaid tend not to go to treatment if it is financed through grants not through the Medicaid system.

He would like to see Medicare and Medicaid paying market rates for treatment. Additionally, looking at results of treatment providers and treatment centers. If the results are not adequate, then people are not getting appropriate treatment and the money is going to places that don't work well. It is a very complex issue Dr. M asserts and suggests that looking to other countries might worthwhile. He feels that the American system is quite broken. We discussed pharmaceutical companies, insurance companies and raising prices for essential medications. Dr. M gives me the examples of Narcan and Epinephrine as essential medications with skyrocketing prices. I personally believe that lifesaving medications need to be very cheap or free including Narcan, Insulin, Vivitrol, Epinephrine for example. I just saw a documentary on insulin in an episode of Patriot Act. Nobody should make money from insulin. It was practically donated by the inventors and it is very cheap to make. Yet, now people are dying from rationing their insulin or dying because they relapse, and they could not afford Narcan or Vivitrol to prevent relapse or overdose. Dr. M also talks about hospitals rising prices and having people pay for services a higher rate to cover their losses on people who cannot pay raising health care. Medical prices become astronomical. We go back to talk about treatment and its effectiveness. I ask Dr. M his thoughts on decreased treatment days. He feels that the insurance companies dictate treatment days and it is not very effective because people keep relapsing and going back to treatment multiple times, which becomes very costly. Since this is a chronic disease, the number of times people need to go to treatment is individual. There are people that don't really want to get clean and just use treatment services for housing and to get better between binge use. There are others who truly want to get clean and after treatment they get back to their home situation where nothing had changed, and they relapse. I ask Dr. M what helped him stay sober. He tells me that the first thing is:" ***willingness to change and do whatever the professionals tell you to do***". He tells me that this is very hard for people to admit that they need help. Continue in treatment. Dr. M has been sober for about 10 years and he still goes and sees an addiction professional every 6-8 weeks to touch base, to get another point of view. He feels very fortunate that his insurance pays for this service.

    Not everyone can afford to pay for something like this he adds. Everyone's story and needs are different he tells me. Not one magic wand would fix all. Certainly. He tells me what does not work. War on drugs is a total failure he feels. Shame and punishment of drug use does not work. Providing treatment for everyone would only work if the individual is willing to do the treatment and willing to make the changes necessary to stay sober. Acceptance and compassion to other people as everyone has intrinsic worth, do not just throw them away he said. We are all children of God he adds. It comes down to love thy brother on the second commandment of Jesus. If we just all did that it would certainly solve a lot of life's problems. He adds that if we just all loved each other instead of saying horrible things about one another life would be much better. We talk about happiness and joy in life. Dr. M feels for some people drugs is escape from misery and poverty. On the other hand, people with a lot of money including multi-millionaires also get addicted. I ask him about his final thoughts. Here it is: ***Just love each other.***

22. Happy Addictions

Kayla mentioned there can be so many addictions and she called them happy addictions. Kayla was saying how about when someone runs a marathon every month. She asked so what is up with that? Is it a good thing? So, they are training very hard she said, and they are really hard on themselves and a lot of people will look up to them and saying how amazing this is and might look at people training so hard as role models. Kayla describes that what addiction is can be really broad and it might be difficult to understand what drives people to do something that could be addicting. When I was talking to Edward he had mentioned running as an addiction as well. Exercise relieves endorphins and can be addictive. Is it a happy addiction? Is there such a thing? Kayla said it all depends on the reason why someone is doing it. Are people running away from their feelings? Or just want to be strong and healthy? It makes a difference. Tracy discusses that people can be addicted to something that is positive, and then it can still take over their lives.

23. Lola's Story

I sit down with Lola in our front porch in a nice summer evening. It is a little chilly, but still nice out. Lola works in the community and has tremendous experience in addictions in her life personally and professionally as well. She is a wonderful person trying always to do the right thing and committed to help others. Lola tells me that her definition and view of addiction had changed throughout the years. When she grew up her parents mom and stepdad did not drink much. Her father did, and she remembers thinking maybe my dad is an alcoholic. He was drinking every day. She stayed there sometimes, her dad would have big parties and they would drink a lot. Now he is 75 and his health declined. He can't drink now how he used too; she thinks he would if he could. He was a high functioning person. High ranking military officer, he had a lot of friends, successful marriage with his second wife. She had nothing else in her family as far as addictions. She recalls some events in college where people were using substances and it was getting a little too much. Her best friend had a drinking problem. She had past trauma. She would be drinking intensely and become reckless. She used alcohol, cigarettes and marijuana. She made strange choices. At that time Lola did not really get what addiction is. Lola was into arts; she was with people who were artist and musicians who live unconventional lives. She was always less inclined to place any judgement on how somebody should be living and what they are doing. She still sorts of maintain that. She went to grad school. She worked with adults of severe and persistent illness with a first few jobs she had.

There was addiction threaded into that she mentions like in any job anywhere. She recalls a memory from college when she was working at this novelty shop and she had a friend there who she describes as a fun weirdo, she remembers him coming over, they were drinking a lot then and she was smoking a lot of pot then. She was 19 years old. She remembers her friend coming over and huffing a bunch of glue. She was going like ugh, she was really freaked out about it. The process looked so intense and she was wondering why her friend is choosing this strange thing. She just that that was gross. It was intense, it seemed too much, she felt like he was really willing to go to a distance with this. It was very intense. Then her friend got into medicated cough syrups, then ultimately, they drifted apart. She does know that he got into heroin. Lola describes him as a sweet, innocent, goofy guy. Lola thinks he was able to get out of heroin after a few years. It looked different to her, this experience, looked a little dark. We go back talking about Lola's best friend Helen in collage. Lola is wondering wat kind of conversations they had and with the knowledge she has now she feels they would have had different conversations about addiction and drinking. Lola describes this friend very loyal and someone who gets very defensive and angry if they feel that there is something that is disloyal to her. It is sometimes hard to bring up difficult issues with Helen because she portrays it as betrayal. They are still friends. Lola just knows more now; she describes to me when she was younger, she just wanted to expand like little kids spinning around. Experience the world a different way, a different reality. Lola gets that and she thinks there is a space for it. She is not against most things. She does feel that people have to be careful and intentional about it. When she thinks about addictions mostly now what comes up for her is the clients she works with and her last two relationships. Both relationships were about 4 years. The first relationship she got into they worked together, it was unexpected, Dave ended up being super compelling. Dave was handsome, she got pulled into the chaos, not realizing what is happening, she had not had this experience before. Lola did not realize that for Dave that was his constant reality. Lola feels that if she would have had a better understanding of addictions, she would have realized that this was not a temporary thig.

  Dave lived in constant chaos all the time. She remembers going to his apartment and he had signs all over for himself. Notes would say if he stopped drinking this would happen in his life. He had been addicted to substances since he was 14 years old, he started pot even younger than that. Dave was using meth as a teenager; it was given to him by his mom. Dave lost a sibling to meth. Dave was able to stop meth but not drinking. He was able to stop drinking for periods of time. He got pulled back to alcohol. Lola feels it helps him twist his reality. He would ask what is really an alcoholic. Lola would say, well if he was not one then I am not sure what one is. The way she said this it made me laugh. Lola tells me Dave is a raging asshole too. She describes him as violent, crazy, mean, loses jobs and homeless. On the other hand, he is very smart, talented, very attractive. When he does not drink, he is able to get all kinds of traction, but he just can't get passed that. Lola describes that Dave's primary relationship was the alcohol and her trying to get a way in that was a treat. She feels she was pulled into a swirl. Sometimes she was the primary relationship and there was this weird shuffle that would happen. She got to a point when she would know when he was gearing up to drink. He would not drink for seven months and then Lola would know it is coming or if he had anything to drink, immediately. She was hyper vigilant because she was traumatized by him. There was one occasion where he was so violent and scary that Lola wanted to call the police, but she was too scared to do it. He would corner her, hurt her and threaten her.

He would hurt himself as well so he could say Lola did it. Lola had a lot more to lose, Dave could go as low as he wanted to go. She finally got out of that situation. He stopped drinking for a while then Lola had room to be angry. It was safe for her at that time to have her feelings and she realized she could not do the relationship. Then she fell into another one her current boyfriend Adam, maybe it is over now she was not sure. She at that time come from a very messy place. Adam was quitting drinking at that time too. Then he started drinking again as well. It was a different chaos. Adam would never hurt him. Not physically anyway. He would get mean and sort of shitty. He would become suicidal, he would go out to his car and drink during work, he would not sleep for days and would just be drinking, she would find him in his car crying, unable to move say or do anything. Lola tells me that we are supposed to be able to pull away and not enable someone, but it is very hard when they become suicidal and she thinks they might die. I asked her how all this makes her feel. There was some silence. In a way Lola feels that others might not trust her judgement because she twice in a row fell into these situations. She tells me about Adam, and he is brilliant, funny and super tender hearted. He is good she tells me. He was addicted to things since he was 12. Adam stopped using IV drugs when he was 14. It is crazy she tells me. It truly is. He used heroin, methamphetamine, Lola was not sure what else. He was homeless back then eating out of trash cans at golden gate park. He left home at age 12, did not go back, he lived in a warehouse. Older kids were selling drugs, that how he made his living too. He saw some horrible things. He was a bright kid but sensitive and people did not know how to deal with that he questioned everything. He got labeled as a bad kid. He associated with that message and he also git some bad messages from his parents, believed them and left. He lived in a group home for a while. He went to jail for 2 years as a teenager for drug related stuff. He got out, he was hopping trains and traveling around, then he had a baby.

    We discuss addiction. Lola tells me that addiction and she thinks about the things we do to avoid pain and blanket our suffering. Something that gets a possession of us. Lola used to smoke cigarettes. She had an acupuncturist ask her:" **_are you smoking them, or they smoke you at this point?_** " It used to be that she was smoking them. She only smoke cigarettes when she had a drink. It was an occasional, special privilege. Then it gets to a point where she was not choosing it anymore it was choosing her. Lola adds that it is important to identify that addiction is different for every person. She believes in harm reduction. Lola then tells me a story about her brother and her sister. Her youngest sister become of the age where she started partying, so Lola's brother wanted to make a special occasion to go camping, have her drink something in a safe place. His motto was kept it intentional and special. He ended up making her sister so drunk that she peed her pants. Way to make it special Lola said with such a tone that I busted out laughing. We both laughed for a while. Lola still teases him for this but on the other hand that is how she assesses things for herself. It stuck with her she would ask herself did I keep it special last night? She feels that self-determination is important. People do have a choice. She tells me the importance about connections that it is something that is missing for people who fall into addiction badly. She feels that more compassionate and less punishing systems would be helpful. At this point we have some side conversations; Lola acknowledges that it is hard for her not to run and rescue someone if she thinks they are in trouble. Then we steer toward suicide. Lola feels that many times people would say if someone is suicidal than are not in their right mind. She tends to disagree. What if they are? Who are we to say. It is not our place to say she feels if someone's life worth living. She had worked with so many clients who had so much suffering and there did not seemed to be an end in sight. She found herself silently in her head giving them permission. She would never say this of course, but she would understand if they made that choice. She would forgive them. We talk about assisted suicide and that people can decide on that for terminal illness.

The question is could severe mental health issues or addiction be looked as terminal illness. Is there a place for hospice care? Lola brings up an example a client she has she has so much medical stuff going on now she is just planning to be home and drink herself to death. Could there be a better and more humane solution? She is wondering if we could be more intentional and help people like her client with making a plan that supports their wishes. It is a difficult choice. What is our responsibility here? Lola tells me about an idea for holding space for people. She feels education and helping families and people to know how they can step in and help someone dealing with addictions. What are the right questions to ask somebody? If people do ask that question how they can try to figure out what they are missing, what they need and want. What options and resources are available. Of course, she said we don't have enough resources and options for people now. She does not feel that the 12-step model is the only recovery model. Lola feels that people's recoveries are very individual. We discuss treatment and how treatment might work or not for some people, it is very individual. Lola is telling me about a client when they are deep in their addiction, they do not even seem to be the same person. For some people going to groups and being in a recovery community is all they need to stay sober, they are embraced, loved and become this different person. For other people Lola tells me they have to be around their family and being motivated by family not to drink. We talk about treatment and addiction support. Lola feels that what is in place is not effective enough. She feels like more money needs to be funneled into it. She was not sure what the costs are, how maybe things could be more economical. Creating more intentional recovery communities that are self-sustaining. Lola also feels like we also need support for people who are not able to maintain sobriety. Lola asserts that is very hard for people to get out of the addiction and the community they have around them.

Finding something meaningful might help, creating something and be successful in it. Lola gives the example of art. Be social helps. Lola feels like social anxiety can also throw people into addiction. They might use drinks to be social then it gets out of hand. Lola identifies as a socially anxious person. We talk about food and food addiction for a while. We talk about how food is comforting. At least for a moment then people usually feel crappy. Lola then tells me about a friend who she lost related to opiate overdose. It was Fentanyl. Lola said she and her friends always know this is going to happen it was a matter of when. Lola is wearing this friend's perfume today. She knows that 15 years ago. She tells me about artists and musicians who are very intense people with a lot of energy who got into addictions. Maybe to experience things even more deeply. Lola feels like they needed to expand somehow. I ask her my magic wand question. She thinks for a while. She tells me a few times she does not know. She is thinking about brain changes. Something similar to Vivitrol and Naloxone. Changing a receptor making them work differently so people don't crave things like drugs. Early childhood education to be a good human, emotion management and throughout all school. She feels that would be huge. Emotional stuff and learning how to deal with emotions can make a huge difference Lola asserts. She feels her life would be much different if somebody would have thought her about how to control her sensitivity. She is a highly sensitive person and it makes things different. She did not know how to deal with her emotions and her parents did not know it either. She was so dramatic and emotional; she feels her parents did the best that they could. Lola feels in classrooms talking about emotions more would be helpful. She also tells me that when someone goes through a trauma it makes a huge difference how people react and the treatment sometimes the reactions can be even more traumatizing. She brings up that suffering does happen in life. Suffering can happen every day. It is how we deal with it.

    She tells me about sugar and coffee addition she has. She feels she can deal with the coffee addiction, but sugar is more difficult. She is trying to have more veggies instead of looking to add more sugar into the diet. She is telling me about fantasizing about on her way home picking up ice cream. We talk about natural sweeteners and making ice cream with healthy ingredients. Final thoughts from Lola she feels that realistic education about what addiction looks like would be helpful. She thinks about this idea that she heard before that is someone does something bad people would form a circle around the person and give testimony to the good things and qualities they have. The idea is that they must have forgotten their inherent goodness. I love this. They obviously forgot that they are good because they did this bad thing. Reminding them who they are. It is a great idea. It is protective. At his point bats start to fly around and we have a nice side conversation about them. I show her our bat house. Lola feels positive reinforcement is so important. Exclusion is a problem. She feels like things are going to get worse in the world the way the world is going. Teaching kids to be good people.

24. Technology- Social Media

Kayla mentioned social media and its influence on youth, and how they think they are supposed to look like or act like based on what they see in the pictures. Not eating enough because wanting to look a certain way is certainly a great concern. This had been a great concern of many people I had talked with. Posing an image on social media is very different then real life. There is a lot of addiction and inability to put the phone down, people keep checking their messages, see who liked the picture they posted. Does it really matter how many friends someone has on social media? How many friends people have in real life whom they can count on? Have a conversation with? Grab a tea or coffee together?

Rory describes being terrified for the kids and youth now growing up with the phone in their hand at all times. He describes it as a new opiates and parent being helpless around it. What can parents do? Rory thinks this is it. The next addiction. Social media, smart phones. There are spec scans that are showing how the brain is being changed social media outlets. The kids cannot get off of them. They cannot. Rory said: "we have unleashed a monster" and parents don't know how to deal with it. The clinical community is also not sure what can be done about it. Not enough research out there. When we find out the brain is already been damaged. We had a conversation about conscious choices not to have our phone with us all the time or do not look at our phone all the time. It is ok to miss a phone call; we can call back. I been making a choice not to take my phone in with me when I go somewhere. I don't really need my phone in a restaurant. I want to enjoy the experience without interruptions. If someone has a private practice like Rory, he needs his phone in case a patient needs him. Still it does not mean that we have to be on it all the time.

Tracy feels like technology and social media now is a huge problem when it comes to addictions. She describes technology as being harmful, not as harmful as drug or alcohol. Tracy feels like that the way kids are addicted to technology it is the same as someone else is addicted to heroin, it does the same thing to the brain. It rewires the brain. Takes over. Chloe feels that screens, phones are an addiction that is not even recognized today yet as addiction. She describes people who just look at screens for days don't eat or drink or do anything else. She feels more education is needed about this. Dolores gets this little flash on her screen that tells her how long she had been on the phone. Her voice here is full of surprise when she said oh, really? That many hours in a day. She is surprised. She chuckles. She finds it very interesting. She was talking to a patient who works for a nonprofit and what they are trying to do is have people talking to each other. That is their whole goal. She told Dolores that the world really changed with the cell phones.

Lot of people don't communicate by other means except through text and messages. It is easy to test she tells me. It is easier than having a conversation. Once we start and people go back and forth it can be hard to stop. It can go on for a long time. Dolores sees this a lot with kids, during the day they are in school then they isolate, hide out they don't have any social time other than in the classroom. She seen a lot of those. She tells me a little girl who was having panic attacks and stopped when she went home. Dolores asked what changed. She never went out. Not the best solution. It is a very sad solution. Talking to Bob he tells me that social media is good to use, but people can overuse. He is scared for the kids growing up using their phones all the time. He heard about the brain chemistry changes. He knows it is probably not good for adults either, but more dangerous for kids. He feels we might not have enough research on it. We talk about social media where people check their phones all the time to see who liked their post. Instant gratification. We talk about brain chemistry changes. Scary stuff for future generations. I have a conversation with Danny on the phone.

25. Danny's story

I have a conversation with Danny on the phone. He already knows what the book is about Toni had a conversation with him. We talk for a few hours. Danny is retired from the coast guard. He did 30 years of service. I thank him for his service. Alcohol and drugs were the two major addictions he dealt with from the professional perspective. There is so much presence of alcohol and drug use in the military that Danny had alcohol and drug awareness and training that was mandatory every year. They had classes about alcohol and drug addiction as well as suicide prevention. They had a high suicide rate. He tells me that suicide is closely related to drug and alcohol use. He personally known people who committed suicide because of drug issues. He tells me about one of the suicides. This person started with Danny around the same time in the coast guard. His suicide was different.

Danny is not sure if it was related to alcohol and drugs or not. He had another experience on a ship in the mid 1990's. He tells me on a ship people kind of get to know each other and they are forced to co-exist with each other. He talked with Charlie occasionally. Danny did not know him really well. One day he was in the ship and next day the captain gathered everyone and told them that Charlie had ended his life. Rumors had started on board and it was suggested that alcohol and drugs were an issue. Another time in Danny's career he worked with someone who left a suicide note. He had multiple issues but there was a phrase that Danny never forget that was in the end of the mote he mentioned "mother alcohol". It is a very sad things he adds. Danny considers himself lucky that he had received all this education from the coast guard every year, he feels that probably most people do not receive a formal education about these issues. He describes our society as a frame. I am imagining a picture frame here, then he tells me individuals are in it and we have to look at it from the point that what training and education and support individuals receive in society to help them. I like the phrase he uses next: "To help individuals cope with the demons they might possess in their lives". From a sociological perspective he tells me this raises the question how much local, state and federal governments should get involved in people's lives to help them when dealing with addictions. I ask Danny what he thinks how much the government should get involved. He tells me this is a complex issue and gives me some historical aspects. Since the 1940 he said things had been separate it was people to themselves and government to themselves. America as a nation was considered to be the individual on their own.

    Self-reliance and independence, he adds. It is a good thing he asserts, and at the same time if people fall on hard times and they have to rely on themselves and their families to help them. After the great depression he said the government had to step in and help people for the first time because so many people very destitute. In 2019 the government is getting again involved in people's lives he fells. It comes down to security versus freedom from a sociological perspective. To be free it is a hands-off approach from the government's perspective. The downside is he said that when someone falls into hard times like addiction the government does not help them to get out of it. When a government gets more involved it could help more people to turn around and educate them and give the tools to become a productive member of society. The downside of it is that these programs and assistance cost money. That money has to come from somewhere. The other downside of it is that the government is getting really involved in our personal lives. He tells me that there is a lot that goes with the old saying: "It takes a village to raise a child". He is not the first one telling me this. He believes that we have a lot of problems in our society. Just look at the news Danny said, pick out any one topic, violence, hit and run, somebody robbing a store for example. We have all these issues, immigration is another one, another big topic. He talks about citizenship for example. What does it mean to be a citizen he asks. He talks about the definition of citizenship and the responsibility of that citizen to the country. The individual should be responsible their own actions. He tells me the concept of taking a village to raise a child. From a community perspective. Help our community instead of being in isolation and not doing anything. He feels ultimately the government should be involved, but there is a caveat to that it should be a temporary measure just life welfare and foster care. People need to help the individuals, help them turn their lives around to become a productive member of society where they can stand on their own two feel without requiring further assistance. He brings up foster care as an example. The original idea is a temporary removal of a child until the original parents correct their behavior and economic status so the child can go back to them. How many times do we actually see that he asks? Many kids get bounced from foster care to foster care instead.

  Danny had studied organizational and family behaviors in collage. He studied teen behaviors and circumstances surrounding those behaviors. Including family and addictions. He brings up the point that when we study and learn about complex issues like addiction in society we have to include local and state government perspectives and how to help families change behaviors to get out of addictions. As a child in the 1970's he was raised around these behaviors. He went back to school to study how to correct these things. He tells me his personal perspective. As a child Danny's family was on welfare. They were very poor. His father was a drinker. When Danny was in his 20's he found out that his father got into drug use. He has a sister who is a recovering alcoholic a cousin who is an alcoholic. He dealt with addiction a lot in his family. He told people the way he survived childhood without ending up in prison or in foster care system is beyond him. He ended up drug free and in the military. He heard people say that children are resilient. Danny's father was also a child abuser. His idea of disciplining Danny was grabbing a 2x4 from the back yard and beating him with it. He disciplined him and his sister that way. In his childhood he had drugs, alcohol, child abuse. There was always something going on that the police would come over then they would leave. In today's world he asserts that his parents would go to jail for the things they did. The times in the 1970's was different. His dad ended up going to jail and needed to take classes on childcare and parenting. Danny had a lot of half sisters and brothers, he calls his father rather promiscuous. Danny tells me that all his father knew if what he learned from his father and his father what he learned from Danny's grandfather. He calls it a vicious cycle. Danny stopped the cycle with his children. I ask Danny what he thinks broke his cycle. He tells me the Coast Guard and the education he received there, studying sociological issues in college and seeing what addiction did to his family and others while growing up. He just knew, he does not want to go there. He tells me about rules, boundaries and limitations and how they affect us from a personal and professional perspective.

Danny tells me about his current life. He lives in California, on a nice property with fruit trees. He makes wine from the fruit and likes to drink it. Now he tells me he has to ask himself how much wine is too much. Is there a point of time when the wine would affect him personally. At what point does it become an issue? In the Coast Guard they teach people that they can have up to two drinks a day and that would be still ok. This might be may be or may not be true. He knows that the time might come up when he realizes he need to change his behavior. He hopes he will have the strength to do it. He talks about addressing why do people feel the need to drink in the first place. Danny used to chew tobacco for 20 years. He started chewing when he was a teenager then after 20 years the idea of possibly getting oral cancer from it was too much for him and he stopped. I ask him if he could stop drinking if he wanted. He tells me probably he would have to stop making wine. He feels motivation can help stop addiction positive or negative. For him with the tobacco it was the negative consequence, he has a family history of cancer and he did not want to lose half of his jaw to cancer. He feels like motivation to stop drinking would be based on his health. At his point of course my nursing brain has to tell him that alcohol is a carcinogen. He was not aware of it. According to the CDC drinking any type of alcohol increases the risk for 6 types of cancer. The reason is in the breakdown of alcohol to *acetaldehyde*. Acetaldehyde damages our DNA and prevents our body from repairing the damage (CDC, 2019). The CDC website where this is located is **https://www.cdc.gov/cancer/alcohol/index.htm**. Danny feels that most people do not know this information. He did not know this information. Danny feels that if it would be a high carcinogen there would be government label on the drinks just like on cigarettes. Well, maybe there should be a note on the label. We know it increases the risk.

We go back to Danny's childhood. He tells me his father would many times leave for 3-4 days then come home drunk. He would be drinking he would also be unfaithful to his mother. This is one of the most prevalent childhood memory Danny remembers. His father leaving for a few days then coming home drunk. Then his father and mother would get into an argument and he and his sisters would have to witness that. He had 3 sisters and have 2 sisters now, lost a sister to lymphoma. One of his sisters still calls him from time to time because she has difficulty with their childhood. It affects her adult life extensively. His childhood affected him, and he looks at it like he is 100 percent responsible for himself. He does not want others to feel sorry for him. He does not want to rely on religion to wash away his sins and provide redemption. He relies on himself, his wife and family. He does not want to dwell on the past and on his childhood. He is living his life the best way he can live it. Those memories will never go away. He will not let them ruin his life. He has a baggage. Everybody has a baggage. ***In the here and now he decides how he lives his life.*** This reminds me of a book I read. The Power of Now by Eckhart Tolle. I highly recommend this book. It has a similar concept. Focus on the now not the past or the future. For Danny it is a simple thing. Be 100% responsible for our behavior. He tells me ask ourselves we are ok with who we are. Examine our behavior over a day, a week, a month a year. If we are not ok with who we are then we have to ask ourselves why that is. Then make changes. Redirect our energy toward change. Need to find the strength to do it. He is not saying that change needs to occur completely on our own. If people need help with resources or someone to point them to the right direction, that is fine. He is telling me that the one thing that affects him from childhood is that he is very self-reliant. Because of all the things that happened to him he rarely seeks help from other people. He calls it a double edge sword.

    He believes that whatever problems he faces he needs to get over it on his own. He sees this as a negative thing. He feels people should be able to rely on others when they need help. It comes back to the community perspective. It takes a village to raise a child. No one should have to get through life on their own. People should be assisted and educated when needed. Danny tells me about his life in retirement and his relationship. Danny and Toni have a very good relationship, they been together for 16 years. He tells me that they never had an argument about anything. He describes having a happy great life. He tells me he could not ask for anything more. He does not make a lot of money in retirement. He can pay the mortgage and the bills. It is enough. He is perfectly happy. He tells me that if people want to live the way he does planning in life does help. Sensible planning. He likes traveling, seeing a little bit of the world, enjoying himself, he likes camping and his motorcycle. After retirement in the first couple years he was trying to figure out his purpose in life. In the Coast Guard for 30 years his purpose was defined. He lived by organizational objectives and lived with people who had the same drive and desire as he did. They all lived by the same rules, he had an extended family. When he retired, he was struggling with what his identity now. It was hard for him to figure out at first, but he did he realized that having a job should not define him. He should define himself. He had to be ok with not working. He is happy, he works on the house and that he gets to travel. It is good enough. He had to ask himself if this lifestyle he lives now is good enough for him and the answer is yes. What he describes to me is a lot of self-reflection and asking himself questions what he wants in life. I believe that self-reflection is a very important tool to find ourselves, who we want to be. We talk about family a bit and Danny tell me that he is a better man because of his wife Toni. He feels that she has the outlook on life that everyone should have. Toni is the type of person who looks at things positive and tries to make the world better. He is humbled by the fact that even if his wife could do her life over again, she would go to the same troubles she went through to meet him.

  Our past defines who we are today. When Danny looks at his wife and looks at the things she went through and look at the things that happened to him or others he know and think I am having a bad day, then he thinks of Toni what she went through and tells himself that he has nothing to complain about. Danny never knew anybody before who died twice, come back to life and have the outlook that Toni does. She is an amazing person no doubt. Danny wants to be a better person and have the same outlook on life like Toni does. It gives people a perspective. Danny tells me about his retirement plan and his plans to take care of his wife even if something happens to him. He receives a monthly income and it was hard for him to take his retirement and go from working every day for 30 years to not working and receiving money every month. It took some time for him to get over this. People would remind him that he served his country and he know it and it was still weird for him. He went from working and going to school to have nothing to do. We talk about our school experiences. It is weird for both of us not to have a paper due and what do I do now. He is been now retired 5 years. He is very happy with his life. He enjoys cooking food. He tells me about wine making. He never drunk before his marriage. He was 43 years old before he really had a drink. He tells me about future plans. He talks about taking care of a farmstead in a future and not making wine. He now has a vegetable garden. They grow their own vegetables, hydrate the fruit. He wants to be self-reliant in the future. He likes to grow their own vegetables and bake their own bread because they know what is in it. The wine they make is also organic. He tells me about wine in the store that have chemicals and can cause health problems.

    A lot of people get hangovers and dehydration because of the sulfide and chemicals in the wine that they buy. He tells me want is in their wine. Juice, sugar, alcohol and yeast. He is not justifying making wine, he is telling me this to inform me of their conscious decisions on what products they eat. He does love green tea and tells me he might just start drinking green tea now. Danny tells me that his mom drinks a lot, always smoked and never really took care of her health. He wants to be in better health than his mom now. Danny works out to keep in shape. Likes to walk or do work out at home. He does have a goal of losing a little weight. He tells me about being overweight at his 30's then getting too skinny after that. We talk about sugar in alcohol. He tells me about plans to leave California and moving to Idaho. California is very expensive. They live now in an agricultural community. He tells me about people in San Jose who cannot get a mortgage in a 6-figure salary. He knows someone in the Coast Guard who rents out a single room in San Francisco for $1500 a month. Danny and Toni live about an hour from the bay area where most people are working. Hoping they will be able to sell their house in the future and buy a farmstead in Idaho. Homes now sell in the area where they live in a week or two people moving farther and willing to commute to afford a home. Housing is just unaffordable in the bay area anymore. He tells me about the ***limited number of days we all***

have in this earth and we have to decide how we want to live those days.
      We circle back to define what addiction is. Danny tells me that he thinks **addiction is that prevents people from being the person they want to be.** He tells me addiction can also be defined by blaming everything and everyone around instead of ourselves. It is a slavery, he tells me it binds people a behavior, creates an attitude. Addiction binds people to be a person they don't want to be. Danny tells me that the hard part is breaking that chain, breaking that behavior. Addiction could be anything he tells me it could be chocolate; it could be doing physical fitness; it could be something people consider positive addiction. Nerveless addiction is something people cannot get away from. People want too to get away from it but can't figure out how to do it. Addiction is something that controls us instead of us deciding our own faith and destiny, addiction decided the faith for people. Most addictions are negative addictions controlling people. Breaking addiction is getting control back in our life. Danny tells me addiction is a negative control on our mind, body and soul. Breaking addiction is living the way we want to live not the way we have been living. Taking control of our lives. It is an individual thing. Danny tells me he is super happy with his life now and he does drink alcohol. He does not see this as a negative thing. He is enjoying what he is doing. He asserts that the moment he would feel that alcohol would create a negative consequence on his life, his wife or anybody around him, knowing the person he is he would just stop. Danny knows that in general alcohol is not good for people. If he asks himself if alcohol has control over him, he would have to say it probably does. What a great self-reflection. He is consciously happy with his life, and he also realizes that the older we get the more concerned we have to be about our health. He knows that there is a point where he has to ask himself if drinking alcohol is worth the potential future health consequences he might encounter. He feels no matter what the addiction is we have to ask ourselves this question. Even if it is a positive addiction. There will be a point in time where it will hurt. He tells me he did not get to that point yet. He is honest with me telling me that he drinks. I really appreciate his honesty. Danny does not feel he fits the stereotype that he observed growing up. He saw what

drinking did to his family, his dad, his mom, his sister. He definitely does not want to be like his parents. He feels one day he needs to make a decision. He tells me if that means stopping to make wine and getting rid of everything in the house so be it.

    Danny tells me about a memory of his retirement ceremony. He spent a lot of time with people on the ship. In finishing he speech he said: "we all went through a lot together, we had people we lost, we had people who left the organization because of drugs and alcohol, my advice is to always be aware and get involved". He remembers that suicide he told me about before. He told the junior officers: "Know what your shipmate is doing. If you see something out of the ordinary don't just brush it off, get involved, you can save a person that way". Danny feels that one of the reasons is why people have addictions is because somebody somewhere did not intervene. He poses a question. Can we avert addiction by getting involved in a person's life? By going out of our way to check on a welfare of a person? Being a good friend? Being a good son or parent? He would say yes. Take the time out of our way to talk to a person who needs help. Danny feels that he is lucky that he has people in his life who love and care about him. He feels that **_as long as we get involved in someone's life no matter if it is a friend, a parent, a co-worker we could prevent a lot of addiction_**. He goes back to the concept it takes a village to raise a child. He feels that in the larger framework of society it takes people in all stages of life to help each other. No matter who the person is. He tells me that as a public servant he feels that he must do good by others. Do good by the people who put him to the place where he was and where he is now. It does not mean overreaching government. Then he adds if someone needs help dealing with addictions and family and friends or other resources cannot help, we might need to step in as a society local, state or federal government to help the person. He feels whoever runs any kind of program they all need to be in the same page. He feels that page is a temporary situation.

    We are going to help and give the person a good job give them the tools to succeed then after that they are on their own. He tells me that is how it should be. Correct the behavior, help the person in what they need to help with, put them on the path toward success, once they are on that path they are on their own. If for some reason they relapse

Danny adds people can step in again and help them walk that path again. What we run into with government help he states is that they keep helping people and it is to their detriment. He brings up the kids in foster care he mentioned before. Kids going from one place to the next because it takes the parents 5 years or more to get them back. Kids going from one foster parent to the next is not fixing the problem. That is not fixing the parents, it is not helping the parents. He feels that the same thing applies to addictions. We can help a person to be self-reliant and stand on their own two feet. This brings up the same problem Dr. M talked about some people keep using the system for housing and between use. Otherwise Danny tells me they will keep coming back to get more and more treatment and we end up getting people who are addicted to government services. I certainly heard those stories when it comes to our jail system. That is all people know and they get caught up in the cycle. He also brings up government services like welfare. People get on it and won't get off. It is easier to do that then to get a job and live on our own and he thinks that is a problem. He really feels this is the same thing that is going on with addiction. He talks about this endless cycle when it comes to addiction that people go back and think well if I use again there will be services that help me get clean and this creates and endless cycle. I ask Danny if he thinks that there are programs out there now that help people stopping the cycle. He does not have knowledge of them outside of what he knew at the Coast Guard. What he had seen in the Coast Guard it is a combination of disciplinary, medical and psychological help. It is a very stepped program. If someone is doing well, they get their life back and rank. If not, ultimately, they can lose their employment. The incentive here seems to me is keeping their employment and pay. Most people who Danny knows they have done the program and they succeeded. Some people don't. He'd been in that process as a supervisor. He thinks that about 20 % people don't make it. They end up being discharged. At least 80% succeed. That is phenomenal success considering the statistics outside of the military.

    We discuss that how having a safety of a government job and housing might play a role in success compared to the outside world. I saw people who don't have a job, have no housing, can't afford therapy, have no support and they keep falling back to the cycle of addiction. Not surprising. He feels that this is correct in the Coast Guard all these services are provided. He used to counsel young people and he would tell them that when they are in the military any branch of it the military is a way of life. It is not just a job. If they have a problem, there is a mandatory treatment to do. If someone works anywhere else nobody cares about their personal life. Military is completely different. Military owns people and is involved in their personal life while outside of the military this is not the case. Lots of people also have a problem with that there are a lot of kids out of high school who find themselves in the military and there are a lot of rules and regulations that they have not experienced before. I ask him what he thinks about providing that help to all people. The Coast Guard for example in their budget already includes those addiction services and they are paid for. He thinks it would be great for everyone in society to get all the same help, but there is a difference he tells me. In the military it is not a voluntary thing they have to go through the program, or they get kicked out. It is mandatory thing where if someone refuses, they could go to jail. They can go to military prison because they are disobeying orders. In society the person out on the street are not subject to these same rules. To offer these programs would be still good. He does not think you could mandate it. It would be martial law. In the military people give up a lot of personal rights. The conditions are different in society.

There are different motivators in the military then in society. He brings up who pays for this as well. The majority needs to decide if this is something they want to pay for. There are so many factors to consider. Would people go to the programs? Are they aware of the programs? We talk about government programs and bring up the idea for example if there is a kid in foster care because the parent deals with addiction then the treatment of that parent could be mandated. He tells me that sometimes in government the left hand does not talk to the right hand. Different agencies don't talk to each other. Social agencies collaborate with each other by helping the parent so the child can go back to the parent.

26. Suicide

A lot of people whom I talked to and met through my career have been touched by suicide. Difficulties in life, inability to cope with current and past events, hopelessness, addiction problems and mental health problems can lead people down to that path. There are stories in this book of people trying to commit suicide. The story below is about a young man who succeeded. He left behind a lot of family and friends who are still grieving about the loss of his life.

Era visits me, we are sitting out on the porch in a nice Summer afternoon. She tells me a story about a young boy who was her son's friend. His name was Lucas. The boys used to be very good friends. Era worked evening shift as a nurse and her son spent a lot of time at Lucas's house. She invited his parents over for dinner once. She was very surprised because Lucas's mom was drinking a lot of beers. Era could drink maybe 3 beers as a maximum. Lucas's mom continuously was drinking, and Era was concerned. She was not sure what to do because the culture she came from and the hospitality side of her just kept bringing this mom the beers, on the other hand she knew something was wrong. The dad was drinking hard liquor, whiskey. Lucas's parents pushed him to be independent and he moved out of the house, got his own place after high school. Era's son started to hang out with him less and less. In the beginning it was all fun. After the summer ended friends left for school and Lucas ended up just being around people using alcohol and drugs. He was using alcohol for sure, maybe drugs Era was not sure. She has not seen Lucas for a while, she missed him and asked her son how he is. Her other son told her that Lucas and his brother are not keeping in touch much anymore.

One day early morning one of her son's called Era and told her that Lucas hung himself. He was in debt; he was under a lot of pressure. Lucas wanted to be a pilot; he went to a lot of trainings. He had a lot of expectations from home, he was the only boy in the family, he had two younger sisters. He loved trucks. He had a new black truck Era recalls, then he had an accident with the truck. Era felt like that was not him not to take care of the truck and get into an accident. She felt that he was trying to hurt himself then. He went missing so people started to look for him. Close to Era's home there was a motel that was doing remodeling. He hung himself there. He was 18 or 19 years old. He was clean of drugs when he did it or were gone from his system. This suicide hit Era very, very hard. She cried every time she saw the mom, just wondering how a mother deal with a loss like this. Era thinks that there were problems at home with the parents. She was told once they broke up and Lucas brought them back together. That kid is gone, she said and what I can say? She tears up. She was feeling guilty. She wishes she knew something was wrong and she could have helped him. She did have a dream around that time and did not know then what the meaning of it was. Era describes a street with a cemetery she saw in her dream, there was no paved road, she wanted to go through, she was thinking about if she should she even go through. She was on a horse; she saw 2-3 bad guys in cape like clothing she called it pelerine. They looked like people who dealing drugs. Cartel people of Mafia. She was thinking if she had a car, she would be more protected from them. Then, in her dream the horse flew above them and she was safe. In the right side in her dream was the cemetery. This was the same cemetery where Lucas later was buried.

    This is still very emotional for Era; she saw the boys grew up together. The kids were like brothers. Era's son still keeps a photo of Lucas. Era went on a cruise a while back with friends and was thinking a lot about Lucas. Tears started to flow. Then a little bird came by. Maybe it was a sign, maybe a coincidence. Who knows. She hoped that the little bird symbolized hope and healing and freedom of burden. Era's son and his friends had a hard time dealing with the loss. They went out drinking. They get the attention from the Police; they were driving, and Era's son's alcohol level was 0.13, things got very bad from there on. It was underage drinking and driving. He had to be in jail one night, he could not drive for a while, then his car had to have a breathalyzer. Era's son still drinks on weekends sometimes. He never drinks and drives. Era described her and her mom waiting for her son to get out of jail with a Starbucks coffee and sandwich and the police standing there laughing at them. He can still not pass the border to Vancouver, BC because of this incident. He would need to pay money to clear the offense. Era feels like indirectly God have her son a lesson. Era's son never shared the pain with her about losing his friend Lucas.

27. Tammy's Story

Tammy and I talk on the phone for the interview. We did meet prior to the phone conversation and had an in-person discussion about the book. Tammy is the type of person who is there for people and tells them things as they are. Her story begins in her teen years. She dabbled into a lot of different drug usage. She did not use needles. She used everything else. She was one of the lucky ones, she did not have an addictive personality. Tammy looked older than her age. She was hanging out with an older crowd that used alcohol and drugs. She feels this did not help her decision making. Most everybody she was involved with used something. Later in life after Tammy had children she looked back and reflected on choices she made. It took her a long time before she could work in the field of addiction. She had a lot of anger and resentment.

She graduated nursing in 1989 and it took her several years before she applied to a job doing detox. Once she did, she was glad. She brought the experience with her from her first marriage. Her husband dealt with addictions which resulted in the end of the marriage. In the beginning of the relationship there included a lot of drinking and drug use. After Tammy got pregnant, she stopped using any drugs and alcohol. Her partner continued to use. The first time he assaulted her she was 8.5 months pregnant. Looking back now Tammy reflects that she should have ended the relationship then. She was young, she was 17 and decided to stay in the relationship. Tammy now feels that because she was so caught up in the relationship, she did not use common sense. The drug and alcohol use by her partner increased. Just right before she left him there was a party at the house and she caught him shooting up in the bathroom. That was the first time she knows of that he was using IV drugs. He was using cocaine. She decided right then she will leave. Even after Tammy left his usage increased. He was in and out of prison. He died in prison from AIDS. This really affected the kids. Tammy was alone with two small children. At that time there was also a lot of stigma surrounding people with AIDS. This was in the 1980's. The last time Tammy saw her ex-husband he had hepatitis, he had open wounds on both of his arms, he was still injecting in his open wounds. He never had any treatment as far as Tammy knows. It was not something that was offered much back then.

    Tammy made the decision never to take the kids to prison to see him. She felt it was not heathy for them. It took her a long time to get over this experience. During their marriage, he was very controlling. He alienated her from her friends and family. They had moved to a different state and she did not know anybody except his family. His family was not very supportive at all. His family was very religious. In order for the family to come to their house Tammy had to get married first. The family was in denial. They had the belief that marriage is a long-term commitment. Even with the abuse. One time her husband assaulted Tammy in the car, the police came by and he got arrested. She called her mother in law to get the keys to the car. Her in laws would not give the keys to the car. Tammy ended up staying with her in laws for a few days. When she went back to get her stuff, all her things were smashed, taken to the back yard and were burned. One of Tammy's children has problems with alcohol and mental health issues. Tammy had not spoken to her in a few years. All the prior events effected Tammy's life and her self-esteem. She had no self-esteem when she left her husband. She had no job, moved in with her mom and stepfather. It took Tammy a long time to get out of unhealthy relationships. She stopped dating for a long time. She was raising her kids, going to school and struggling to survive. This made her stronger. She knew she will not let anybody lay a hand on her again. She did not want her children in an unhealthy environment. She tells me that looking from the outside many times people don't understand why she would stay in a relationship like that. People stay because they lose their self-esteem. Her ex would tell Tammy:" you are worth nothing, nobody would want you, nobody wants you with two kids". She tells me abusers like that know exactly what to say to keep others down. Sometimes this is all part of the addiction. The person who is the addict they don't want their partners to leave, and they do everything to make them want to leave. People dealing with addictions are very good at lying, saying what we want to hear. They play on our emotions. It wasn't until Tammy was afraid for her children when she decided she has to leave.

I ask her if anything happened. It was at the same party she told me about earlier when, her ex grabbed her son who just started to walk. He lifted him up in the air with one arm carried him to the bedroom and swung him on the bed. She knew then she had to leave. She was not afraid for herself, but she was afraid for her children. Her children did not remember any of the violence that happened in the home. This made it for them difficult to understand why Tammy left their father. Tammy feels that this history had helped her deal with people who are dealing with addictions and mental illness. She knows how it can change someone. It does not matter how much we love them, does not matter how supportive we are. None of that matters. It is all on the addict, she adds. She feels this can be very hard for people to understand especially parents of children. All they want to do is help their children, and all they really do is harming them and enabling them. She many times had to teach people to go against the grain. As a parent people want to try to do everything to help your child. In this instance, **the best thing people can do is nothing.** Sometimes Tammy thinks that all those bad things happened to her that later in life she could help people. It is one thing to tell somebody: "I know how you feel", and they really don't know how that person feels. It is another when someone had been in their shoes and can share their own experiences.

Tammy shares an experience from work that always touched her, and she will never forget. She had a young attractive lady in her 20's come into detox from heroin. Both of her forearms were abscessed. It had to be treated. Her arms looked like somebody used an ice cream scoop and scooped meat out of her arms. Tammy used to have to put a wet to dry dressing on the wounds every day. (An open wound need something moist to prevent sticking to the flesh) The patient screamed when Tammy put the Kerlix (big gauze roll) in the wound. It scared Tammy. She realized that the water was too cold, and she need to warm it up before putting the Kerlix into her arm. This young patient really touched Tammy, it really showed her what addiction can do to someone and the person cannot just stop. Here was this young woman with whole life ahead of her, yet mutilated. She tells me about another patient. A man in his 40's. She describes him and depressed and lonely. Tammy got to know him well. After a very complex detox Tammy told him that he is killing himself with his use. Tammy told him he might as well shoot himself. She said this statement to him to shake him up and make him think about what he is doing to himself. He was the kind of guy who needed to hear this. He looked at Tammy as said: Well, that would be cheaper and quicker wouldn't it? They both laughed. I laughed too. It is not funny but it kind of is. The way she said it imitating the patient it was funny. Tammy did not see him for the longest time, she was even looking in the obituaries. The guy was in and out of detox before for years. A few years went by and a man come up and tapped on Tammy's shoulder. She initially did not recognize him. He told her that probably she does not remember him and at that moment it clicked. She could not believe it. He been clean for almost 2 years, he had a job, he had an apartment with some roommates. It was not the best job, but a job regardless. He was sober. Since then over the years when Tammy sees people who are struggling just like this patient, she had she tells them: I know I can't do this. She would tell them his story. How he never gave up. From the providers perspective it's been difficult for Tammy to work with pregnant addicts. Especially the patients that were treated, they had their baby then they come back using drugs and pregnant again. That was really hard to take care of someone like that and keep personal feelings out of it.

    She tells me when we talk about addiction, what is a better example than a woman who keeps using even that she knows what that does to her fetus. It is a pretty strong case for addiction she adds. I ask Tammy how did it make her feels seeing the women pregnant and keep coming back? She tells me a mixed feeling, angry, sad, helpless. Every time somebody came back it made her feel like she failed. She would wonder why the women would not get their tubes tied. She would be upset that there are not enough places for the women to get help. Tammy feels like that if there is an option and the women does want to get their tubes tied, they should be able to do that. It is a fine line she tells me. If a woman had been pregnant and her baby born addicted, ok everyone makes mistakes, even in two times, but if it keeps happening 3-4 times someone should be able to step in at least talk about options. Tammy has a lot of anger and resentment against religions. She feels like churches are all against abortion, yet nobody is there to help someone raise a child. She feels like if people with a Christian faith are concerned about women having abortions then they need to step up to the plate. Tammy never felt that there was help from people about abortions yet there are so quick to pass judgment. It takes a lot to raise a child. It is always easier to judge then to step in and help. She tells me that at least an opiate baby has a chance, if they get through the withdrawal, if they get a loving home, if they are raised right, lots of if's. They have a chance. There are very little side effects from opiates. There is a genetic component of course. With an alcohol baby there is nothing we can do. With Fetal Alcohol Syndrome (FAS) the damage is permanent. Tammy feels that addiction treatment is essential for pregnant women. Even if they had left and used drugs or alcohol and come back. At least while they were on the addiction unit, they were clean. Every clean day counted. She wished there would be more places for women and more done to prevent in the first place.

Tammy thinks that addiction is uncontrollable urges that people have to fight every day, whatever is drug, alcohol, food, gambling, sex, whatever the addiction is if people are able to recover from it, it is a lifelong struggle. There are so many people who have addictions and don't even realize it. Anything that people do that is detrimental to themselves or anybody else. Tammy tells me she does not have a drug or alcohol addiction; her addiction is food. She looks at it from that context. Especially when she is trying to eat healthy and come upon a bakery with some cannoli. She would stand there looking at them. She would tell herself standing there that this is terrible, she wants them so badly. She is trying to eat right; she knows it is bad for her. She wants to lose weight; she wants to be healthy. She wants to be comfortable, but she tells me: I want that f***ing cannoli. It does not matter what the drug is, she tells me it is the same thing. She thinks of her mother who depended on insulin, but she could not control her eating. Her mother knew all the problems diabetes would cause and Tammy used to fight with her, yet she would still hide chocolate bars in her nightstand. That is addiction. Some people just don't have the self-control and it does not matter what the addiction is it can get people physically and mentally. Tammy tells me that when it comes to food, she is the worst addict. In her mind she can talk to herself why it is ok if she just has one that tomorrow she will be back, or she had a rough day she deserves it. It is whatever is in our mind that we can talk ourselves into. That is the addiction, she tells me, it is always there; it is always this little voice in the back of our mind. It does not matter even in years go by. Heroin addicts used to tell her there are certain places they cannot go near. They cannot go down a certain street because it is the corner they used to buy. It triggers their brain. It is a struggle every day. We discuss food addiction and some of the pathways. Tammy tells me they also push all that stuff on us from a very young age, it is all over TV, no matter where we go, we are ingrained to it. She asserts that this country is the worst. This country is all about making money. They don't care that the food they are putting out is unhealthy or even dangerous as long as they are making money. It is the same thing with the tobacco industry. They can put a warning on the package. Still selling it for a profit. Food is a big one. We all have to have it. It is a saddest thing for her to see these young elementary school kids that are so fat that they can barely walk.

She feels like that food and alcohol are the addictions that people are more accepting of. We discuss that alcohol is everywhere. Tammy feels that education about addiction needs to start at a very young age. She compares the education that needs to happen to when she was young and they were teaching kids about littering, there were commercials on TV, groups of people got together to clean places up, it was involved in every aspect. Now it is seldom to see littering out of the car, people are more aware. This was thought when people were young and each year in school kids were thought more. Tammy feels that by the time people are in high school they should know everything about drugs and alcohol, the good, the bad and the ugly. None of it should kept quiet. Get them young and engrain it. Smoking is been a battle, a hard one with the fight with the tobacco industry. Getting the parents involved as well. There will be some parents who might not want their kids to be told about addictions, and we still have too, she adds. Tammy also feels that in healthcare it should not be up to the insurance companies when someone needs treatment. She feels we should have more follow up care. It does not do any good to detox somebody then send them back to the same environment. She does not feel treating addictions is a priority still. She feels like nobody wants to spend money on drug addicts. Tammy feels that both addiction and mental health are taboo subjects. They are always going to be the red headed stepchildren. People just don't get it that prevention is the only thing we can count on. There should be more options for people, have Suboxone more available for people financially and by location. The government doesn't really care. The government looks at how much it costs to cure yet they don't look at the overall cost of not doing anything. She is not sure what it would take for the government to make addiction a priority. She tells me about the 1970's and the 1980's with cocaine affecting the minorities. Nothing was done then. It was oh well, people are going to die. More being done now, and still it is too little too late. Tammy does think that education is the key, and that the fix will not happen immediately. Education needs to start in elementary school. More option for people who want to get help.

    She gives me the example somebody coming in with opiates to the emergency department and she would love if she could just pick up the phone and say I am sending someone over, and it is going to be the real deal treatment with follow though. Without early education nothing will change. This way eventually they will meet in the middle. No quick fix. Tammy feels that addiction can happen because of family, environment, socio economics, classes. Heroin is a poor man's drug. It is everywhere. The majority of people who have addictions also have mental health issues. The two kind of goes together. It is hard to know which one starts first. The problem is so much bigger than alcohol and drugs. We also have to look at mental health issues. It is overwhelming. We have to look at both mental health and addiction to help people. It is very complicated issue; we need to treat the whole person. She tells me about PTSD, interpersonal relationships, family problems, so many things that can go wrong to bring someone to addictions. I asked Tammy what helped her in her food addiction. She tells me she come to the point to eat less and exercise more. We just have to make up our minds and do it. She sometimes looks at food as enemy. She is not sure how healthy that is. She would look at the cannoli as a temptation that would set her back on her track of becoming healthier. Try not to put herself in a situation where she is forced to make that choice. Try to plan ahead. It is a mindset, not get the fried, get the baked food. She feels this can be different for everybody, what is the last straw. Some people never get it she adds. I ask her if she has any final thoughts for me. Tammy tells me that over the years she changed her opinion on some things. She never used to think that weed and alcohol can lead someone to start to use heroin. She feels like it is not so much the usage of the beginning substances but the people around the person.

The environment plays a big role in the development of drug usage. She would educate more on friends; who we are socializing with what do they do for fun. If someone is with a group of people who drink and use drugs a lot, they have to be aware that they are more susceptible to use drugs and drink. It is inevitable. She feels that in the younger years the big part of it is the peer group. As people get older with more responsibilities if someone has not developed addiction, they are not an addict. The peer pressure makes a big difference. People who use together that are sharing something special. Heroin addiction is a culture. They just know by looking at each other.

28. Being the Provider

A provider can be anyone. It can be a nurse, doctor, counselor or it can be a friend, family member. Being a provider is someone who takes care of a patient, family or friend who is dealing with addiction. This is no easy task. Providers just want to help. Beth described that patients are always different, she felt there is a sense of entitlement. She is always careful not to judge her patients. She said:" I treat them all because I want to save that one person". Trying to be a resource and provide resources that are out there, and also setting firm boundaries. One of the difficulties is when the person who deals with the addiction does not want help. Beth told me if they don't want help, she makes them lowest priority because she has other patients to take care of. She had too many people who walked away against medical advice. Sometimes it seems impossible. It is impossible to offer that help, not enough time to do the extra step. I remember those days too; I had too many walk always as well. It was heartbreaking to watch, then I wondered will they be back? Will they be ok? Will they be found dead somewhere? Sometimes we knew right on admission that this person will not stay. Just hoped that they will make it. Somehow, by some kind of miracle.

    Beth describes that in the medical field many times there is just not enough time to care for a patient. In doctor appointments the providers are stressed for time and people are lucky if the providers spend a few minutes with them. The question is if that is enough to really take care the whole person or is it just enough to quickly diagnose something and stick a prescription in someone's hand. There are so many matrixes to meet, charts to fill out, referrals to follow up on many of the providers I met in my life are overwhelmed and overworked and don't have a lot of time to actually spend with patients. Beth alleged that when she goes to work, she takes care of people who are addicted. She does need to pay special attention to people with addiction if they have an intravenous infusion going on because of the chance of using, have to monitor visitors, cannot have anybody going in and out. The rules have to be very strict because of the chance that they are going to use a substance. Have to take all of the patient's belongings out of the room. Beth is not mad at them or angry at them. She knows they have a problem. She would love to be able to help them. She is so busy at work. Beth also very busy in life working 2 jobs, going to school, taking care her children. Beth would love to help even that one person and she has respect for those dealing with addiction. She still has to create a healthy boundary at work if someone is disrespectful to her, she will not tolerate that behavior. She describes that a lot of people in addiction they are feeling that they are entitled to whatever. As a nurse taking care of patients Beth tells her patients:" do not beat up your body, just don't beat yourself up. What you put in your body is poison". She asks people to stop dwelling on the past, let it go, hoping that this will help them cope and they stop using.

  Dr. Tedd Levin told me a story about his private practice in Portland. One of the hospitals he admitted his patients to required that all the primary care physicians take call for their Overdose Call list. When patients were admitted through the Emergency Room with a drug overdose, if they did not have a personal physician who practiced at that hospital, they were assigned a physician through the overdose call list. He describes that generally the doctors did not like to be on that list. The reasons being he said that the patients were just not the nicest people to be around, they were rarely appreciative of the care they had received, swearing, being" nasty", just not being very nice people. Additionally, the doctors many times did not get paid for these complex cases where they had to work very hard to save someone's life. Dr. Levin describes events where drug dealers were arrested who swallowed the drugs that they placed in condoms when the police come. Swallowing the evidence so they can get off. Then they would get arrested and admitted to the hospital to watch to make sure they don't overdose at night because it was uncertain how much drugs they have swallowed. Dr. Levin would get called in to admit the patient and then he would have to watch them until the condoms come out, this involved many laxatives to create loose stools, then the police would take them away. We also had a discussion about the limited time doctors have in clinics to do health care appointments. A 15-minute appointment is very short to do health care screenings, treatments and interventions especially when it comes to something so complex as addiction. Dr. Levin describes that people he knows who were dealing with addictions don't take care of themselves they are not going to go to regular appointments they will go to urgent care when they need too. He shared a story of working in urgent care and having people come where he drained abscess caused by using drugs. He describes a case in 2015 at an urgent care clinic where there were a lot of people go who were poor or had OHP (Oregon Health Plan).

He has seen cases where people who were dealing with addiction started to use their muscles for injecting drugs because they have used up all their veins and the veins are shut. He calls this "muscling". He describes getting out a quart of pus of someone's thigh. Normally when he does a procedure like this, he describes yellow pus coming out but, in this case, he also had black tar heroin coming out of the thigh at the incision and drainage site. He describes that additional diagnoses also need to be treated when we talk about addiction because majority of people dealing with addiction have dual diagnosis or triple diagnoses. They don't just have the chemical dependency, but they might also have bipolar disorder and ADHD (Attention Deficit Hyperactivity Disorder). Dr. Levin feels that if the other two diagnoses are ignored, then the success rate of treatment for their chemical dependency will not be good. In ADHD, if not treated the impulsiveness can create opportunity for relapse. If things are ignored like bipolar, depression, anxiety, people will continue the drug use, he recommends all co-morbidities (co- existing conditions) need to be treated. There are a lot of contributing factors he explains if this is happening now or not. Based on insurance, the doctor, the patient. Not everyone with addiction is willing to see a therapist. People dealing with addiction, Dr. Levin describes are so busy trying to treat their addiction they have no time for anything else. He also talked about when he was a Preventive Medicine Resident, he worked on with an obesity group at the University of Arizona and the success rate of losing weight and keeping it off after 2 years was less than 5%. Most people lost weight but regained the lost weight within a year. He describes a very well-rounded team for the study group with a psychologist, preventive medicine doctor, exercise specialist, and nutritionist. Still it did not work well. Food is complicated he said, people eat for so many reasons not just because they are hungry but because they are anxious, depressed, lonely, every human emotion can be associated with eating. He also describes trying to treat thousands of smokers in the past 30 years with low success rates. They are still higher for smoking cessation then for weight reduction. During our conversation Dr. Levin said we have to eat to survive. Food is the toughest one.

Tracy describes that addiction is a problem at least 85% of the families whom she works with. She works with families who have welfare background. She had seen cases related to drugs, alcohol, gambling, sex. She describes the addiction grabbing her clients and slowly tearing their families apart. She works with mothers who had their children removed because of addictions. The moms not being able to function well and make good choices for their families that creates danger for the kids. The addiction takes over. Tracy asserts that it is not them, it is not the person it is the addiction that is the problem. She feels we have a societal responsibility to take care the children. She feels that the family unit gets kind of lost in all this. She describes how the parents just get blamed, and her role is to get in there and try to support that parent and provide information on resources available for them to get help. Tracy tries to remind people who are dealing with addictions who they were before the addiction got a hold of them. She tried to pull them out by providing guidance and support. Tracy feels like she is doing this at work because she was not able to do this for her family. Diana had been working with a lot of families through her work and volunteering who are having problems with addiction. She is part of a DHS review board that reviews several cases a month where parents are at risk of losing their kids or have already lost them. Michelle describes her work with families who have already been affected because of addictions. She sees families who are either trying to come back from being affected by addictions or in the midst of the consequences because of their addiction. Consequences she sees are the inability for people to control things in their lives including financial issues, poverty. Their brain being affected that decision making is difficult even just to live their daily needs.

Joel describes experiences through her work that she saw struggles with addiction, mental health, housing, trouble with interpersonal relationships, families breaking up, family units being isolated. Joel mentioned that if someone comes to the hospital or clinic and in their chart, there is any time of addiction noted, it is assumed that they are there seeking drugs. There is an assumption that is made:" That they must not really hurt, maybe the hurt is not so bad, people can't see the hurt so since there is not a big gaping wound on their leg, they must not hurt". People assume that any person who has any addiction in their past just want drugs. We discussed the difficulties of pain, feeling it, assessing it, not making assumptions about it. The fact that someone might think that they are in pain, their brain telling them that are in pain, are they really in pain or is it just the brain trying to get something? Joel said we created this; pain become the 5th vital sign that a nurse would have to assess. People would get a prescription for antibiotics and a take home pack of Vicodin she recalls; we created this situation. Now, we have aging adults who are physically addicted to medications. Now they can't have the medications they were originally prescribed; it has just been taken away. We created this. Was this all purposeful? Yes, for big pharma she said. She talked about pill pushing and pharmaceutical companies going to doctors' offices pushing them to give this pill or that pill. Also, the fact that it is easier just to give a pill than try alternative methods first. Flower describes working in an addiction recovery unit for 10 years as a nurse with pregnant moms. She describes as a regarding work.

  Brenda had seen many people with addictions in her work life. She had some great success stories. She has been able to help people to make the determination to seek help and overcome the barriers to get treatment. Brenda is telling me about a patient who she was able to get into detox. Unfortunately, after detox he ended up in the street, he was homeless, there wasn't a treatment bed open after detox. Him being sober lasted about 2 weeks then he ended up drinking again. He had a significant addiction where every time he tried to quit, he had seizures. He could not just manage this outpatient. He got back into detox, this happened about 3-4 times. Each time it went longer in between him falling off the wagon. Finally, he was able to go to treatment after detox then coming back to the area. This patient had a lot of trust issues and throughout this process he was able to make connections which become very valuable. He learned to trust his new connections. After about 2 years he ended up drinking again, and then he initiated his own entry into detox without Brenda even knowing about it. He is now been sober for about 200 days, he is working and helping others become sober, he is managing a safe house, he is thinking about going back to school and becoming a counselor. This is one of Brenda's best success stories. He is very appreciative, and Brenda just keeps motivating him to continue to make connections because that replaces the old habits and create positive things in his life that support and creates stability. Another patient of Brenda's just got out of the hospital again, he has severe cirrhosis (late stage of scarring of the liver) of the liver, (big sigh here from Brenda) jaundice, (yellow skin color indicating liver disease), other issues. Brenda last saw him a year ago, then he was missing in action for a while. A year ago, when Brenda was trying to get him help, he was not ready, then he lost his mother, a month later he lost his father. He started drinking again. Brenda is helping him deal with his anxiety and depression, without using alcohol. He is seeing Brenda and getting connected to counseling to help him cope with anxiety and depression without covering it up with alcohol. Brenda is hoping building new connections that will help him. Brenda tells me about another patient who has a history that is complicated by a brain injury. The brain injury makes it difficult for him to deal with life and more difficult to deal with addiction. He is a very wonderful and good-hearted man with a very complex issue. He is kind and friendly and had difficulty following directions because of the brain injury and would easily get frustrated. He is on vivitrol now Brenda tells me which is wonderful news. He has been in detox for a few times, he has been out for a while, he had a slip recently and come back right out of it quickly. He is back on his medication. Learning how to manage daily life and addiction and diabetes. It is very complicated.

    I talk to Dolores on the phone. We talk for about one hour. Dolores tells me she does not have much personal experience but does some work experience on addictions. She does feel that one of her sons is dealing with alcoholism, but she does not see him much. She had experiences working in a treatment program many years ago (about 40 years ago in the 1980's) in Pennsylvania. It was an alternative to incarceration program for youthful offenders who were addicted to heroin and they were convicted of crimes and sentenced to the treatment program instead of going to jail. If they did not succeed in the program or if they did not cooperate then they went back to jail. It was a very interesting experience Dolores recalls. It was a residential treatment program for both men and women16-24 years old. The program was run by the Abraxas foundation and it still exists today. It was a long-term program that sometimes took years, not like a current 21-day treatment program. They worked with the addiction as well as addressing the underlying issues that caused the addiction. Dolores asserts that the underlying issues in short term treatment programs usually don't get addressed. This was before addiction was looked at as a disease. They have found that underlying issues like sexual abuse played a role. This was the first time that Dolores was exposed to research and it was very interesting for her. It is quite amazing to think of it, she was in the forefront seeing this which is now being thought that childhood trauma can be the underlying cause if addiction. She saw this 40 years ago.

    Dolores tells me about another experience when she was an intern and worked in a dual diagnosis treatment program in Portland, Oregon. She had worked with people having addiction and an additional mental health problem like depression, anxiety or PTSD. This was about 25 years ago around 1996. At that time, she tells me they had a lot of very successful hospital based dual diagnosis programs. This ***dual diagnosis program worked very well when people had enough time to be in treatment.*** I asked Dolores if she thought staying longer was helpful. She said yes, especially if the person needed medications and adjustment of medications. Dolores felt it was very helpful to keep people in the hospitals until they stabilized on their medications. Now she tells me doctors have to make educated guesses and hope for the best. If it would be me or someone's family member, I would want the doctors not just guessing. Get people as stable as possible before discharging. Dolores knows it was more expensive, and she feels it was a lot more success having people in a longer-term treatment program than now. Many people I talked with feel the same. Dolores then chuckles and tells me that frankly, she feels 21 days is ridiculous. The brain does not even have enough time to readjust. Nor is there time to discover and heal lifelong wounds.

Dolores shares about kids and youth entering job cops for education and training. She feels that there is a push to get them in right after treatment and she does not feel this is a good idea. She feels people will fail because the access is so readily available. Even if there are no drugs allowed on center people can get it outside any time they want. Now people can get marijuana, it is legal and if someone is an addict it is poison for them. Dolores recommends going to an outpatient program first and survive 3 months, then go to outpatient treatment and AA meetings and then come back to job corps. She had seen kids fail when they had gone to job corps right out of treatment. They fail big she said, and it is very sad. Dolores feels like it would be a good research to look at programs we have and identify how they work what is the success rate. It would be a great NIH project she feels. She was not sure that with the current political climate if there is any type of funding available for research. She asks me what I know about this. I can only tell her what I had observed and heard throughout the years. There is seemingly a cut back continuously on mental health and addiction problems.

Programs struggle to stay open, to provide services, applying for grants to try to make it. Facilities and programs close because they don't have enough money to stay open. We talk about the opiate issues and she feels that they are saying there is money for it, but we have not seen it. I was wondering even if there will be some money how long it will last. Is it just a Band-Aid again? Or will there be money to look for root causes and create preventative programs. Dolores describes that she knows parents whose kids are addicted and struggling with it, they are in their 20's and 30's. She saw people in her practice who have problems with drugs. She tells me that she feels that they had problems before and once they started using all the problems become consolidated around the use. It is devastating she asserts. Dolores feels addictions have been around the long time, and it is more obvious now because of the level of opiate addictions and the deaths.

Then, Dolores tells me that she is a little resentful of the control over pain medications for people who genuinely need pain medications. She gives me an example from a personal experience. She had to go get some Tramadol (also called Ultram, mild opiate pain reliever) she called for a refill and found out that her insurance company would only pay it for a week at a time. She felt frustrated that the insurance company would do this. Her doctor did not do the limit, she never abused drugs. She got the paperwork on it which made it look like Tramadol is a very serious opiate. She knows that there is a little derivate of opiate in there, not much like morphine she asserts. She feels like now it is a little over controlled. She had to give her driver's license when she picked up at the drug store. She said, really, oh ok. I can understand her frustration and also understand the need for regulation. It is an opiate and with so many people getting addicted and dying it is one step can be taken for trying to control use and monitor use. Dolores does not feel that the issue is there, I ask her where she thinks the issue is and she chuckles and tells me she does not know. We had a discussion if it is also a societal problem and we both felt it is. She also felt that people who get older do have physical pain and it is difficult to manage that and they do need it. Dolores brings up kids getting into a medicine cabinet. Very true; many places it starts like that. Dolores feels it is pretty hard to figure it out.

29. Healthcare

What are people's experience when it comes to healthcare? I often wondered what is my role as a health care professional in our society, as nurse, a public health professional, a mother, a spouse and a responsible person who tries to help people, patients or anyone who suffer from addiction? I walk into the room, walk in the street, work in my community and hope that I can add to the change to any small way and save the life in front of me. Chances and odds are against me many times. Sometimes when I walked into the room, I already know that this person will relapse again and all I can do is give my best and hope they will survive and come back again to get help. Many don't. Why? Addiction is a chronic very terrible disease as it gets hold of the person's mind and does not let it go. It is a lifelong suffering circles of relapse and recovery. Once the brain learned the shortcut to the pleasure center it tells the individual to use drugs or alcohol more just to feel "normal", to be happy. It is very difficult to break the cycle and many people had told me they felt like they will die if they do not take another hit even that they did not really want to use anymore. It is hard to try to break addiction when the mind knows a path for drugs and the person using is trapped in the cycle. We need to make sure to take care of ourselves. Take some deep breaths, take a nice walk, imagine a beautiful picture, have some water.

The hardest part is when we know someone personally or a patient who is trying to get clean and break free from substance abuse will go out and use again. I know they are trying. I can see it in their eyes, words, expressions, behavior that they are not ready do not have the skills, the willpower to quit yet. How could they really? How would they know? Sometimes I know before they even have any idea. It hurts to see, there is nothing I can do just try to encourage and support the best I can and hope that they will survive and find the way for a healthier life in the end. Do they have a chance? Could they fully recover after all the trauma they have been through? Did the drop of knowledge, kindness or caring make any difference at all? I hope so. I can't stop thinking of the families who also suffer, the mothers, fathers, sons, daughters, brothers, sisters, aunts, friends, grandparents we talk on the phone and try to offer support and encouragement, but also help them set boundaries for their health. Why does it matter? To me it matters a lot. It means everything. We are talking about human beings. Nobody chooses to be an addict. It is not a life goal. What could be more important than support and help one and other in times of distress, disease? We can change the world by helping people one person at the time. Help people understand, that addiction is not a choice and an addict suffers like anyone else from any other disease. People suffering from addiction need people, communities and government to support and break the cycle just like someone with heart disease, Alzheimer's, diabetes, obesity, disability or anything else that changes our life any kind of disease or trauma. Addiction is a disease; people who are in the disease process need all the help and support we can give them to survive. What can we do to help?

People way too often just look at the individual not necessary all the impact the illness of one person might have on a whole family and society. Looking at societies and how they influence people I see a lot of examples in the area in addictions. People becoming depressed because of economy, do not have jobs don't have the means to take care of their families and start drinking or using substances to self-medicate that creates a major problem in the US today. This problem exists all over the globe. Addiction could be prevented, yet not much is being done. The US spends so much money on interventions that do not work and not enough on prevention and treatments that actually work. Why these things do matters? Addiction destroys families, neighborhoods, communities and claims many lives. Anyone can see it walking down in the streets, it might be a person, trash, used needles, camps. It could be something else. Way too many lives have been lost to count. Claims the people we know or might not know it could claim our friend, brother, mother, child, friend, sister, co-worker, boss and many more. Part of it is not caring, or not knowing what to do, since it is just an addict right, they could just stop drinking or using drugs.... only if it were that simple. People relapse. Sometimes it is a partner that is using, a mother or other family member, or the neighborhood where they live in where everyone using. It could be the stores on the way home that all advertise alcohol to drink or the corners where drug sales are present. Unfortunately, our brain remembers all those places that are part of the drug use and anything can be a trigger to use again.

There is so much more that could be done to help individuals with addiction and provide support and caring that is currently not being done. It breaks my heart seeing people dying and families being destroyed. This could be changed by caring for the individual as well as for the family and community and providing compassionate loving support as well as well-designed interventions and preventions; to decrease or eliminate the need to be in the fog, to be so desperate to use drugs or alcohol to decrease the pain and suffering people endure. What can we do to change things? What could that drop in the sea to change the color of addiction to bright blue from the red and black of blood and death?

Sheila describes that healthcare should be provided for addiction including prevention including diet, incentives for exercise, resources, especially because addiction can lead to so many health problems so helping with addiction is preventative. Bottom line addiction is an illness and it should be treated. When I talked to Beth, she felt we do not do enough, she said it is harder to get into treatment centers, she said she is grateful for Obamacare, because there is more treatment available. On the other hand, the treatment centers are overpopulated. She was wondering if we need more treatment centers and more help to deal with addiction treatment. She had called it an epidemic, a battle. It is everywhere. Beth described a visit to Seattle where she saw a young girl at a corner and was not sure if she was dead or high on something, people walking by her smelling like pot. It is everywhere.

Mary shares her feeling about treatment centers. She feels people walk in and they are a pathology with a lot of suspicions. When they get a dirty urine, get thrown out when they need the help the most. Mary feels like the behavior of coping which is using substances is criminalized and people lose hope. Is it right to send someone out of treatment if they have a urine that is positive for a substance? In one way they need help. Another is the effect on others who are in treatment. Mary feels this is an unfair punishment. Mary also feels that the way systems are set up to help people who are addicted are not correct. It is only helping people who fit a certain model or check in the box. Mary gives an example: a rehab facility is not taking someone who is diabetic because they are high risk medically. So how those people who have other medical conditions and considered high risk supposed to get out of addiction. Aren't they the ones who are most vulnerable and need help? Whether it is diabetes, inability to go upon stairs, behaviors or something else Mary feels that there are too many barriers for people who are dealing with addiction to try to get into treatment. It all comes down to money basically, Mary explained who are our funders willing to pay for? For profit, non-profit, it is ultimately very sad to see that many times if someone has money, they can have treatment if they don't fit into the box that need to be checked they don't. This means that some lives are valued more than others. Is this right? All lives should be valued the same. Mary feels that education and talking about addiction is part of the health care role. She talks about the health care system wanting to know all details about people's personal lives but then do nothing to change it. So, if the healthcare system asks about alcohol and drug use Mary says then they better be prepared to help with those issues when people want help. Access to treatment, access to care regardless if someone is an addict or not.

    Dr. Tedd Levin describes the health care system's lack of functioning when it comes to treatment, there is not that many evidences based good treatment models out there to help people. Additionally, he describes lack of coordination when it comes to treatment programs, there is a lack of follow up. After treating people with overdose many times, they were out from the health care system in 1-2 days and their addiction was not treated. He describes this as a "revolving door" where people will keep coming back again and again, and if they are very unlucky then dying on the field. Availability of Narcan helps asserts Dr. Levin, it can save some lives, but still got to have a treatment program. We cannot just save someone's life from overdose then kick them out to the street or send them to jail. He compares trying to quit substances to smoking where for the average smoker it might take 6-7 times to quit smoking. Treatment for addiction is not like once it is done the person cured. People live with the disease for the rest of their lives. Dr. Levin discussed that people have to figure out what coping skills serve them the best, some people like the 12 step programs, other people are turned off he explains by the "quasi-religious aspect" of the 12 step programs.

Angel talks about the healthcare role. She said: "our healthcare sucks, it is horrible, it is horrible, even if you are insured it is horrible". She talks about her son who had anxiety starting at an early age and the difficulties navigating the health care system. They were both educated parents, with a decent income and good insurance and she still describes that it was "horrible" trying to find resources for their son. Navigating the system for many people who might be making less money or not as educated based on what she seen happening to kids in the school system, she describes as it is "nearly impossible" task for people. She recommends that health care be more streamlined, more user friendly, and fairer. She described kids with rotting teeth because the kid's parents don't have dental insurance.

Paige feels the mental health access needs to be provided to people who need it. Also providing tools that help battle addiction when they see a therapist. Paige's clients shared many frustrations with her that when they go to a therapist, they listen to them but not give them any tools or guidance what to do. Paige has been recommending to her clients to ask for tools and suggestions from their therapist or provider. Tell them what they want to work on and ask for help. This can be very difficult for some people. I saw people struggling to even make the appointments for mental health sessions or prescriptions and to ask for help can be even more difficult for them. It is one of those things that can be very hard for people.

Chief Jason mentions that healthcare seems to be a constant battle when it comes to addictions. Jason feels that the root of the problem is not addressed when it comes to addiction. He gives me an example of treating heroin addiction with putting in a methadone clinic. It does not resolve what is really going on with that person why they started using in the first place. It is a band aid that covers up the deep rooting problems. He sees methadone just as another addiction that many drug abusers fall into. It does not cure the disease just changes what they are addicted too – Jason said. He feels that having more treatment and mental health support would help and having treatment centers more centralized.

When Kayla and I were discussing healthcare, she felt that healthcare needs to be more inclusive, look at what is going on with a person when they come in, to assure the whole history is checked before prescribing someone opiates. **<u>Understanding someone's history and taking the time to talk to the person.</u>** Be educated about what is out there as different forms of medication and offer different options of pain relief. Kayla feels that health care providers including doctors and nurses need to do more education about mental health. Looking at a whole person not just a piece of the puzzle and prescribing a pill. Nowadays the providers are too busy to look at whole person and find out what the real problem is. She feels this is very upsetting. Universal healthcare for addictions. I grew up in universal healthcare. To me it seems more natural not to have to worry to go to the doctor about what insurance I have and how much this will cost. That is what our taxes are for, not building barriers between us and other countries.

Rory feels that the healthcare role gets muted by another question which is the first question he asks a new client: "What is your insurance?". What insurance we will be using, or oh, they do not have any insurance. Ok, he said:" then I can put you on my sliding scale". He offers this option as a courtesy; many other people in the community do not offer this option. Sometimes the sliding scale is still too out of reach. If someone does not have insurance, they do not get treatment. Period. Any facility should offer a percentage of their bad to the community at no cost. He recalls that in his county and surrounding areas there used to be about 200 beds in treatment, yet we could not get someone in from the community if they needed care. They would just not take them. People would just get turned away. Rory feels that the opiate crisis will dissipate and that is when strategic planning needed what to do the next time when the next substance comes up, he describes alcohol in the 60's, cocaine in 70's and 80's, methamphetamines in 80's and 90's, heroin in 2000's. What is the next one he said, we don't know it might have not been invented yet? He talks about designer drugs in the far east with chemical letters and numbers without a name. He feels that people will always seek drugs out.

Tracy feels that the healthcare system contributes to addictions we have in our society. This might be changing now. She gives an example of going into the emergency room for an earache and getting narcotics. Prescribing narcotics after surgery for 2 weeks. Some people are more sensitive and can become addicted fairly quick. Tracy describes then how the body adopts and want more medication by creating other illnesses, like headaches, back pain or big toe pain, it could be anything really and it is not necessarily a conscious thing, all the body and the mind knows that the drugs felt good. It wants more. It is not the persons fault asserts Tracy; the addiction is already taking over their body and mind. She saw this with her own grandparents. They got put on pain medications long term. Grandparents got addicted to pain meds. Tracy feels that the healthcare system helped create the problem either because drug companies wanted the money, or maybe it was intentional. Hard to know. It is connected for sure. Now, Tracy feels that the health care system needs to offer more to help people get out of addictions.

    Diana feels like it all starts with the education of the future doctors and providers to have more information that is taught in medical school about addictions. Audits on the prescribers, who can prescribe what to who, she asserts that prescribers would not like that. She feels that some of the providers just: "hand out stuff" and don't worry about the effects. We had a conversation about pain and how a provider would know if a patient is in pain in the hospital and how much pain medication we should provide. It is a difficult topic. Pain is subjective it is what the patient feels like, of course there are signs like elevated pulse, blood pressure, facial expressions, body expressions. It is not easy to know what pain is, and how much pain can someone tolerate. We discussed techniques that maybe could be taught from a young age how we deal with pain. From my nursing experience in the hospital if a patient was in pain, I gave them the pain medication the doctor prescribed. I would give them as much as I could to alleviate the pain. In this case we are talking about quick onset pain related to surgery or injury which is very different from chronic pain. I just talked to a previous colleague Dolores yesterday about this and she mentioned that as we get older, she is close to retirement age now, things hurt, she has some pain that she occasionally takes a medication called Ultram (It is a schedule IV medication) and now her insurance company controls this and only gives her one week worth at a time. She has not been abusing the medication nor has a history of abusing it. So sometimes things can swing to the other extreme and people have to go through extra burden to get what they need. Dolores mentioned to me things just sometimes hurt. Old people as she called have pain. So, this can create a great conflict because we also discussed pain medications in grandma's cabinet that a youth can get a hold of Diana mentioned alternative things for pain like acupressure, acupuncture, alternative medicine options, muscle pain relief, pain clinics that don't use medications but other ways to alleviate pain. Helping people making the right choice about pain relief especially if there is any incline that this person might abuse medications Diana asserts.

    Michelle describes the health care role as addiction services are covered to some extent but there should not be limitations on how much help a person can get when they struggle with a disease. It gets complicated she said when we look at finances, policies and what is available as a resource. So how we are going to do this. Then she mentioned that because of the big financial burden is why she tends to focus on prevention What could be done before addiction hits. Create conditions where addiction is not as likely to happen. So, at this point our conversation went into wishful thinking. If Michelle would have a magic wand, then a place is to start is awareness. Having a conversation. Janett feels like that some addictions are not taken seriously enough like methamphetamine. She feels like it is a very serious addiction that could use more support. It is way worse than smoking she asserts, but she heard people putting meth use in the same category as smoking before. She feels like there are no resources to help people who are addicted to methamphetamines. It is like with any other social resources, Janett thinks resources need to be offered. Hard to get cured if nothing is offered. Even if only 10% gets cured more than none. She feels it is worth time spending the time and money. Yet health insurances don't agree with this, don't think this way. Better mental health services could prevent people getting to the point of addictions in the first place Janett feels. A lot of addiction stems from mental health issues. If people would have other options to deal with their mental health difficulties, then some people might not get to a point of using substances as a coping mechanism. Janett feels we need more mental health and recovery programs, early intervention things. She laughed and said this is all I have. I told her it is ok; we are not trying to fix the universe here just having a conversation and I was curious what she thought.

Bernadette asserts that people when they are ready to go to treatment, it should be available to them. Treatment should be the same if someone has insurance or not, private or Medicaid. Money should have nothing to do with the quality of a rehab. She feels like it is up to the individual to get treatment or not, it is a hard thing to do and she feels like most people decide not to have treatment. She had experience when she was working in a hospital how difficult it was to get somebody into treatment. Could not find a bed or insurance did not cover it. Funding could help maybe.

Do people have the right to be cared for?

The short answer is from most people I talked to yes, of course, help them. Save them all. Beth said, oh yes, for sure. It is a disease, so for sure she said, but she admits: I just don't want to care for them. She feels like they do have a right just like everyone else to be cared for. The question is how do we do it? Beth asks how we can change someone's mind who is dealing with addiction to allow us to care for them? What can we do so they accept the care? She felt this is very challenging. Very interesting thing healthcare is. It should be everyone's right to get treated and have a healthy life. Is this happening now? It is interesting to see how rules and regulations can affect what seems to be a basic human right to value life and help others get healthy to the best of our abilities. Who has the right to say that we can only do so much, and this is it? We will treat this disease or give funding for another disease, but we don't care about certain diseases or certain populations because they might be less productive than the others. I got a phone call last week. It was a family member who was trying to find a treatment center for her loved one. Not the first time. The loved one was homeless, had died many times and brought back to life yet since he was homeless, he could not get into a treatment program and could not get the support he needed. I assume that probably some programs tried to help, and he left those programs, but still, is it right to say no to this family? At what point do we stop helping? I talked to a friend recently who has a son struggling with addiction. Even if he could get into detox to get the toxins out of his system, there are no treatment beds, he would just relapse again. She had tried everything she can think of to save her son. Running out of options at this point.

Mary, Kayla, Janett, Albert, Susan and Edward said absolutely all people with addiction have a right to be cared for. When they are ready and when they want treatment, knowing that treatment can take multiple tries. Additionally, Edward mentioned that all people have a right to be cared for. Angel also felt that people who are addicted absolutely have the right to treatment. No matter how many times it takes. She describes addiction as a physical, mental and spiritual change to the body. It is no different Angel said then when somebody has cancer four times. If people are willing to try, they should always have that opportunity. Paige feels that she is split with this question about 50-50. It is complex. One side as a taxpayer she feels frustrated with people not trying hard enough or not having the incentives and motivations to clean up and become taxpayers on the other hand she sees all the families who are trying everything and getting into great debt. She was unsure which I can totally understand. Chief Jason feels that yes, people with addiction have a right to be cared for. He states that unfortunately it is an endless cycle when people fall into addiction. He feels that especially with the cost of health care, addiction need to be dealt with because it will ultimately cost more in the long run. I would add to this that the ultimate cost is someone's life or disability that is caused by addiction and all the pain and harm to family and friends.

Rory said, not sure if it is a right, but we should provide care. Now, how that looks like he was uncertain. He describes frequent fliers in the treatment community who use treatment as a hotel. He describes some people who were tired of paying rent and went to use to get into a place that is more sounded like a spa then a treatment. Place with horseback riding, masseuse, swimming pool. He thought. Damn girl. Laughter. Going back yes, he thinks people should be treated. We now have no way of screening the frequent flier. He said we don't know how to handle people who say oh yes, I relapsed for the 400th time. Then they are in treatment again, but they know everything, will leave early. We still take them in, he said because all treatment is dollar driven. Again, it is all about money, right? Rory: "remember all of this treatment is attached to a dollar in someone's pocket". How sad. People's life is at stake and others make money out of it. Makes me sick. A friend told me recently that nothing gets done about it because powers at being are too removed from the everyday people, they don't have any idea what is going on or they don't care. Not until maybe one of their family members has an issue. Maybe then they do a little something about it. Rory describes a treatment facility he worked at where the facility got $43,000 dollars for every person in a bed. No matter if they provided good care or not. It was crazy money how he called, and it was run not by therapist, psychiatrist or addictionologist, but by businessman, hedge fund managers. He is resistant to say yes everyone needs treatment, yes, they do but they only get that option until they run out of insurance. We need more uninsured beds to ease the suffering. What if people cannot afford the medication they need? Rory describes insulin costing $500 per vial, and people dying because they cannot afford the medication. Then people can go across the border to Canada or Mexico and get the same medication for fraction of the price. Is having affordable medications our right? Chloe said yes all have a right to be care for because anyone can have an addiction. She can have an addiction tomorrow that she did not have before or did not realize she had. She describes people not realizing they have an addiction problem. Michelle said yes of course they have the right. To her it is just being human to care for someone who might need medical or emotional support. She feels no matter what if it is addiction it is irrelevant. It is a person who needs help.

  Joel thinks healthcare is a fundamental right for everyone. She does not think we do well for caring for people now who are dealing with addictions. She feels people are being cared for with judgement. She describes a story of someone she interviewed recently for a job. She was working at a hospital and received a report about a homeless patient who was high on drugs and was told use peppermint oil. She decided to go in give him a bath wash his feet and get clean clothes for him. This way the problem was fixed no oil needed and the patient got his dignity back. Others might have just left the patient and the previous shift did leave the patient. Use our compassion, she said. Do we have enough resources I asked her? She felt yes if we use them right. Joel felt that our resources are terribly misallocated. She asserts that we have money and resources in this country but that the money is just not used well and not used for the reasons it should be like taking care of our own instead creating a go fund me page for a border wall. She feels like a lot of money could be reallocated; it is the mindset. We tend to be selfish and narrow focused; she feels. Have a conversation with people who are having the problem. Open our eyes she suggests and have a hard conversation with ourselves, she does. Discussed wages that are low for people who are actually working with people who deal with addiction or can support preventing addiction like teachers, social workers, counselors. This would be a whole another conversation she said. Janett feels we should always provide the opportunity for someone.

    Albert feels that healthcare plays a big role, hopefully when people need help, they would go to their doctor or mental health professional. A big role also been played in the last 20 years the health care field helping people getting started on that kind of stuff. Albert feels we have to be very careful on how people prescribe, monitor those better, helping people get out of situations caused by prescription drugs, having more contact with people, knowing people better and see people more often. Again, he asserts if someone doesn't have health insurance, they don't have a doctor. They don't go see them. Maybe they go into the emergency room or urgent care. People don't have a practitioner that they see often so people don't have a doctor to build a relationship with. Albert mentions at least have an opportunity for people for care, they might not take it. We can't force people to take it, we can't force people into treatment. People have to be ready to do it. We have to keep putting that handout for a chance. At this point I ask him if he feels like treatment is the right answer. Not always he said, he saw treatment counterproductive sometimes where people forced into groups or forced into things, they are not ready for or not right for them and it puts them into a whole different space that is not necessarily good for them. Generally, he said it is good to have somebody to walk people through it and point them to the right direction. He saw people going through treatment program after treatment program and keep failing, then something clicks and all of a sudden now they are doing it on their own. It happens he said, it depends on the person, depends on the situation. We discuss treatment centers and the fact that many of them are for profit, Albert heard secondhand stories from people being in a program before it was being shut down, and the treatment place being not so helpful just wanting to fill the bed so they can bill insurance. ***The for-profit motive puts it in the wrong mind space to start out with.*** I love it, and I could not agree more with Albert. Treatment should not be for money, but to help people in need. There are people who are there for the right reasons of course. We need to wonder about the administrators Albert said, the owners, who know maybe nothing about treatment and just care if it is making money or not if it actually works for the people who are trying to get better. Very twisted isn't it? He thinks so. Does not make any sense Albert asserts. Healthcare should not be about making money but helping people. He discusses maybe having incentives or outcome driven payments, just for housing someone for 30 day just to get released and use again or end up in jail is not beneficial for everyone. People need follow up after treatment Albert states. We cannot have someone in a structured environment where they tell people where to be every hour a day then just say ok now goodbye and good luck check back in if they relapse. Just not right. This is not to say that there are not wonderful programs out there who do the follow up and a hard program, and support people in their recovery.

Flower was telling me about treatment, it is a chronic disease, people will potentially have relapses. She gives an example to someone who is a diabetic. If they eat a piece of cake they will not die. If someone is an addict that piece of cake (which would be the drug of their choice) can kill them. The consequences are more dire. The consequences with CPS for example if someone relapses can be that they are losing their child. The consequences of it are so much more severe that the support and recovery is essential. There needs to be enough support that people can reach out. Flower feels like the families also need support whose child or loved one dealing with the chronic disease of addiction. The less stigma is the better, there are so many people and so many people are affected Flower asserts that we do not have the luxury of stigma. Continue the conversation, show love and compassion. Addiction is no different than diabetes or heart disease, she talks about the parents of children and how much they suffer from addictions. I saw that for sure both parents and children suffering, families and friends suffering. Flower also gives me an example that if someone would have a heart attack the hospital does not make them wait and check for insurance before performing troponin levels (indicators of heart muscle damage) to have the heart attack intervened on. When it comes to alcohol treatment she tells in a very unhappy voice, insurance demands that someone be in withdrawal that puts them into risk at seizures and delirium tremens before authorizing treatment. At this point she is pissed. She does not swear usually, and here she said:" I think that is so f***** up". It is crazy. It is exactly how insurance is adversary to care she adds. She feels like insurance should just pay for it. Insurance should not be able to be an adversary to care. Flower thinks that there is never going to be a perfect system of healthcare because there are just too many layers of bureaucracy. When planning a system, she feels we need to adjust for the urgency when someone is ready to go to treatment, we need to send them. The nature of addiction is that when people reach out is the moment of opportunity. She compares it to a moment in a domestic violence situation or suicide ideation and they are reaching out. Need to grab that opportunity, if there is no help it could be a potentially disastrous outcome.

    Dr. Beatty explains that public health is a paradox shift, it is time for public health to focus on prevention of mental health issues and addictions. Need more prevention type information. Public health and healthcare responsibility are to have treatment options, services, more than the emergency response team coming in and providing naloxone for overdose. A better response from the prevention's standpoint and then it needs to be more funding from the healthcare perspective. Focus on prevention. Prevention is so important. It is much harder to fix something once it is broken then to try preventing it in the first place.

    Brenda talks about the disconnect between health care entities. She gives me an example of someone getting to the emergency department with addiction, they keep them there until they are stable, then discharge them. Brenda feels like it would make so much more sense if there was a central place that they can call or reach out to the provider to help make arrangements after discharge. It would be great to have some transition where a person who is struggling can get from point A to point B without falling back on the street. How do we do that, Brenda was not sure because so many different entities communicate with to each other. We have to do more than sober them up and kick them back out to the street asserts Brenda. Susan felt like regulating substances could help decrease overdose for people. She told me she does not know. She also does not want people to be in pain and cut down their pain medication. She feels like a lot of people had suffered from that. She feels like it is a tough one. She feels uncertain. I ask her my magic wand question. She felt like natural medicine could be implemented more instead of just prescribing a pill. There is not money in research for those she tells me because of the pharmaceutical companies. I can feel the frustration in her voice. She tells me about acupuncture and how it could help with addiction. Working with naturopaths. Looking at the whole body not just one thing. Looking at the mental state as well. Treating a whole person should be the standard treatment instead of just giving a pill for one thing. She is telling me about a research she read about that shows that our bodies keep a score. The author talks about trauma and the body and how the body is holding onto pain. Susan feels like when pain medications are prescribed other things need to be looked at like mental status, because covering something up can create more likelihood to addiction. We discussed the current health care system and how providers are trying to treat patients in 15 minutes. It is quite impossible to treat a whole person in 15 minutes. Susan gave me an example for this. She saw a nurse practitioner when she was having bad anxiety, she was her PCP. This PCP was prescribing her Adderall and saying:" this will take your mind off anxiety". She is still appalled by this. She felt that medication would just make her anxiety worse. The practitioner did not investigate why she was anxious, she just wanted to give her a pill. Susan did not take the pill, she went to therapy and worked through her anxiety. She felt like this was a good example where health care could be better. The provider only saw her for like 10 minutes and did not even ask about what was going on in her life. This still bothers Susan. Susan also had hurt her knee and asked to be referred to a knee specialist. The provider did not want to do the referral, she just wanted to give Susan cortisol in her kneecap every six months. She felt that was just a terrible idea. Susan stopped seeing that provider shortly after that incident. Susan felt that when her brother was forced to go to treatment it was not helpful to him. Once he hopped over a fence to get away from a treatment center. She recalls when her brother was in transitional housing people were using drugs there. Susan feels addiction can happen to anybody.

Dolores feels that the healthcare for addiction should be free. Help people to overcome addictions and support them. She tells me it is hard to envision how this can happen with the way's things are set up now. She thinks all healthcare should be free. It should be just something people have available to them. She feels we could do this. The insurance companies do not have to make the money they are making now, then that money could go into helping people. She thinks that Medicare works, and we can do it for the whole county. She really feels strongly about this. Insurance companies are not doing better than Medicare she tells me. It cost a lot to become a doctor and she thinks that doctors should make money, but they don't have to be "bazzillionares". Dolores tells me that sometimes when she sees what the doctors charge, she is shocked. Dolores gives me an example. She went to the eye doctor and they did a test with a machine. The office charged Medicare $600 for the test. Medicare did not pay that much but they still charged that much so if someone does not have insurance or have a high deductible they would have to come up with that money. She tells me a lot of people now have such high deductible that no matter what they would pay out of pocket anyway. That is a lot of money. Dolores feels that the pricing system seems unfair. Dolores has a private practice. She used to take insurance but not anymore. The insurance took away too much. She does not overcharge. Her patients pay her, then they send the bill to the insurance themselves. It became too complicated to work with insurance with all their regulations. Now she just does an invoice.

I asked Fuchsia about the role of healthcare. There was a long pause. She said: "I don't know". She felt she does not know enough about it. Then she tells me that she thinks there should be more funding to treat addiction more seriously. People should not have to pay so much for healthcare. Not pay for healthcare at all. She believes it is a basic human right to receive healthcare. Universal healthcare, nonprofit. People should not make profit from about others who are sick. It's very backwards, she said. She is not sure how to get there. Then we got into politics, cost of healthcare, universal healthcare, not covering eastern medicine acupuncture or naturopathic medicine and had a nice conversation about it, compared experiences. Personally, for me it was weird to have to pay for health care and school because I grow up in a system where people did not have to worry about these things. In my conversation with Bob he felt that healthcare could definitely play a bigger role when it comes to addictions. Provide more advice how to deal with things. Provide programs that are more accessible to people. I ask him if he feels like they are not right now? He tells me that he personally does not even know where he would go to look for something like that. He would imagine that they are specialized expensive facilities. He is right they are. Then we talk about treatment. He thinks educating people, offering classes how to live a healthier lifestyle could help. He would go to a class like that. Teach how to deal with stress and societal pressure. Healthcare could open up. He thinks that the rehab model might not be effective. He feels it is an artificial setting, then people go back to where they are comfortable, it is not really working. He thinks that the healthcare system is not really effective and open for people. It is expensive. He does not have health insurance. I ask him how he feels about that. He cannot go to the doctor. He has to prioritize where he puts his money and his health does not go to the top all the time. It is very uncomfortable. I ask him what a good solution could be? He thinks. He is not sure. I asked him if he heard about other systems? He tells me it would be good if there would be a way to figure out healthcare without having more taxes which a lot of people don't feel good about. When he gets his check 50% of it is already gone on taxes. It is stressful to consider. Maybe a more efficient way to allocate resources without more taxes. We talk about government provided healthcare that already exists, Medicaid, Medicare, VA system. Why just not provide it for all? It is kind of interesting. We talk about treatment centers and they are for profit, it does not seem to work well. Could we make healthcare about the people not about money? Other countries have done it.

30. Government

What is the government's role is when it comes to addictions? Health policies and delivery of care can be changed to focus on prevention of harm to the current and future generations by looking at family and community units and how they are affected by substance abuse. Addiction can emerge because of depression, anxiety, mental illness, being in a wrong place at a wrong time, growing up in a violent neighborhood or in a neighborhood with low income. There are ways to create caring environments and places where people can turn for support and mentoring and change ways of living. Additionally, being less materialistic, so more people can be family and nature focused, decrease advertising of harmful goods and emphasize the beauty of living. Creating a community and country that focuses on health and wellbeing not on profit and how much money is going into some pockets. It is all about money isn't it? Who makes the money? Companies and individuals by selling products that are harmful to others. Why for profit and why not? Why would people and organizations who make profit care about people dying and families falling apart? They have their profit and can take the vacation they want, buy their next house and live well. Why would they care about an individual suffering? People can offer one small change that helps others. What could help? One option is: Having families treated instead just an individual. Providing more support in the community for people who are suffering instead just prescribing a pill to aid the richness of pharmacy. Another option could be: Creating policies that encourage strong communities and focus prevention would be very beneficial for the population. I believe that addiction needs to be treated. It is a disease. Thus, treatment is necessary. It helps if the person who is stuck in their addiction want a change. Treatment should be a holistic approach. Not just detox and sending someone home. Detox, then treatment, then follow up, including lifelong support. The same way we just don't drop someone at their door after a cardiac surgery.

Sheila asserts we have to make sure everyone is covered so everyone can be treated. Automatic coverage. So, if someone need a treatment, they can be treated. Private insurance? Federal or state insurance? Do people's insurance cover treatment? Is there a treatment limit? Should there be a limit? What the government could focus on? During my conversation with Beth she had mentioned that she feels that the government should focus on schools, she felt that the school system is just as broken as the health care system. She felt like we need to look at what other countries are doing, especially look at mental health. Funding, health, mental health, schools, general health insurance. These are areas where Beth believed that the government should step in.

    Edward felt that the government's role includes providing safety regulations for opiates and other drugs that could be addicting and cause harm. ***Holding the companies who created those drugs responsible and require them to pay for the treatment of people where they caused harm. All of the people.*** However, that might look like. When someone causes harm, it is not ok to get rich from it and have others suffer. Dr. Tedd Levin describes experiences in the Multnomah County jail in 1979-1980, where people with addiction were just thrown into a cell and had to suffer withdrawal without any support of medications. Now, fortunately, at least there are treatment protocols in jails and prisons to deal with drug withdrawal and addictions. Dr. Levin feels addiction should be treated the same way as cancer, high blood pressure or diabetes is treated, treat addiction like a medical disease. He thinks there should not be any barriers to treatment.

    In my conversation with Angel she brought up immigration. She said nobody who had come to this country as an immigrant has ever taken away anything from others. We all need a hand sometimes. Angel emphasizes that we don't lose by helping people, we are gaining by helping people. We have to be willing to help, Angel said, not just with addictions, but with our kids, with the elderly, with people who are sick. Angel feels like that the government has a huge role and an absolute responsibility to provide addiction services that are accessible and now they are not. Now this responsibility is placed on the individual. The problem is too big to be an individual problem it is a societal problem and we need the government's help. She shared her visions of using tax dollars wisely, and instead of paying for parades, paying for addiction treatment. She feels that we need to have a government to help. Our government currently is not doing that. Pay it forward, she adds, have higher taxes and not have to worry about healthcare, housing, safety, food, maternity or paternity leave. Angel thinks we lost those important pieces in our current system. We had a discussion that with better care and security of resources all quality of life would improve, and less money would be spent on chronic diseases. Prevention can do wonders. Just invest in people she adds. Paige feels we need higher standards of care when it comes to mental health and addictions and the government could help with this. She was uncertain how this could look like. She described that having health care coverage is helpful. Governmental health plans help cover treatment even better for someone who is on Oregon Health Plan for example compared to a blue-collar worker who is trying to send their kid to treatment and having to come up with $15,000 cash out of pocket to make it happen. Families cannot afford this especially because treatment usually does not work just one time, it can take a few tries.

     Chief Jason describes the government's role as providing more education and treatment. Additionally, there is a need to stop pulling programs and funding from education and programs that teach kids about not using drugs. He feels like programs are pulled based on not being successful. He is asking what a successful program is? Even if 10 kids don't use drugs because if a program in the school, he considers that to be successful. He talks about the D.A.R.E. (Drug Abuse Resistance Education) program and how he has not heard any kid coming out of that program and saying I want to do drugs. Controlling things like prescription process is another way the government could help, asserts Jason. Pharmaceutical companies are charging so much money for life saving prescriptions, Jason feels that there should be a tax on that for the companies and that money should go to creating treatment programs. Kayla when discussing roles for the government, she said, well yes, the government has a role. We both busted out laughing. Sometimes we just have to laugh. One of the things that come up is providing healthcare for all people. Including all people who are dealing with addictions. Universal Healthcare. Overall, she felt that there is a lot of work that need to be done to be more transparent, about having resources, letting people know what the treatment options are available, making it available for all people. Talking more about it, not shaming people because of the situation there are in now, incorporate talking more about addictions to our educational system.

Rory describes difficulties to access treatment if people don't have insurance or money. People simply will not get treatment and those people will die; he adds. He describes a kid he is working with. Even if he is on a state health plan and could go somewhere else the wait is very long. Rory feels that there is not enough treatment available and there is not enough pretreatment work being done. We are lucky to have some great organizations like SAMSHA and NIH, unfortunately they are losing a lot of funding. Rory feels that the government's role is to share the best outcomes, what has been working, how does that look like. What are the treatment outcomes? He feels there could be a clearinghouse for all the research being done and give people the current relevant information. Give it back Rory asserts. Tell people what the research says, what does not work, so we can stop using a model that is not effective. He gives examples of Matrix, Trauma informed care, DBT and said that unfortunately there are people who are doing some of the trainings and therapy who are not trained well. Maybe they have read a book one time. Not really effective. It does not work that way, Rory said. He gives another example. EMDR (Eye Movement Desensitization and Reprocessing Therapy). We know it works, he said. The training is $5,000. No one is going to send their employees into a training that cost that much. Tracy wonders what the government support could make things less appealing to kids like marijuana. She describes the big push for tobacco, then the big push against tobacco. Tracy wonders how the government could apply methods that worked in the past like with tobacco reduction to new things that come up and are being addictive.

Diana describes the government's role (after a big sigh), she thinks that they somehow need to control the pharmaceutical companies, make them responsible for starting programs that address drug addiction. Giving them subsidies for setting up the programs that deal with drug addiction. Require education about drug addiction. Diana adds: "It is a business. What are we going to do? Just hope it does not affect our family". Hope that it won't affect any families. It is not reality now, and we can strive to change that. There are already so may bad things out in the world that can hurt people. The question is: Where is the ethical and societal responsibility? I had to take an oath in nursing school to do no harm and was proud of it. It feels to me that ethics is so important in our lives. There are people who just want to make money and don't care about others. Greed in companies, governments, businesses. For profit. Why does it take so long for the government to act when people are hurting? - asks Diana. She brings up the coal country and how much time it took the government to step in. She describes it as a horrible situation with all the oxycodone. The government finally did step in in a few places. It will take a long time to reverse the effects. Diana feels that there needs to be more options available to those who want to get clean. She asserts: "I don't know the answer". This is a conversation. We've got to start somewhere. Diana also bring up problems in small counties that are rural. There might be one or two places to go if people need help. It is not enough. Even for those two places, not everyone is eligible to go and be cared for. She is thinking a nonprofit would be good where people can go and get counseling. Healthcare for everyone would be better. It works in other places. If people need help, they should be able to get help – she adds. Why is treatment for profit? Why are people allowed to make money out of another people's suffering? Should for profit treatment centers be allowed?

Michelle talked about kids education in general. She had noticed that kids educational experiences are focused on discipline where to sit what to do, tests and limits. School is a lot of hours of someone's childhood. If kids do not fit in, that can cause problems down the line and not everybody fits in a box and can sit endlessly all day to do schoolwork. Learning styles can be very different. Kids can be so much more creative outside and doing interesting projects and learn that way instead of sitting in a classroom. She describes that so many school aged kids now have depression and anxiety. So how can we raise our kids to be self-confident and feel supported by society? Make recommendations to the wider society. How did schools function before all this technology and fast pacing world? What people used to do before television? It should not just be the parents; Michelle asserts that it is everyone's responsibility to support a positive change for our next generation. Janett felt that as long as there is a want for drugs, drugs will keep coming. She thinks we need to stop the big shipments of drugs and stop the criminality of it. Janett thinks people can be addicted to anything that releases oxytocin in our body. Examples she brought up included tanning, pregnancy, food and Oxycontin. She also discussed fermented fruit and animals liking the fruit. There are videos online that show drunk animals after eating too much of the fruit. Albert feels that the government can help the situation by regulation of drug companies, prosecution and improving the criminal justice system. He feels that the drug war been a disaster, did not help addiction issues in the country. Use enlightened data driven approach he adds, to figure out what is going on, why is it going on and try to get to the base of it. This is the only way to do it. Albert adds that we cannot punish people out of addiction. Sometimes jail works for people to get sober, and sometimes it does not. Sometimes people tell the court:" give me as much sentence as you want 30 days, 60days 90 days I am just going to go out and use again as soon as I get out". It depends if the person is ready or not. I asked Era what we could do to help people with addiction. She responded that even though we spend money on addiction we have to do much more, maybe 10 or 100 times more. Add more nurses and more counselors. Too many alcohol shops she asserts, they are in every corner. Not to use additional chemicals in alcoholic drinks might also help.

    Flower feels that more treatment facilities could be opened, offering reimbursement for places and having more education could be helpful. She feels like the counterculture is the culture that is not using. People that are sober are the counterculture. She has people in her family that don't drink and that is not what she sees in the culture at all, there is a lot of marketplace behind alcohol. Dr. Beatty asserts that the government's role in this is to provide a universal type of care like in some other countries and have some type of policy to support it. The government's role is to provide universal or affordable care to all in this county under our constitution to prevent addictions and mental health type issues. All health care should be provided by the government.

Brenda tells me this is a giant problem and there is no perfect solution. She does like the fact that the government is bringing opioids into the forefront. People learning and having more understanding is helpful. Doing MAT (Medication Assisted Treatment), and decreased barriers around that has been helpful, for most people it is not a barrier anymore to get into MAT. She describes this problem as the rare fish in the giant ocean. They are trying, but there needs to be more emphasis, more awareness that is brought to the forefront to be able to decrease the stigma. Then, Brenda asks: What do we do with those people who don't want help? And the people who might want help, but now become disabled because they killed their brain cells? Then they can't function in daily life. She has no solution for some of those things and hopes that someone will come up with something. Prevention is a huge piece in the puzzle- she adds. Prevent rather than treat. It is kind of like nursing. Prevent injuries, prevent bed sores and prevent infection. If we can all do that in the hospitals maybe, we can all do that in our communities. Prevent addictions. Could we do it? How would we start?

Susan describes recently going to a city council and talking about tobacco licensing. The members were asking why they are even talk about tobacco why they are not talking about opiates. I asked Susan what she thinks about that? She felt that based on what she had heard so far, yes, it is needed, she feels like it takes time to build out something. She thought we are doing a good job about it but that was not the council member's perception about the issue. They perceived opiates as a much bigger problem in the community. I asked Susan if she thinks it is enough what we do now? She had a lot of uncertainty in her voice, she was not sure. She proceeded to tell me that she knows it is difficult, and she did not think it is enough, need to couple the support with mental health. She felt for example that harm reduction is a good program, but it is not enough; it needs other pillars to support the stopping of addiction, especially addiction to heroin. Susan gives the example of her brother. She felt like her brother was lucky because their family had money to send him to rehab and was very supportive, but she describes this as a rare case. Susan felt that people need more resources to put it all together. Susan also feels that:" addicts should not be treated as criminals". She brings up Portugal and their choice to decriminalize drugs that turned out well. Provided more support for people with addictions and provided connections for people in their families and communities. It would be more helpful then criminalizing addiction. Creating more strict policies to help with addiction. Provide more support in equity she added.

Bob feels that the government could have a role in providing programs, he is not sure if they should have more role. Educating people and offering resources. Limit prescribing opiates and know the effects of the drugs. Pharmaceutical companies need to be better regulated and inspected because now they are doing things they should not be doing. Bob thought that the government does not know what to do about it. Pharmaceutical companies should be held responsible. We are paying taxes to have a service he tells me; people should be cared for. We discussed that people can go to the hospital for care, and it is not affordable. People get care in the emergency room yet does not mean that people get the treatment they need.

31. Violet's Story

Violet and I talk on a phone for about an hour and a half. Violet is a provider in mental health. She has some wonderful experiences in the mental health field. We discuss struggles in rural mental health. She shares some stories about her family. Addiction runs through Violet's family. Violet's grandfather was an awesome man when he was sober which was about 10% of the time. He was very violent at other times, there was a lot of domestic violence in the home, a lot of poverty, a lot of emotional and sexual abuse. It was all related to alcohol use. Home was never a safe place and there was a lot of trauma. Violet asked her mom if it was so bad why didn't they just leave? Her mom looked her and laughed. Violet:" you don't understand this was the 1950's in America". Nobody could leave, women could not hold a credit card, women could not own land, could not get an education beyond high school, if they did work the jobs being available were to be a teacher a nurse or working in a shop. Women were home and took care of the family. They did try to leave. They went to the neighbors, he hurt all of them, then they went to family, he hurt all of them. Then they went to the church and he hurt the preacher. There were no laws against domestic violence, women were pretty much property. They could not get help, there wasn't public assistance there were no shelters. They were stuck. Violet's mom was adamant about telling her that there is alcoholism in her genes and don't test those waters. It is there. She did test those waters through college. Now she would occasionally have one or two drinks, she knows not to have more. She had training in mental health and in her master's program in their addiction course the teacher was begging the students to please work in addictions even if it was just in their internship. The teacher wanted them to see how much addiction and mental health intertwined. Violet added anything to the addiction list that is maladaptive including gambling and sex addiction. She got trained in seeking safety which is a dual diagnosis program. It is a beautiful program, she adds. It talks about trauma and the addiction and the cycle it comes with it. If someone had trauma and uses addiction to cover it up, they are more likely to be traumatized again. Nine out of ten times law enforcement is involved when there is a physical altercation or sexual violence including alcohol. Violet's first job in Utah was working with co-occurring disorders. She learned more there than anywhere else in her career. When Violet did her first group and listened to stories that people were telling her she realized that the only difference between them and her is that they got caught. She had 2-3 drinks before and got behind the wheel. It could have been her. A jail commander told her that people can drive 200 times drunk on average before they get caught. Even if someone got behind the wheel once drunk it could have been them who got incarcerated, got the legal charges against them, that ended up with a felony. Violet has her private practice now. She worked with clients who have difficulties because they are required to work, do probation, do UAs. They can't drive, and things are far from each other and it puts them into an impossible situation especially if they are on parole in more than one county. Violet feels that there is much shame and judgement and disparity in our criminal justice system around substance use. It would be nice to simplify things for people who just made one mistake to help with all the hoops they have to jump through. There is a difference between a person who just has one DUI and one who had many she adds. Failing can create more stress and lead to more drinking. Violet feels that substance abuse is a symptom, it is how people are trying to function and manage things. It is a coping skill. Not a good one. Many times, the only one people have. It becomes the matter of finding someone a better crutch then the one they had before. We cannot just take the crutch away she adds, people will fall. People need a comprehensive recovery map.

  She tells me a metaphor: the ditches on the side of the road and the roads themselves can be dangerous and people need to know what to watch out for. This way people can be more prepared for their life and what it brings to them. Some of the addictions are related to intergenerational substance abuse. Violet's grandfather's grandfather also was a drunk. Things get passed through time including the good things, and the challenging ones. In her master program the same professor who was telling them to work in the addiction field told them that not everyone has the same expectation about life. Some people are thought by their families that they are going to graduate from high school and go on and get a degree and do something meaningful, save money, and others were thought that we go to prison and fight the system or use substances to manage the stress in life. Having law enforcement and CPS in their lives regularly is just what happens in their lives. Violet adds that if we could all acknowledge that that we don't all get the same upbringing that our culture, our background and our generational differences play a part then we can start to look at what we want to change.

Violet also worked with Native Alaskan populations for about 15 years. She tells me this was more "proof in the pudding" that when people get targeted, labeled, alienated, abused, displaced and come away from the goodness and the fabric of their cultures and families things get more challenging and people tend to move toward addictions. Providing culturally appropriate and meaningful care is profoundly important. She became really aware of the disparity in care that was available. This also goes for other areas as well especially in rural communities. She tells me if someone needs mental health services it might or might not be there. If a person needs substance abuse services insurance may or may not cover it. People need to choose what to: do they move to a new place, leave home, family, job so they can get treatment then come back to the same environment or do they sit tight and stay under the thumb of addiction, legal issues and crime. Violet describes that part of her work became transferring skills and identifying areas in people's lives that are working. It is not all a loss even with substance abuse. "Man, if you deal drugs you got some serious skills". Including building a community, networking, math, understand timing of business and organization and if someone can transfer all these skills to something healthier, legal, more productive they don't have to start over. They can use their life experiences and build on them. Great examples of this are some of the stories in this book including Kevin's and Doug's story. They worked hard and turned their lives around. Don't throw the baby out with the bathwater so to speak she adds. People make mistakes and they can pull from it. Learn from it, be resilient and move forward in a meaningful way. Violet recommends the work of Brené Brown on shame and vulnerability. In substance use shame is a huge piece. "you are an addict, you are a felon you are a criminal, you are an abuser" – all these labels that we can slap on people who are having problems creates shame that attacks the identity of the person – Violet adds. It hits people in their core, it makes them feel stuck and they don't know how they can change now.

> *Violet's advice: Instead of I am a mistake have a healthy sense of guilt that I made a mistake.*

    She tells me about the separation of people feeling that they made a choice that was a mistake versus the feeling that they are the mistake. Violet tells me more about Brené Brown's work and positive thoughts instead of societal judgment. Lot of this sound familiar to the findings that are collected in this book based on people's stories and experiences. Judgement is a huge piece, and it is everywhere. If we could just stop judging people, right? Violet tells me about pieces of our lives and how we can pick them up and restore them despite of whatever mistakes we made. When she tells me this, I imagine a forest and some of the trees died and some of the trees are fallen down, some rotted as well, and there are new young trees growing and there are some bushes and old growth trees. We are a forest of old and new growth and all of us have some pieces of our past that is not so green and not so beautiful. I had talked and met so many people in my life who had done some horrible things in their past and now they have beautiful pastures growing and young trees that are not just beautiful for themselves they also support others when their forest is in a dark place. Violet gives me an example of gambling and addiction and if someone loses all of their money. That can be looked upon as they made a mistake instead of them being a total failure and I am out of this friendship or relationship. Violet had worked in the crisis system in the last decade. She had learned a lot about addiction and suicide. Shame can play a huge role in suicide. A lot of people who gamble end up killing themselves. People who are getting so many charges that they are feeling that life is over and end up killing themselves or attempting to kill themselves. There is a lot of life savings that can be done in treatment, she adds. Violet is passionate about saving lives and working hard to support people in need as a provider.

I ask Violet specifically about her experiences working in the Native American community. She shares some beautiful stories with me. She had seen how people can suffer when they are ripped away from their culture. She tells me about a young woman who was born with fetal alcohol spectrum disorder. In Alaska there is a big effort and movement to educate about FAS (Fetal Alcohol Syndrome) because there is a high rate of alcoholism. People use alcohol for coping skills for depression, darkness in a mal adoptive way. Some of it has to do with a lack of other options including treatment and meaningful activities. In some places in rural Alaska the only options are something that has to do with a religion, which may or may not resonate with people. Another option was to go to a bar. It is a factor in a community and what people choose to do. There has been a huge focus on nature and having nature help the healing process. In Native American culture carving canoes, carving totem poles, painting them getting out and doing canoe journeys can be helpful. People used to canoe from village to village to trade, connect with others and to marry and intermingle. Water is a huge part of Alaskan living, getting out to fish, crab and berry picking. It is incredible there- she adds. She tells me how different that is from a city life where people may or may not see a tree or may or may not walk on grass. ***"If people would just get back outside"*** – Violet adds. This is a huge piece, the connection to each other as human beings, to nature, animals and plants in our environment.

    Violet talks about blueberries, collect them all day, eat them while collecting them, then go home and make blueberry syrup and blueberry pie, blueberry muffins and blueberry pancakes and dry blueberry fruit leather and that keeps people busy. During winter when people are eating these things, they think about all the time they spent out in the field. Violet has been reading articles about this generation being called the inside generation because literally they are not accessing the outdoors. She tells me about Native Alaskan videogame that has the culture in it, it is beautiful it looks like an artistic movie. If it is there, the games she adds how we can make them that it would show our history and pride and it is meaningful. Alaskan life is rich she adds, she had learned so much there. She had worked with one young woman who had FAS and was living with her mom who continued to drink alcohol after giving birth and made some challenging choices, some out of necessity, out of fear or just out of what is familiar. Familiar is not always good or healthy it is just what we know. It can in a false way feel safe. Familiar is not always safe she adds. Her mom would drink and would bring abusive men in the home and this young woman was molested by multiple of her mother's partners. This young woman become profoundly angry and compulsive. She was a high risk for substance abuse because of the trauma and FAS disorder combination. It is all she known. She had multiple children with multiple fathers all of them being removed from the home a few weeks after being born. She had continued to perpetuate the domestic violence that she had known and experienced. It is one of those cycles that many others described during our conversations. Violet worked with her on impulse control and seeking safety.

Violet describes addiction as survival brain:" I don't care about the consequences I want to feel better now". Violet thought her a lot of very good breathing exercises. "If we breathe deeply, we are taking ourselves out of flight of flight response". The brain measures threat from an actual threat to a perceived one by the amount of oxygen flowing through our blood stream. Violet gives me some examples of real threat like a tiger attack or perceived threat like stress from city traffic.

Violet recommends:

Simply learning deep breathing and taking 10 breaths with moving your belly in and out as you inhale and exhale you bring enough oxygen to your brain that it tingles. It is almost like a high. It tells the brain it was a false alarm, there is not really a threat. - Violet

Once people are relaxed, they can synthetize and make choices. They are out of the flight or fight zone of their brain. It allows people to see a big picture. Violet did education around this and provide practical tools around breathing. Build up coping mechanisms. Violet tells me that at first, she does not need to know what the trauma is the person had to help people develop healthy coping skills. The young women she worked with first focused on diet, exercise, nutrition, reconnecting with culture and art. She was phenomenal in beading. She beaded things that Violet's jaw just dropped. Violet makes me laugh by saying she could not crochet a straight line to save her life. The things this young woman could make were beautiful ornaments, trinkets, key chains, wraps and the stiches and patterns were specific to her culture. She did this with a lot of pride.

    Violet worked at the South Alaska Native consortium for health and that was a profound experience. They offered a sweat lodge, a talking circle, drum circles and a basket weaving group. Women could get together and talk about their coping while developing a very culturally important bonding with each other. They would take their woven baskets home as a reminder of the support system they have. They also did beautiful regalia that were specific to their clan. All these programs were already present when Violet was there, she did not create any of them she referred people to them. The young women got better, she got one of her 3 children back and now keeping her 4th child. The other 2 are staying with their father and it is a good, healthy thing she adds. She has her coping skills now; she draws on them when she needs them. She needed to find ways to cope. She cannot go to family for help and support. She lost weight, she got healthier. Violet tells me ***it is possible to heal and not to lose hope***. "A big piece of recovery is reestablishing awareness and trust in our internal resources". A lot of people with addiction feel that they cannot trust themselves, they cannot trust their intuitions. If something does not work the sooner someone can admit it, the sooner they can change to do something that does work for them. Sometimes we shut that down because of what we are familiar with or what we have thought. Intuition tells us it does not feel good. She does not know why. She feels that it is just as a human being reaching for something else that feels better. Reawakening that personal drive for achievement and creative living. Choosing to draw on what is healthy and available and create something that people can do from there. It is not simple of course; true recovery is a lifetime event. Even addiction aside we all are recovering from quite a few things. We are recovering from our government failing us, from funding a programing not working, having too much plastic in our environment.

Humanity tries to create solutions for things. Plastic cups were created because we felt that we were destroying too many trees with paper ones. Sometimes we make errors trying to fix errors. If we can decrease the chaos and increase how connected we are within ourselves, we can make those active steps to make good things happen. Connections are lost many times in today's society because our society is very individualistic. People get lost in it. It is too much. Violet feels that addiction means that people are trying the best they can with the resources they have at the time and with what they are familiar with to make sense of connecting with the world. Trying to feel safe and comfortable, happy, loved and connected. This came up over and over again through the crisis work that Violet had done. We can label people all we want, like they just want attention she adds. She saw a post recently stating: "if you shift your own label for a child from attention seeking to connection seeking- see how that impacts your perception". Things like that, she adds, blows her mind, the difference one-word can make. The power of our speech and thought. She feels this is profoundly important in our work. Addiction is that:" I got far away from myself or maybe I never even knew myself. I still wanted and deserve to be connected she adds. I will do this the best way I can". If people feel isolated and awkward, so much of addiction comes from wanting to fit in socially, to have a connection. Feeling of boredom, awkwardness and embarrassment. Violet had seen some very powerful movement with youth. She herself has a 14-year-old and thanks God that her child so far did not seek drugs for thrill or excitement. Finding more meaningful and fun things to do is important. She tells me about the adrenalin rushes available. If people have the means and they want to do skydiving, it is a big one.

Trying new experiences, surfing, horseback riding or any other experience that teaches the brain in a healthy way that fun can happen without substances. It does not have to be expensive; it could be a new hike in the forest. She feels that exercise is a big piece of that. When we use substances, it is because we just want to feel good. **All the natural endorphins that make us feel good get released through**

exercise. Getting people engaged in physical activity and artistic pursuit and anything that is thrill seeking can all help. She tells me about a commercial that advertised beer for breakfast. She was appalled. Why are we teaching in public television that this is ok? Why do we even have alcohol and smoking, and vaping advertised in television? Why is there a cotton candy flavored vape? Who is that targeting?

Next, Violet tells me about the show Patriot Act on Netflix. The show highlights some of the discrepancies in society. There is one episode about related to opiates. It is so sickening she adds. The major company that created Oxycontin and ended up being slammed and fined for it also created Suboxone. Basically, they created the sickness, perpetuated it by getting doctors to prescribe even getting doctors things like lap dances. We discuss Suboxone and its own set of problems. Violet tells me about a family friend who lost his life. He used heroin. He got off of it, got on Suboxone, he quit the Suboxone abruptly, went back to the same dose of heroin he had initially used. He overdosed and died. It is so common for people to do that, she adds. It is an epidemic and she is glad that there is some funding, but the funding is not enough. She tells me about Fentanyl. Now the same company who developed Fentanyl is working on a drug that is 10x stronger than Fentanyl. I wonder why on earth we need such a strong pain medication? Not enough people died already? Beyond any comprehension. It is horrifying Violet adds. We are seeing a wave of deaths with Fentanyl already, and people are not knowing they are getting it, or they know, and they are getting too much. Violet tells me that law enforcement has been touching Fentanyl without knowing and dying from it. She feels this profoundly affects people whether they are users or not. It impacts us.

Violet tells me about all the potential that is lost related to addiction. It leaves devastation. People don't just lose their life. Each person had several loved ones, several different facets of life, people who knew them. A lot of people get affected. Violet feels that addiction in a way is a commentary on money, power and influence. The more we can speak up about it, destigmatize addiction, make treatment programs readily available, accessible and understand the truth the better - she adds. The fact that with like the needle exchange just as many family people are driving up in their suburban vans as homeless people walking up.

She brings up her favorite topic and gives me the example of diabetes as many other people before. People with diabetes get their treatment simultaneously with counseling. Nobody tells them shame on them come back when they are ready to quit sugar. MD's would lose their license if they do that. So why is it that with addiction we don't to do the same? This is a disease; this is a struggle. It is not a choice. People still think addiction can be a choice. How about diabetes, is it a choice? Does somebody want to be a diabetic? I don't think so. The same way nobody wants to be an addict. Yet, we don't punish people eating sweets and cakes and becoming a diabetic. Why are we punishing people who become an addict? It is ridiculous she adds. She tells me the difference between people who get addicted. It is like if we were on a boat and we would sink, and some people had a life preserver that others didn't. Then the people with the life preserver have a much better chance of living. Even if they get hypothermia probably, they are not going to die. On the other hand, she adds some don't have a chance because they don't have the protective factor in place. In this case the life support. Do not blame the person if they did not have the life vest. Someone can't just say why did they get on the boat without life vest. People have to look at things from a different angle.

She jumps back to Fentanyl and asking the question: "why doctors are even prescribing it for anything more than terminal patients". I do not know. It was never meant for anything else. Violet got a lot of training in Alaska for alternative therapies for pain instead of pain medications. She describes pain as something we can't see or measure. Even a scale from 1-10 can be very different in accuracy for people. Is 10 what people thinks now really the worse pain? Is someone at the point that they cannot walk, and they must have a surgery and the doctors all agree and they are in the hospital? If not, let's not call it a 10. What is a 9, 8 or a 7? How can people learn to cope for the next 20 minutes? Tried alternative methods like walking, ice pack, and elevation? Pain does exist, and it is also ok for some level of pain to be there. Violet feels that people can get very dramatic with pain. She feels very specific measuring tool is needed for pain with nonpharmacological interventions at first. This can also work for other things like depression, she adds. What can someone do for example in the next 20 minutes to feel better. She gives me an example how this scale could be used for addictions as well. She also tells me about harm reduction and the lesser of two evil sorts of speak. She does not care if somebody is playing a video game if they stopped taking opiates. Find what works and capitalize on that. Give ourselves credit even just making for the 20 minutes. Even if someone uses after 20 minutes, she adds, it is not a failure. They attempted a coping skill, they thought about it. It is a step into the right direction. It might be 40 minutes next time, or the person might smoke opiates and not inject it by IV. Good for the individual that they were able to do that instead. Giving people credit. Helping people to see small victories, she adds, because we can't just say people are failures that does not take us anywhere.

    A big piece of addiction and working through it is not setting people up to fail. Letting people know, they will not be going to get through all of this in a month, or 6 months. This is a lifestyle and a lifetime of finding to be present. Violet feels we get so far from being present. Very true. We try to look to the future or the past and compare things instead of focusing on the right here, right now. Violet quotes someone she used to work with, and they described addiction is an attempt to create a shortcut to enlightenment. Violet just thought that is it. People want to feel Nirvana, want to feel peaceful and blissful and connected and aware and one with a universe. It is all have to do with love and connection. Instead of doing whatever that hard work is to create it we go for the quick fix. She tells me the example of food. She adds that she is so guilty of that. She had been in McDonalds in the last few weeks. Survival brain being hungry, angry or tired. We want to feel better right now, so we don't care what we are putting in our body. We don't think about that we just want to feel better. If we would start to normalize this and educate around it; it would be helpful.

    Violet brings up the example to have an emotional intelligence class in high school. We need to start emotional intelligence classes before kindergarten and keep teaching more every year. There are so many people still today who I met, and they think that if another person in their life is angry or behaving a certain way it is about them not about the other person. We can't control how others behave. We can only control how we behave. We need to arm kids with knowledge on emotions and how to control them and cope with them is a wonderful idea. Violet tells me a study about hunger. The study looked at domestic violence perpetrators and about 78% of them had low blood sugar when they acted out, based on the answers. When we are hungry, we are going into a different part of our brain. This is where food comes in, she adds. If we are in a place where we don't feel safe, we overeat. Back in the cavemen days people ate everything in site because they did not know when they get to food next, we still have this instinct today. Violet adds that this and flight or fight does not excuse the behavior, yet it is part of the puzzle, part of the explanation. Part of therapy is how to get out of that fight and flight brain and make better decisions. Violet also does a lot of couple's therapy. She tells people to check in with themselves are they irritable, tired or hungry? If they are, it is not a good time to have a conversation. She brings up people who smoke. Ask them: why do they smoke? Is it to build connection and community it others? Is it to have an excuse to take a break and go outside? Is it just to do something? She recommends people who smoke to create a new activity, not smoke during their break, instead take a breath through a straw, have a popsicle or blow bubbles. Do something else with their mouth instead of smoking to please their oral fixation. Get outside and take 20 deep breaths. Violet believes we can heal and fix a lot though doing things intentionally and meaningfully. She loves things like this, and she is highly passionate about this topic. Wanting to connect, wanting to feel love and wanting to find what works. Be in our brain and our body, then we can deal with what is making us anxious more effectively. She lets out a big sigh, then laughs. I love it. I love her passion and compassion toward others and her desire to help.

  We discuss coping skills and emotional intelligence a little more. It is a big piece; it can be easily overwhelming, she adds. It is so big that when she looks at it sometimes, she gets overwhelmed and shut down. Then, she remembers a woman walking on a beach and throwing a sea star back to the water. A man walks by and asks her what she is doing. He added that there is so many, she cannot make a difference. She picks another one up, then another one. It made a difference for this one, she answers. Violet feels this is important when we talk about emotions and coping skills. Everything will be different for each person, each family, each location. Living rurally, in Washington is a challenge. To get to a big city is 5-hour commitment. It is a challenge even for somebody in middle class. Violet looks at all resources for her clients including searching Facebook for ideas. She also looks at what had worked in other communities and how could she adopt that work locally. How can she connect a particular client to resources that are meaningful. Then, maybe that option could be a cookie cutter for someone else.

    She used to work in Colorado to help with people who had mental health problems create independence in their lives. It was on the patient's terms. They know what is meaningful for them. She had to make sure that this person's home with a mental health disability was clean. She got there and the home was spotless. She told her client that her home is cleaner than Violet's. Her client was so proud. Violet asked her how she did it. She shared that her last worker came every week and showed her how to do the cleaning and they did it for 3 years. Then she decided she liked how her house looked. Violet asked her what else she could help with since she did not needed help with cleaning. The next thing she wanted is to have a job, to have more money. Violet asked her what she wanted to do. She wanted to sell Mary Kay makeup. Violet does not wear makeup. Violet did not think that she could do it. She did it. She made more money from makeup then what Violet made from being a case manager. She is still doing it today. Her story and determination impressed Violet so much. It was an example that anything is possible. She brings up vocational rehab that helps people trained if they have a mental health or substance abuse disorder. That program is invaluable, it is a success that the government created. When there is the right person they need to be connected with existing programs. Violet feels that:" When we connect with somebody, and they can work, their self-confidence gets better". Violet always tells people about those available training resources. Violet likes to remind people that they always have something to give. "Any ways that we can find that people can give back to the community form natural connections and boost confidence"- she adds. Violet gives me some examples of the elderly and how many people who are older have no one to talk to. Volunteer to clean up a beach for example instead of watching TV, make a difference. We meet people and it can change our life. Supporting employment is also a great resource to help people who been out of work for awhile. Creating resources within each local community can be a great grassroot effort. We discuss trauma stewardship and that working in mental health and addiction is hard work. The average length people say in the field in 5 years, she adds. She feels that the trauma stewardship piece needs to be brought in more. We are interacting and treating each other as professionals. If providers are not functioning well as a community, as a society, in a meaningful authentic way, then how can they even pretend to give people the help and support they deserve. How can we keep people in the field? Retention and treating each other in a meaningful trauma informed way is not just a problem in mental health. In many fields there are a lot of trauma. First responders for example. It could be in McDonalds or anywhere else. It is indiscriminate. It can be anywhere and can affect anyone. I can hear her passion through the line. She adds we have to be there to catch the people who are falling. She is also passionate about how society can create a less traumatized environment. Keeping the checks and balances in place and remind each other appropriately when we are out of balance. Violet try to effect change. She would not stay with an organization that is not ethical and supportive of their clients and staff. It starts with each of us. Consciously choose to get out of flight and fight to be in a calm, creative, empathetic mindset. Schedule time for ourselves. Take care of ourselves so that we can take care others. Self-care is very important. It is a constant checking in with ourselves instead of checking out.

32. Society

Imagine our society as a forest. In a forest there can be many different types of trees and other plants, animals exist and collectively they create a habitat that is livable for all. There are other outside conditions that the forest cannot control like storms, rain, sun, earthquakes, hurricanes that tear away and hurt the forest. Therefore, forests have to have a strong a balance for maintenance and recovery to prevent animals and plants to die out. The same way we have to have a balance in our society. What is society's role in general and what is the role what it comes to in addictions?

Sheila thinks that in our society we all should be there to help when the person is ready to receive help, including having free resources. Similar to smoking where there are free patches available. Resources should be available for addiction. Beth thinks bringing people together would help in our society, and she describes that this is very hard. Beth feels that our society is broken. It is just broken, there are pot stores on every block, one of the things she describes is not supporting pot stores. Maybe coming together and creating a whole new system for addiction. Creating a group for families and people who are dealing with addictions, something more modern. Beth also had mentioned to create change society, in a way that it is not all about money. It is all about money now. She feels people do not care about others who are addicted to drugs, they just want to make money. It is a sad thing Beth said, it could be their brother. Maybe changing the society where people care about health like in Great Britain, they put health first and income last. That would help, we should all be united in that way. It is a disease Beth stated, and she was getting pretty mad about it. I saw many people who are mad, sad and upset because they have family, friends and know people who are going through addictions and it is very emotional. Mary describes that maybe one thing we can do is talk about addictions differently to remove the shame, talk about it, what is addiction. Educate people on what is addiction. Mary brought up a great point. There are communities where people's livelihood is depending on making and selling drugs, providing hope for these communities that there can be other things that provide that income can be helpful in our society. Changing the conversation about how we talk about addiction. Edward feels if addiction is viewed as an illness in a societal level, more assistance can be provided.

In my conversation with Angel, she felt that people on our society in general don't have great coping skills anymore. Additionally, she thinks that people are not being very comfortable about being uncomfortable. She feels that being uncomfortable "sucks" and people don't have a lot of tenacity to go through it. While it is not a negative thing Angel feels that people start self-medicating because they want the uncomfortable feelings to go away. Instead of being open to the experience, no matter how it makes people feel. Go through it, feel it she recommends. Be in the moment. Learn from it, grow from it, which can be really hard for people. Angel feels like the whole social media has been a huge contributing factor especially for kids. There is a view that everybody's life is so great which is false from reality. This can create an idea that if someone is struggling then there must be something wrong with them, and their life. Angel said, no, we all struggle, this is part of living, growing and maturing. She also feels that society today made it really easy to be detached from each other. Angel sees kids at school who are struggling with drugs, alcohol and other stuff. She feels that the kids are experiencing loss and don't know how to cope with it. Angel was also talking about the idea that we just need to help each other and extend our hand toward others instead of being afraid that we might lose something if we do so. She brought up the example of immigration. Kayla describes our responsibilities as having people who know how to work with mental health and addiction problems. We just do not have enough support Kayla feels and also mentioned that she is beating a dead horse here. Many people I talked to say the same thing, that there should be more support in mental health and addictions that is available. More providers, more treatment, the list just goes on. It is difficult everywhere, and in small rural communities there is a need for more support.

Rory feels like everything is very mixed, depending on who people talk to and what funding they have. He feels like most treatment facilities are phony, fake. Do a sloppy job at best. He wonders how anyone comes out of them sober. While are some great facilities out there, there are hundreds of what he calls mom and pop shops that just tack the shingles on and call themselves a treatment facility and doing a bare minimum to get qualified. Nobody supervises this. He describes a treatment facility he worked at before, which is closed now, that that was a problem. Nobody supervised this. Nobody supervised from the owners or from the state and they get away with stuff that was illegal. I worked for one of these places, not for long left pretty quickly I could not bear what was going on. It was all about money not the people. Even though I did not know what was going on in the background, it just felt wrong. Turnover of stuff was crazy high. Nobody could take this long. Many places trying to treat addiction without looking at the mental health component. Rory laughs, and tells me that this does not work. Now, maybe someone is not addicted, and the mental health problem is still there. So, the cycle many times will begin again as the root cause was not addressed and dealt with. This is like putting a Band-Aid on something, but not actually treating the deep wound or injury. It might superficially heal for a while, and it will open up again with yellow or green pus coming out and creates a life-threatening infection. Need to treat the cause. Otherwise it won't work. Just put the Band-Aid on? How many times? He also talked about needle exchange programs, the need for safe injection sites. He feels a methadone clinic is not a solution. He describes his training and the goal to titrate people down, not to keep them on high doses of Methadone or Suboxone. He so far has not met someone using Suboxone who had been titrated down. It is just not done in the community. He feels this is not happening because the lack of set up of doctors, nurses, case managers and peer support.

    Tracy feels like we are where we are in our society today because of addictions. She describes a conversation she had with someone recently about the homeless problem. She thinks that homelessness is also caused by addictions. We can also link this to mental health Tracy describes, and it is a full circle. Is it mental health or addiction first? In her job she feels it comes down to addictions, homelessness, lack of housing and resources. Tracy asserts that one of the problems is for people trying to keep sober is that: "There is more quantity of the addictive things out there then the supportive things to stay sober". Very true. Tracy describes our societal responsibility as providing education for our kids and education that starts at a very early age. She describes kids' education similar to "stranger danger" and "bullying", used to have the D.A.R.E. program for drugs. She was wondering what the success rate for these educational efforts had been. Then she asserted that keep with the education, do not just do it when they are little, keep going into teen years. Also don't make bad things appealing to teens. Tracy wonders if our society is really in the worse place now then it's ever been, or we are just more aware of it now than we ever been before. Tracy describes her not having the internet when growing up and not being aware of what is going on. The same thing happened growing up in her family, she lived with addiction and she did not know it. Tracy wishes she would have been educated as a child about addictions. She gives an example about the "pot shops" she is thinking about her kids now being raised and thinking it is normal to have a pot shop in every street corner. What this will do to them? How this will affect them as adults? Also, everywhere people go there is alcohol.

Diana feels that there is too much acceptance, not enough resources. Addiction goes on too long before people get help. People having trouble identifying what is going on. Leniency and acceptance of the social life that people have is not helpful. She thinks people are not careful enough and don't think they can get sucked into addictions. More education about addiction would be helpful. Mental health and addictions intertwine, she adds. Teach kids to say no and recognize what could be a bad situation. Our conversation went in all kids of direction, and we ended up talking about homelessness. There is a lot of connection between homelessness, mental health and addiction problems.

Michelle describes that one of the societal responsibilities is to recognize that addiction is an illness. It is a disease; it is more than just someone's decision to use whatever they are using. It is not a moral failing. Providing services for people is essential, create an environment that does not push people toward addictions. She gives an example of alcohol and tobacco where they can be sold and how they can be sold. Providing a way for people to have a chance to be better fulfilled in life. She feels that a driving force behind of addictions are that people do not have ways to cope with everyday things in their lives. She feels that society is set up to allow people to have lives that are not fulfilling when it comes to basic needs, jobs and activities in their lives. As an example, she talks about postpartum depression. She feels part of this comes from pressures put on families including being alone when people have kids. There is just no sense of community where everyone looking out for everyone's kids and support each other. It is just the individual and if anything goes wrong, it is their fault. It is how our society is structured. People moving away from where they grew up, away from aunts, uncles, grandparents. To get the best job or whatever it is, and now people don't have their families around. Missing a support system. She feels this is like a contributing factor. She feels this is a societal responsibility that we should pay attention too and try to make steps toward making it better.

Ron thinks that when the movement to help people with addiction went to therapy, treatment, counseling it is ok, that there was a miss of the root problem. Why is this happening? Why people are turning to drugs and alcohol? Ron feels that we don't have the foundation of support, love, music, joy, and without this people turn where they can feel the support, music, joy and it is the deviant addictive cyclone. Even now in detox it is a struggle to get people in, the place is far away and then after 5-7 days the rehab is not available for 3-4 weeks so what will people do? They will go back from where they got there from the first place a homeless shelter, a friend's place and all the triggers are there again. The expectation of the community is now that they will somehow survive this return to the warzone and wait for a month then do residential rehab. It is a cycle. People Ron sees keep trying and failing and trying and failing. We are trying to solve the symptoms he asserts and not the root cause. Ron feels that our schools need to touch on sex and drug education, depression and anxiety. In our community there is a need to do more prevention not just trying to fix the problem. Ron feels families are disconnected and jobs don't support the community and the community does not support the work force. It's just going to keep happening Ron stated. People want to escape; they want to feel they belong to feel better.

     We need to fix why people feel they don't belong, and why they don't feel good, and want to feel better, otherwise this will just keep happening. What can we do? Do individuals feel they belong in this society? Can we fix it? Ron thinks we need to change politics to pull communities together not being divided and living in fear. Ron wish he knew what the answer is, he would be writing a book too. All we can do is to put information out to others and see what the response is. Is anyone willing to do anything about this? Are there enough people to make a change or demand change? I asked Ron my magic wand question. He said: one unified government and one unified government for the world as well, all-inclusive for all races and cultures. His dream is to release patents that could save millions of lives, unify the world, take down walls instead of putting them up. It is all about money, resources and land. We had a conversation about how much stuff we need in our life. Ron feels that stuff we have, and buy is what drives the money, greed, depression, anxiety, fear and lead into addiction. The need to destress so we are not fearful and stressed. It is a societal problem. There is little mental health support. Ron also discusses politics and the need for a political climate change. We are all people on this earth. We are all in this together. Why are we separating, dividing and conquering? Ron believes a unified world. Decrease access. We need a do over he said. Why can't everybody just get along Ron asks? Can we make a switch where love, piece and community are more important than greed, advancement and power?

Joel feels like as a society we are doing a terrible job of supporting people, supporting each other. She feels that there is a great responsibility in our society to help with any situation, but we are doing a terrible job. She talks about isolation, living away from family, instead of growing up and take care of people like the elders will take care of the children, the children will grow up and take care of elders and have a common situation, more focus on family. Joel feels that we have an obligation to help one and other the best we can. Also, to recognize when we can't. Joel feels that addiction is something that everybody is vulnerable too and people don't want to look at it and admit they could also get there. Joel asserts that we need to care about each other to make it better. Offer education and support. Joel feels like there is so much judgement in our society about anything. Joel thinks that society is just broken right now, it is terribly fractured and in it trying to get people to hear anything is very difficult. She feels that people do not want to look and see, they are clouded. Joel recommends talking about addictions and other issues, not hide it, the more we can acknowledge it exist he less likely it will spin out of control. When we hide things, it is more likely to get out of control. Joel describes people worrying about that something will be taken away from them. She describes that: "it is not like if you feed the child the soldier does not get money". Joel feels that right now in our society there is a line of division between the people who have things and the people who do not have things. We talked about fault lines, fractures in our society that could be fixed if we spend money on families, housing, basic needs to make us healthier, stronger, happier. We discussed socialized medicine and first come first served options instead of making 15 minutes scheduled time appointments. We talked about taking care children in length and Joel recalled that when she grew up, they got a vitamin and fluoride at school every morning. I grew up in Hungary, we had doctors and nurses coming to the school for health checks, immunizations. In a rural county where I live some schools decided to give breakfast free for kids, they realized kids are not doing well because they are hungry. Why do we have hungry children in America?

      Janett feels like we should have universal healthcare that includes things like addiction counseling, support by people who are qualified to help. Chelsea feels that more education would be helpful, she recalls when she grew up D.A.R.E. (Drug Abuse Resistance Education) was in schools it thought her to be very scared of drug use. She feels like it did not teach her how to have conversations about it, what resources are available, if for example if she would have decided to binge drink what would be her resources. Having more open conversations in schools or wherever the classroom is Chelsea suggests. Be more honest about it, addiction exists, and these are the things we can do about it. Albert feels that losing the judgment is a big part, people are already ashamed of what they do when they use drugs and alcohol. He sees addiction issues through the court system. It is hard to get help. It is hard for people to pay for urine analysis, treatment or counseling sessions. People in recovery usually not making money he asserts maybe $1000 a month they can't afford to do a lot of stuff they are required to do. The response they get is that they got to or they go to jail. He feels like if the court orders all this thing for a person to do then we should offer more services to people to not have the barriers. Albert feels that there is a societal benefit to have people not using and healthy, contributing to society. It is not just for them but for everybody so we should be stepping up and help people make things possible instead of creating financial barriers where people can get stuck on. Making drug and alcohol treatment no cost, making mental health treatment no cost. Making all healthcare no cost would be a good idea. It is a societal benefit; we should pay for it. It is good for us, good for them, we want this it is much better than paying to keep people in jail. Other countries can do it Albert said, He does not know why we can't. It is possible. We can't save everybody he said, but at least we can try to do our part. Era feels like we need more love in our society. She feels parents kick out kids too early at age 18 from the homes. She feels human contact is very important especially to people who struggle with addiction. Not stay alone. Have friends, help, family to be close to them to help. Era feels like both alcohol and opiates are deadly for people.

    Dr. Beatty feels that media and the political climate really control society. Everything is influenced by the media, the news, politics. The issue of addiction needs to be supported by the media to get attention so society can embrace it. Be more open in TV shows, that is where the change comes. Social change presented in a way that is visually accepted, open and liberal. It will take some time. Not every state is open. There are still many conservative places in the country. There are still places where being gay is not open people are not accepting and whispering about it. The media has to portray this in a positive way and over time gain acceptance.

    Brenda feels that the cost of addiction is so high that society has a responsibility to help in prevention. The biggest improvement would be helping people prevent to becoming addicted instead of treating people after they become addicted. Prevention is the key. Bring prevention into the school system, Brenda feels like as a community we have the ability to do this. It is a complicated issue, no easy solution she asserts, we need bright ideas to help prevent it rather than help on the other hand by reacting to it. Susan feels like people in society could have more compassion toward people dealing with addiction. She felt like people just "throw away" people who are dealing with addiction. Be more understanding and supportive with helping people with addiction. She feels that a different perception is needed. She asserts that people dealing with addiction are "still a person". She feels that many people dehumanize addicts. Dolores feels that society does have some role in developing entertainment and things that people can do and places that are without addiction. More family friendly and youth friendly places. Grassroot movement that pushes for substitutions for addiction, healthy things to do. Putting money into creating places and activities for youth without substances.

    Fuchsia tells me that society hasn't done a good job about the conflicting ideas about how normalized our drinking culture is and how pervasive an issue addiction is. She feels the individual is still blamed. She gives an example of the me-too movement. She tells me she has a unique perspective on this. She went to an all-women's college for a couple years. She was around a lot of pretty aggressive left-wing feminist. The part that bothers her about the me-too movement is the whole expectation that there is a behavioral change that is needed without the recognition of the alcohol industry playing a huge role in it. She said we are talking about feeling safe going out and getting drunk we should not have to worry about that as women, but she asserts that she knows men who had been date raped too. That is another issue she said, let's just include everyone, why are we separating men and women. She is saying that if both people are drinking and losing control how can we expect good behavior? She tells me everyone knows that when people are drunk, they cannot make a good decision. Why is it shown that drinking is a fun thing and why is it accepted that being drunk is ok in our society? Fuchsia asks. Being with someone who was in recovery made her realize how pervasive is the culture of drinking is and how it is everywhere. On every billboard, and there is not a lot of fun things for young people to do outside of that. As a young person who does not drink Fuchsia tells me she got a lot of grief and people saying:" about oh, you don't go out you don't party, oh let me show you how to be in your mid 20's". There was a lot of peer pressure. She still has this at work. She has a board meeting at a brewery. She is a small person, if she has a beer in a local place she would get buzzed and she does not want to be like that in front of other colleagues. She gets grief for that. Her voice is upset about this and raised up a little. Why there is even a board meeting in a brewery? She feels that now alcohol is such a part of our social network that it is hard for people to accept others who don't want to participate. Hearing hear again just makes me feel sad and upset, here is a young woman who is choosing to do things right and she is getting grief about it. Very sad and annoying. She is asking me if I had experienced this too? Yes. Our house has no alcohol. I had people trying to bring alcohol to a summer cookout party we had. I told them they can take it back to their car. It is nothing personal. Once someone brought wine, I told them we will not drink it he can leave it and I will give it away or take it. He left it and I gave it to a friend who sometimes drinks some wine. Fuchsia brings up that she does not pressure people not to drink so why are they are pressuring people to drink. Fuchsia feels people might feel uncomfortable when she does not drink. She is wondering if it makes people self-conscious or thinking that they cannot have fun without drinking. There is all this weird cultural pressure and people get uncomfortable when someone does not participate. Fuchsia feels we live in a country where we have a lot of privilege but also a lot of backwards policy about things like health care and mental health acceptance. She feels the acceptance is growing and people are becoming more aware, but we still have a long way to go to break down judgements and pressures society puts on people. Not enough funding. When she brings up funding. I ask my magic wand question. She tells me it has to start before the behavior starts. She feels people work so hard and healthcare is so unaffordable. She feels that we think we have this great health care system and it is very terrible. Fuchsia gives me an example of a friend whose husband is from Senegal West Africa. It is a pretty poor country and her friend got sick when she was there, but their healthcare system is so much more affordable. They are saying they are not going to have another kid until they move back because they don't want to have a child here. They have a daughter who was born in Senegal. She does not understand why socialized medicine is even an issue, she kind of laughs saying this it is a frustrated laughter. She is asking why so many people are not in support of it. Fuchsia thinks we are technically a welfare state and compared to Sweden or Germany we have nothing to offer. I ask her why she thinks that is? She says be because of capitalism. It is all about money – we said this at the same time. Then she tells me it is because we live in an individualistic culture, we don't take care of each other. She tells me that the American dream is to support ourselves and our family, get our white picket fence. I ask her if she really thinks this is the American dream of the people? It is her biggest fear, she feels a lot of people fall for it. Fuchsia does not want to become a soccer mom and not thinking for herself. She tells me we are living on an individualistic society where the definition of success is being on our own and living on our own. She describes two of her best friends from college who are from Philippine families and it is a completely different expectation. People are supposed to come home, take care of the family, live in an intergenerational household. Seeing that is easier, cheaper, people help each other. It is very materialistic she asserts; our culture and the way success are defined. I ask her if she thinks people are happier because they make more money. No, not at all she asserts. She feels a lot of people don't know how to be happy. Fuchsia tells me about a certain Christian sect belief that depending on how much good people do on earth is how big of a mansion they get in heaven. She feels this is so materialistic and shows everything that is wrong with our culture and society. She is laughing in disbelief. Are they kidding me she asks? She heard about this a couple years ago.

 Fuchsia tells me something she learned about 15% of the people who apply for military service in this country get rejected because of their IQ is too low. It is a high number for people with a low IQ. Bob tells me that our society should be more active when it comes to addictions. He feels there is not much being done about it on a large scale. I ask him what he thinks we can do about it? He tells me he does not know. A lot of things are prevalent, a lot of things are designed that way. I ask him like what? He tells me games, food, it is a product. We talk about regulations and what kinds of things people could regulate. He tells me we can't really ban candy bars. Maybe we don't need to ban them. Maybe we could use natural sugars or honey in them instead of corn syrup or sweeteners. Better education. Educate young moms. Bob feels better education would definitely help. I just read an article this week on Iceland and how they decreased youth alcohol and drug problems. They changed their culture and added more activities for youth. The article title is: "How Iceland fixed its teen substance abuse problem". Bob also tells me that he had seen a lot of people with family issues, not having a family structure, having family that is unreliable, he thinks that not having a firm foundation compromises a lot of people.

33. INDIVIDUAL'S ROLE

What can we as individuals do to help people with addition problems? Sheila thinks that knowing resources that are easy and accessible would be helpful. Additionally, she describes that we can help people by making it easier to come for us to help. Being nonjudgmental When we are judgmental or just people who are dealing with addition might think we are they are less likely to seek out help. We don't judge people with heart disease or diabetes, we help them every time they come to the doctor, hospital or cardiac rehab. Shouldn't be the same with addiction? Beth describes that we need more role models, she told me be a leader, be a role model for others. Don't go out to drink. Beth describes that an important element is to set a good example for others to follow. Be honest.

Mary feels like individual responsibilities include taking care ourselves, some might have more choices than others, or have limited choices. Self-reflection and thinking of who we are in this world. Who we want to be in this world and how we want to be in this world? Mary describes if our basic needs are not met it is very hard to think beyond that. Edward states that individual responsibilities by not being greedy. He describes people who are creating drugs that others will use and become addicted to just to make money. Ignoring warning signs during the research, moving forward anyway because they are greedy, and they want money. Coping skills on an individual level. When I asked Paige what she thinks the individual responsibility is. She said it is a very tough question. She was not really sure. Maybe to communicate and get up when people fall down. On the other hand, she mentioned that she has seen families trying and it is so difficult to navigate the system and know what to do even if someone is a trained professional. Imagine how difficult it is when people don't know much about addiction and what to do with it. Kayla mentioned that as an individual she would like to do more for people who are dealing with addiction. Because she is a mandatory reported she was not sure how could this work how she could help. It all starts with having a conversation. Extend our arm to those who need it. If people can't at least be educated about it and don't go out all judgmental.

Tracy feels like as an individual it is her job to teach her children and other people, share her knowledge with other people about addictions. Tracy is trying to go to places with her kids where they are not exposed to alcohol all the time. She recalls having so much exposure and trying to change this for her kids. Chloe talks about individual responsibility:" do your research, make sure you know what things addictive are". Be cautious, she said. If someone knows their family history, don't try the stuff that made them addicted. People have a higher likelihood to be addicted because of that. She also reminds us that just because something can be addicting it does not necessarily mean that people get addicted to it. Except she mentions drugs, people might get addicted to drugs.

    Michelle describes personal responsibility, it is difficult where to draw the line, is it the drugs or the person how much they are responsible for the decision what are the causes in the person's live. There is still some element of where people could have stopped and decided not to use substances. It is hard to think about she said. What is a right path for a person? What are all the factors that caused the persons decision to use drugs or keep using. Joel talks about empathy and how important is to be empathetic toward others, not to use labels. Support people instead of judging. Do not identify the person to the disease. So, she said instead of saying" alcoholic, meth head or drug addict" say their name as a person and then what they deal with. Joel said, do not make assumptions. She described how crazy this makes her. It is so easy to make assumptions. Janett talks about treating people with equal dignity and respect. Support others, but don't make them feel judged. Individually try to be healthy, support others. Era feels people are selfish and stay inside a capsule a capsule of protection. People think that bad things cannot happen to them like rape, home breakings, addiction. It happens more often than we think. Era shared multiple stories just from her life, she feels we should help people, not judge people with addiction problems. Era feels that just like her when she was drinking some wine to go to sleep, she was really covering things up that happened in her shift while working like short of staff, hard work. She feels there is a lot of monopoly and everybody wants money and the individual gets crushed in the process. She feels like there is a lot of judgement about addiction and a lack of acceptance, but addiction is strong. ***Addiction is stronger than we think***.

      We live in a capitalistic society Flower asserts and people are allowed to make money if they want to be in the marketplace. Flower thinks it all comes down to the individual because no one is responsible for us. She feels like with all the lobbying it is hard to picture things to be less available. There are huge, huge, huge lobbyist groups she said, and they make a lot of profit. She feels that the individual has to recognize and protect themselves within the environment they are in even if it is hard. Flower adds: "This is the unfortunate reality". If someone can't buy something don't go to the store. The advertisements and stores everywhere make this very hard she said. We have to be very strong to resist buying things we don't need and be informed and educated at the same time. Dr. Beatty feels the biggest thing is acceptance, he is very tolerant, people are different and have different needs. He tells me he is addicted to perfection. He likes to go above and beyond to help people. He feels like what we do comes from our experience. He experienced people not helping him, so he goes above and beyond to help others. He describes his experience as an English teacher. He originally had difficulty reading. Reading was a serious task for him. It was horrifying to stand up and read in front of the class. So, he kept practicing and become very good in reading and standing up in front of the class. He became that guy in the English department to read in front of others. He turned his weakness into success. He wanted to do a good job. He still does, he does right by his students. He found out later he had dyslexia meaning he did not see the words the way they appeared on the paper until he saw them over and over again. He describes himself as an overachiever. To help others with addiction Dr. Beatty describes providing resources and understanding on what people are going through. He feels that counseling as important, discuss problems with others. He feels social media groups might help. It can be anonymous. Then people can openly talk about their issues. It could be an app on the phone. Brenda feels that because we are human, and we should care for one and another to reach out to those who need help and support the people who succumbed to addiction. Brenda also thinks that we have to hold some people with some accountability into what their addiction is to help them reach out to themselves. This would help them value not being addicted and being sober. Accountability can help prevent automatic fall back to people's addictions asserts Brenda. Overcoming addiction can be achieved through community, through individual reaching out and support people who are interested in overcoming their addiction.

 I asked Susan about individual responsibility. She thought about it for a little while, then said hmmm, after a pause Susan told me that she feels that in her personal life if she knows somebody who is struggling, she can help them steer toward a right direction, because she had experience with her family. She was always drawn to addiction and mental health area when it comes to public health. She does not really have a specific idea, but maybe developing some kind of program or contributing some way to help a community that is struggling with addiction. She brought up maybe contributing to research. Dolores feels that everybody needs to be responsible to control their own self. It is on us. If we lose control on our body, job, family, relationship because of addiction. Ask Bob about the individual's role he was not sure about this one, he told me everyone is doing their own thing. He asks me for clarification. We have a discussion about individuals and responsibilities. He tells me people on average can be more open about issues other people have. It is hard to know sometimes he said, people might be doing things for any number of reasons. Being less judgmental toward other people. He feels people judge all kinds of people for all kinds of things. Can we as humans can be truly free of judgement if we want to be? Then he tells me something that "learning not to care about it is very important; ***people put a lot of value in other people's perception how things should be***". He tells me nowadays people judge others for all kinds of things. Judge if we drink or not drink too. Have confidence in our own decision, in the life choices we make. Being open and not to judge.

34. Doug's Story

    I learned about Doug from Neal. Neal's story is also in this book. After some e-mails and a phone conversation we decided to meet. I drove down to Tillamook in an early September day. It was foggy and rainy, only sprinkling. It was a long, and beautiful drive. By the time I got to Tillamook the weather cleared up. Doug welcomed me in his home. We ended up spending about half a day together with Neal joining us at the last hour of the conversation. When I got there Doug offered me coffee and showed me around the garden, they had beautiful flowers and a nice vegetable garden with volunteer pumpkins and a lot of other veggies. There was an apple tree with ripe apples and Doug gave me one to try. There was also a sobriety garden with rocks Doug used to collect from his addiction days and beautiful succulents that his wife planted. The house looked busy. I found out that Doug and his wife are foster parents. Doug also has a son who now lives with them. We sit down in the living room and start the conversation. Doug also has two small dogs who keep us entertained. I tell Doug about the purpose of my book; he asks me some questions then we begin. Doug went through drug addiction and now he is helping others as a recovery mentor peer support specialist. He had helped a lot of people. The story will go back and forth in time as Doug remembers things.

    Doug tells me about a lady he has been working with whose nephew Jim is in jail on criminal charges. Not the first time. All fueled by addition, all surrounding drug use and mental health issues. Jim is undiagnosed with his mental health problems. His mom is bipolar with extreme highs and lows. Jim experiences similar things. Jim could sleep for days or be up for days without any medications, he does things he regrets later. There is a plea agreement hearing today that Doug will be attending to support him and speak on his behalf to try to get him treatment rather than putting him in jail. We discuss jail and pros and cons of it. Doug tells me that the institutionalization that people learn while in jail becomes part of them, and they became part of a cycle.

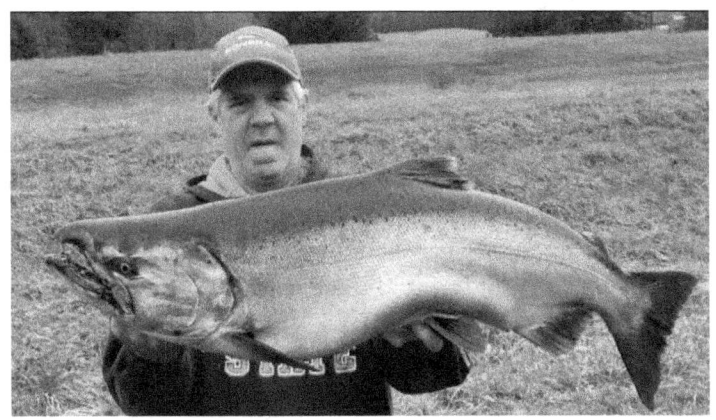

Doug with a 42" salmon

Doug gets up to show me a picture to set the stage a little. He brings in a big framed picture of the family farm. It is a huge farm with lots of buildings including houses and farm buildings for cows, and equipment and storage. The family still has this farm, it is about 600 acres. This is the farm Doug lost his inheritance to because of the drug addiction. He said those words with a heavy heart.

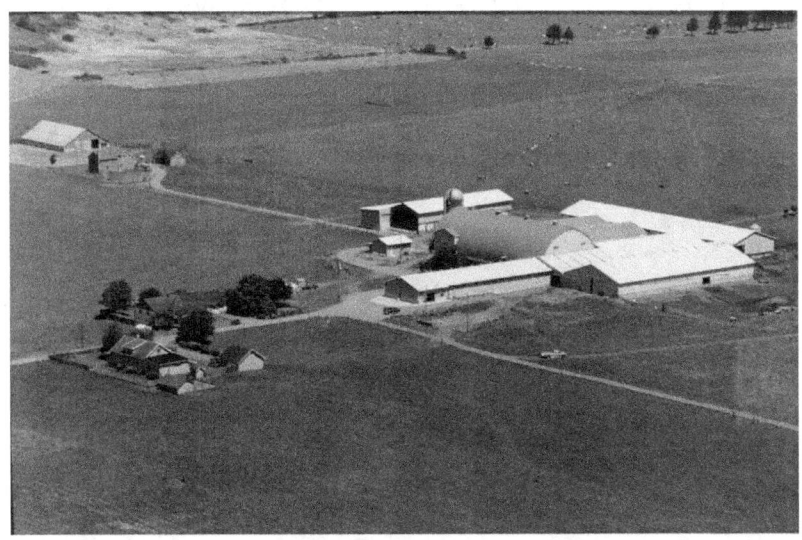

Doug's parent's family farm Tillamook, Oregon

He stole a sheet of corporate checks, the corporation is all family owned, he stole 3 checks out of the back of the book one day. He went to one of his friends with the checks to forge them. Doug had a brother Denny who was adopted just like him and who is no longer with us. There were also two cousins who were two years apart. They all grow up together on the farm. The farm was going to be theirs; they were going to run it. He stole the checks, and his friend Amber, she got into drugs too. He just thought here Amber, let's take some money. They signed out two checks one for $5,600 and one for $5,400. Doug cashed them on two consecutive days at the same bank. The second day when he came with the big check, he could see people in the bank looking at the check, comparing signatures at a desk in the back. He was starting to sweat; he was trying to stay calm. The bank personnel got on the phone, the phone rang and rang, and nobody picked it up. Ultimately, they decided it looks like Irene's signature. Better cash it and so they did. Later he was sitting in jail for some other charge, he called home and he was talking to his mom when his mom said:" hold on your father wants to talk to you". This was a surprise, his father never wanted to talk to him when he was in jail. He asked him if he is comfortable in there? The way Doug said this he made me laugh. The family got the mail and discovered the missing money. He got out of it, he did not do any jail time, his grandmother forgave him. His grandmother told him, don't do this again, honey. She lived to be 101 years old. He stops to show me pictures of family.

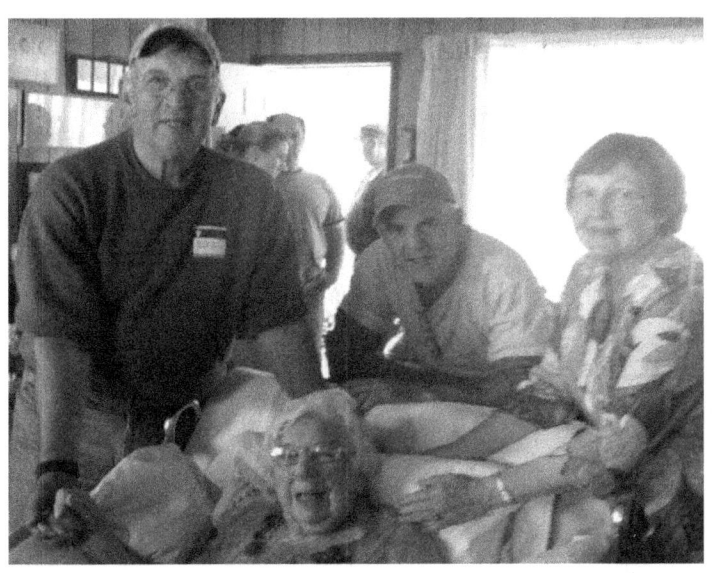

Doug and his parents with Irene his grandmother at age 101

I am seeing a beautiful picture of 3-year-old girl with lots of curls in her hair. Doug tells me the story behind the picture. Sounds like it was a wonderful camping trip. She will be going back to her parents soon. Next, Doug shows me pictures of his son and another previous foster boy. He was actually adopted by his sister in Spokane. He became from his foster son to his nephew. He shows me more pictures of foster kids. They are in a process of trying to adopt one of the foster kids. He shows me a video of one of the girls singing. I could see how much Doug loves the kids. Doug tells me some difficult stories about a foster child mom and her behavior. It is hard to hear, and it is difficult for Doug to tell. The mom of the little girl has been trying to undermine all the good Doug and his wife Tiffany been working towards for about 4 years. Her mom would tell lies to the little girl like Doug and Tiffany tackled her mom and took her from her mom that is why she was living with Doug and Tiffany. The little girl would tell them all the bad things her mom would say about Tiffany.

We circle back to Doug's story. I ask him how things started. He was adopted at an early age and given every opportunity to succeed. He was two weeks old. He grew up on a dairy farm. He had everything he wanted. He had a beautiful family, he had a job, life was great. He was very athletic in his youth, he loved football, basketball, baseball. He loved fishing and hunting. He calls fishing and hunting his passion. Growing up he had the opportunity to go fishing any time. He started working early, when he turned old enough to drive, he bought his first car. 1979 z28 Camaro. He tells me he first got stoned when he was in 6th grade. It was peer pressure; they were hanging out with some older boys. He was just wanted to try marijuana. He did not get into the hard stuff for quite some time, not until high school. They smoked a little pot, they also did it to be stupid, to be goofy. Drugs would not become a habit for a while. In the summers he would go to sports camps. He really liked it. Doug was popular in school. In high school, he is well known. Tillamook is a small coastal town, and everyone knows everyone. He tells me he was related to half of the town and just knows the other half. He had a cousin who was his ideal growing up, he wanted to be like him. He started to hang out with an older crowd at times. All of his cousin's friends were also his friends, they were in the same group. His cousin was 4 years older than him. He tells me stuff about football. Doug got into high school and started to smoke a lot of pot. He would buy it, he would smoke it, he would sell it. This was the time when a lot of weekend and partying began. As a consequence, Doug's grades started to slip. In his sophomore year he was training in track. He never pushed himself at track, he never really pushed himself for anything, he was naturally gifted. Doug easily made friends with others. He ran the high hurdles; he ran 100 yards. He ran this one specific high hurdle at a relay meet where he ran a very good time. He practiced a little, they went to St Helen's high school and he broke the school record. His head started to swell a little. He started to skip 1st and 5th period, smoking pot, working at the farm. He had not thought much about the future.

    Growing up on the dairy farm they had a lot of state cops that would go to their place and go fishing. He hung around a lot with them during the fishing season and thought that fish and game cop would be cool. He thought about it as a career option. As a junior Doug was getting a lot of letters of scholarships from big colleges across the nation who recruiting for track athletes. He was in the 7th place in track at that time in the state of Oregon. Recruiters would show up at the meets. He liked the effects of pot, he could smoke some and check out, forget about everything. This was a turning point in his life. His girlfriend at that time was a statistician for the high school track team. They had a fight. Danny wanted to show her, and he hooked up with a buddy from the track team to smoke some pot. Doug did not run his preliminaries yet. They got stoned. He gets back from his preliminary race the gun goes off and he was stuck, he was high, all the other guys were way ahead, he did not qualify to go to state. He was using pot not to feel. He wanted to escape how his girlfriend made him feel. He was mad. This cycle continued. Half through his senior year the athletic director called him into his office. He told Doug that his attendance record is not good enough to graduate and he will need to attend night school. Doug asked if he can still play sports. He was told no, not with OSAA rules. Doug dropped out of high school and went to work on the farm. His little brother was 2 years younger than him. He was wiry, he was a really good worker. That summer there was at a party at Tusk river park. It was early afternoon; Doug and his friends were playing horseshoes in the sun. Doug was working at a fish plant in Garibaldi at this time. He is been on and off working on their dairy farm as well. His brother Denny surprised him when he come to visit him with a friend.

Denny's accident

Denny had a little Toyota pickup and also brought his motorcycle up to the park. His brother was drunk so Doug took the motorcycle from him and told him when he needs a ride, he will find him a ride, he cannot drive. It was a very windy road right next to the river. 15 minutes later Denny fired up his pickup and took off from the park. In about 15 -20 minutes one of their friends come back screaming that Denny wrecked his car. Everyone jumped in the back of a pickup and headed to find Denny. Denny went off the road about 150 feet, his pickup turned upside down, his knees were up to his ears. It was like he was sitting on the cab of the pickup. He missed a corner and flew off sideways. The pickup landed on top of him. He was conscious when Doug got there. They tried to push the truck off of Denny. It did not work. By this time the paramedics showed up, they got there quick were up at the park at another event and heard what had happened.

    The paramedics freed Denny out of the wreck and got him up to the ambulance. Doug and his friends were helping to clean up other stuff like Denny's motorcycle. The paramedic who was a friend told Doug that he might want to go down with them it is pretty bad. His brother told him: "I am sorry, I can't feel my legs". He kept saying that he is sorry and that it hurts. It is still hard for Doug to tell this story; it brings up a lot of emotions. I can hear it on his tone and see it on his face. He describes his brother as someone who had never complained of pain before. Denny passed out during the ride. When they arrived at the hospital his parents were already there. Doug went into the chapel and prayed for his little brother. Next, he noticed that the helicopter came, and life flighted Denny out, they took him to Portland. Denny was paralyzed from the waist down for the rest of his life.

    3 days later Doug went to see Denny. He was in a rotating bed with his head strapped down. Doug lost it in there. He felt that at that moment he had to grow up. His dad and mom had to spend a lot of time at the hospital. He went back to work on the farm. It was a long process for Denny's recovery and Doug started to use more and more drugs. He started to use cocaine, crank, crystal meth, pain pills, whatever he could get his hands on. He stayed away from heroin; he did not like to see what it had done to his friends. He did end up trying heroin a few times, he never took to it. Doug felt that sitting in the easy chair nodding off did not seem like fun. His brother went through this rehabilitation and surgery where they put rods in his back. The rods were screwed together to fuse Denny's backbone. A few years later the rods were taken out. Denny went back and worked at the farm; the family got hand-controlled tractors. Denny bought a 4-wheeler that was all hand controlled. He started to live a somewhat normal life. In Doug's life at this point the farm paid his rent and insurance and his paycheck went to drugs and alcohol.

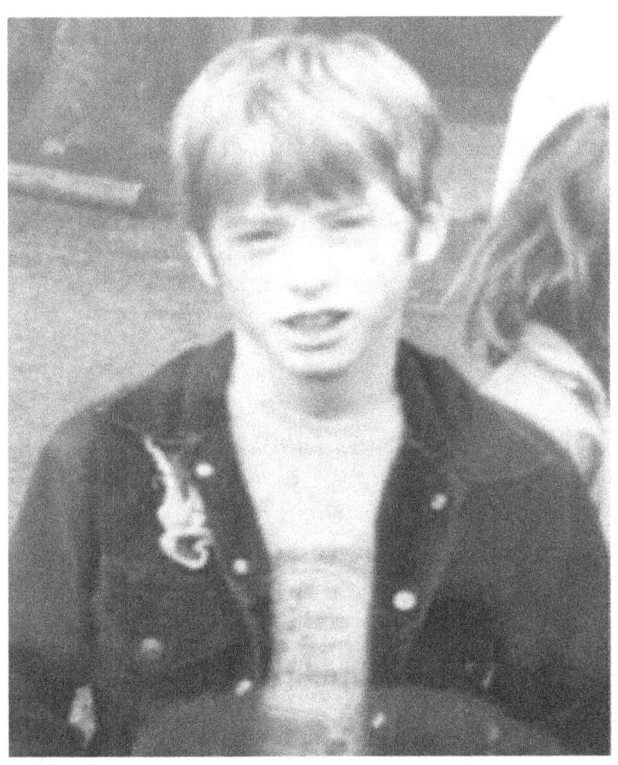

Doug's brother Denny in grade school

Doug started to do a lot of traveling and soul searching. He describes his grandmother as his rock. Doug started to move around a lot, he had been all over the country, he describes this as was running from himself. The first time he did cocaine he was a freshman in high school. There was a party by a river and most of the boys were about 4 years older than Doug. He was called into a room with a bunch of guys and one of them handed him a straw for a cocaine and asked him if he wanted to try it. He said ok. He hated it. He liked the taste of it, the numbness and he hated the uncomfortableness in his own skin. He could not sleep; he drove around the farm all night long. He hated life. Then he had to get up at 5:30 am to change irrigation pipes. He was raised in the church, in 6th grade he had this little bar for 7 years of perfect attendance to Sunday school. His dad said at that time that if the boys do not want to go to Sunday school they don't have to go.

This is when they then went to the farm working and Doug started to smoke pot. This could be a coincidence in timing, and it might not be.

Sometime between 1982-1985 Doug sold a cow. Doug tells me about raising cows. He knows everything someone needs to know about cows, how to raise them, take care of them. His first cow's name was: Round Oak Red Apple Elevation Linda. His cow Linda went on to be the top producing 2-year-old for milk and butter fat. Doug still sounds pretty proud talking about his first cow. Linda was a grand champion and a state champion. Doug sold her when she got a little older and he got $5,200 for her on an auction after commission. Getting that much money for Doug at that time was not a good thing. He and his buddy took off on an 11-day binge and spent all that money on drugs, alcohol, gas and motels. He ended up in Seaside, Oregon at a bar. Later he found himself at a friend's house. The next morning, he realized that he is about $500 overdrawn on his account, he had no gas, no cigarettes, no cash, he was hungry, and he had no way to get back to Tillamook. His friend told him, tell you what you come and check this place out and I get you breakfast and cigarettes; and send you on your way. He was still hung over and in a daze. They got some cigarettes; they stop for breakfast then pull up in front of this place which was a drug and alcohol treatment center. They pull up and people come out greeting him, hi, you must be Doug. Doug was looking at his girlfriend who had this big smile on her face. This was an intervention. She told him that he promised he will check the place out. He goes in and the treatment personnel showed him around. At this point Doug's wheels started to turn in his head. He was thinking he just spent $5,200 how will he explain this to his parents. He thought, oh, I am an alcoholic, I stay here for 30 days then I get back to the good grace of family and friends. He did the treatment there. That was Doug's first treatment center and for the next 30 years addiction become his life. About every 10 years he would find a new drug and a new way to use it until he would get to the desperate place where he was done. His second treatment center was in 1995.

Doug would work in various places, he traveled across the eastern states selling an all-purpose cleaner with a traveling sales company. He was living well, traveling, going to hotels, smoking pot, going to high rises, he was making good money. He was making

$2000 per week. He gave up selling the cleaner. Doug ended up in San Antonio with this guy and they were digging ditches for footers for foundations in a mobile home park. They did it by hand. They made big money. One day Doug and his work friend went to his friend's dad house. The dad was a major drunk. He came out the front door and with a gun in his hand. He shot the gun 2 times, click, click Doug recalls, the gun did not go off. The gun was aimed at Doug's head. It was very lucky that the gun did not go off. Doug looks at this as one of those things in life a chance, where the situation could have gone very wrong. He could have died that day. Doug has a little trouble staying on track. I tell him it is ok. Doug reflects that during his addiction the only people he stole from was his family. His parents bought a safe to put all their valuables in because Doug would go through pockets, steal his dad's rifles to support his habit. At one point in time Doug had a pickup truck, a 4-wheeler, he had a huge collection of hunting rifles and shotguns; he had it made. He tells me slowly but surely, he started to sell off everything he owned. At some point in his addiction he ended up in Alaska in a lodge in the 1990's, he was growing pot and was hunting and fishing with a buddy. He got a job to fish with people even with some very famous people who stayed at this 5-star lodge. Working up there was one of the most amazing experiences in Doug's life. He loved it. Catching fish all they long.

  He came back to Oregon, and sometime there he started to use cocaine intravenously. He tells me it was one of those things, somebody he sold pot too was also an IV drug user. He sold him a little coke one day and they were "banging it with heroin". This is called a speed ball. He was like, no thank you. Until he had a very bad day, and he wanted to get really high, he told this guy: Dude, fix me up a hit no heroin just coke. He showed Doug how to do it. He had a whole bunch of coke; he was living by himself. Doug had some weird experiences. One time he was watching a TV screen and he just "banged a big old hit of coke" and his TV come to life. What he had seen in that TV was his life, he saw an ambulance pull up on his driveway he saw people get out with a stretcher, he was hearing language from emergency room. Emergency personnel picked him up, he still had the belt and the needle in his arm. EMT pulled the needle out of his arm and placed him on the stretcher and hauled him off.

Then he was back on the couch where he was. He was like; "what the f*** did I just see? "he made a decision after this experience to stop using. He took all his paraphernalia and dope out to the burn barrel, soaked it in lighter fluid and burned everything.

Doug called a friend from Portland who he helped get sober previously. He needed help. He asked his friend and his wife if he could come and stay with them a few days, he wanted to find a treatment center. They said:" come on up". Doug checked into his second treatment center in Newberg, this was around 1995. After that treatment he stayed clean and sober for about 18 months.

Doug tells me about crank that is form of speed. He did not like crank he did it only for a little while. It was a methamphetamine. Back then someone would strip batteries and make methamphetamine. Methamphetamine was made in bathtubs. It was an un-pure form of speed. Nowadays, crystal meth is the "shit". Doug started to do some methamphetamines here and there. He did not like snorting it, it burned like a "Son of a bitch". He could stay up on the meth for days. Somebody showed him how to smoke it, then he thought: yeah, this is my baby". Doug would smoke the meth and get very high. People showed him how to make a pipe out of a light bulb, how to make a pipe out of a piece of glass. He tells me that there is so much of his life he cannot account for. He has no clue; it is a fog. He does not know where he was or what he was doing. He made a name for himself in Tillamook it was not Doug Beeler but Doug Dealer. His mom and dad started to drop out social events. They got tired of people asking how Doug and Denny were doing. His brother also battled his own demons.

Somewhere around 2003 or 2004 Doug got a letter from Alaska. A friend of Doug's just got a motel in Anchorage. They asked Doug to manage the hotel one of his friends was going to be a handy man at the motel. They were all ready to go when they got turned back at the Canadian border because they both were felons. It was one of the scariest thing Doug ever been through. In the blazer they had 2 pounds of pot, a bunch of meth, paraphernalia. They were getting high all the way there. They did not realize what they are going to get into in the Canadian border. They give them their ID's they handed them back and pulled them aside for inspection. Doug and his friend thought they are done and going to prison. About 2.5 hour later the inspector let them go. Doug and his friend could not cross the border because DUI's considered felonies in Canada. The border patrol inspector did not find the drugs. Doug come back home to Tillamook. I ask Doug where the drugs were hidden. He tells me all over the place, under the floorboards, in plumbing tools, bags, it was a long time ago, he did not remember all the hiding places. The Alaska trip never happened. Luckily, they did not go to prison that day.

Doug was back in Tillamook for a month when he got a letter in the mail. It was from a woman who was looking for her brother. Her brother was adopted from Portland Oregon. Doug's mom remembered his birth mom's maiden name which was the same one this young women wrote. Doug just found out he had a sister. They talked on the phone and his sister said ok, I am coming to meet you I will be there in 8 hours. They met in Salem. At the time Doug was a 140 lb. He had sores all over his body, he had started shooting up crystal meth and crank. Doug did not like himself very much. He would get loaded and check out. People who he hangs out with were acquaintances. He hot into IV meth use by selling drugs and he just could not escape by smoking or snorting anymore he needed something more.

"My life was a big giant wave behind me that was continuously growing and getting ready to crash on me"- Doug

When Doug was telling me about this feeling, I imagined the waves crushing behind him. A few weeks later my daughter was asking me what to paint. I told her I would like a painting for the book with dark waves on the beach. She created the painting below. Now, I look at this painting and think of Doug and the crushing dark waves that were chasing him.

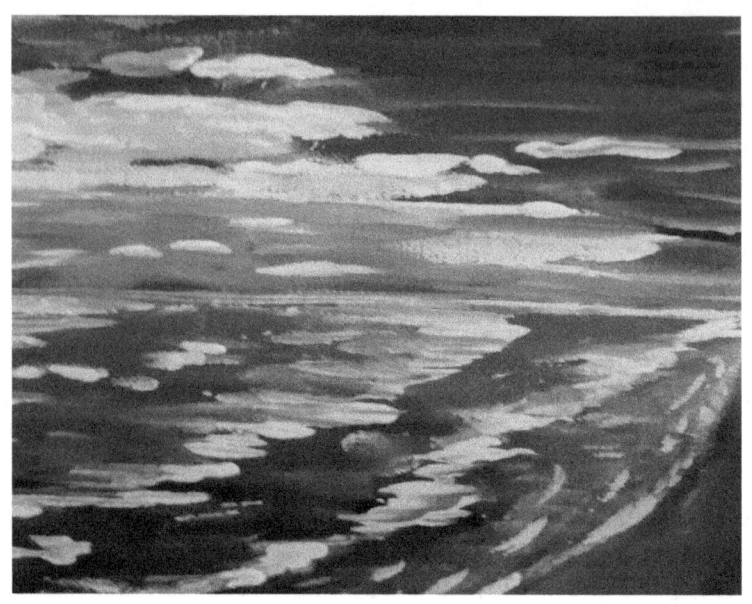

Waves – acrylic painting by Andrea Mihaly 2019

He could feel it. He felt the weight of his life and was looking for a new drug to outrun his life. He did not want to face life; he did not want to be crushed by it again. A "junkie" a friend of his who is now clean fixed him up with a small dose of IV meth and Doug was in love with it. We jump back to 2001 when he is telling me about a time when he was up for 14 days and he was driving back from Sandy Oregon he fell asleep by the wheel and hit a tree with 70 mile/hr. He remembers nothing about the trip. He was driving an old ford pickup. He remembers lifting his head seeing the sky and the outline of the tree. Next thing he remembers was an outline of a hand. The truck kind of turned into a horseshoe.

Doug survived with 4 stitches and a sprained thumb. He walked away. He tells me that his mom and a lot of friends been praying for him because of where he was in his life. Doug truly believes that God sent him an angel to save him that day. One of many times he adds. The gun story he told me before he believes that that was an act of God too. He woke up in the hospital with a drug nurse sitting in the hospital next to him. He had needle tracks all over his arms. She was telling him that he needs to go to treatment, he got a list of AA meetings, NA meetings and all the list of things they found in his system. His mom came and got him. He went home and continued his life of addiction until he got that letter from his sister. He did not really want to meet his sister. He was really excited that he has a sister, he called up a buddy and wanted to celebrate and went to the liquor store to get ingredients for a drink called dog farts. It is made from Baileys and cream, Kahlua and another drink; pour in the shot glass and layer it. He also picked up some meth and picked up some pot. His friend came over and stayed 3-4 hours then he went home. It was now 11pm and the next day he is supposed to meet his sister. He is trying to find this happy medium where he is comfortable. Not really high, not really drunk.

Doug was searching for something; he was so uncomfortable in his own skin. He tells me he smelled like "cat piss". A byproduct that the body produces it is like a formaldehyde from using meth. He had all these sores and the meth coming out smelling like urea. He was wondering why anyone would want to meet him. He got to the meeting place early and he went to one of his Indian buddies in the area who he knew for a long time. They were smoking pot and drinking, Doug was out of meth, he was really high. He told his friend; he cannot go to meet his sister. Doug was 5 minutes away. His friend chewed him out and told him he needs to go and meet his sister; she just drove 8 hours to meet him and has been looking for him for years. He made a big cup of alcohol and on his way over there he spilled all over him. Now he smelled like alcohol and looked like shit.

He pulls up next to this little blue car, they are hugging and crying and then somewhere in a middle of this Doug's sister steps back turns him around and said: "honey I like you to meet your birth mother". He did not even know somebody else was in the car. They found a quiet side logging road, put out a blanket, they chat for a while. His sister had to go back home, they made plans for Doug to go up and visit. His sister also had another brother and Doug met him as well as his sister's two kids when he went up to visit. Doug found out that he was a byproduct of a one-night stand. His mother was not willing to talk about it. Doug left Tillamook, OR on the 2nd of July to go there and did not get to Spokane, WA until the 4th. He would drive a few hours then stop to get high. When Doug got to Spokane he realized after that his truck had big leak of green liquid under it. He had blown both of the truck's head gaskets. He drove the truck to his sister's house and parked it. It was going to be 2 months before it can get fixed. He just had a little pot with him, he was coming down from the meth. His sister was talking to his parents in the background about getting Doug into treatment. She found a treatment place for him Sundown River Ranch in WA. He tells me it was the best treatment center he had ever been through. This was in 2004. This was his 3rd treatment. He was on the Sundown ranch for about 60 days. He had a few come to Jesus meetings there with his parents.

Doug's parents would come up every other week from Tillamook for family meetings. It was one of those times where he first seen his dad cry. His dad told Doug that he pretty much gave up hope.

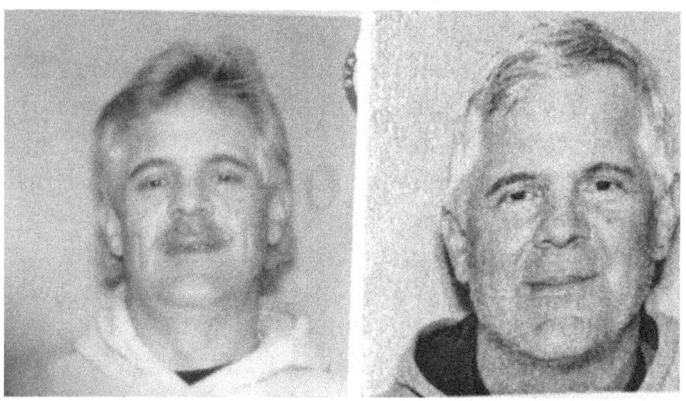

Doug 30 day sober in 2007 and 10 years sober in 2017

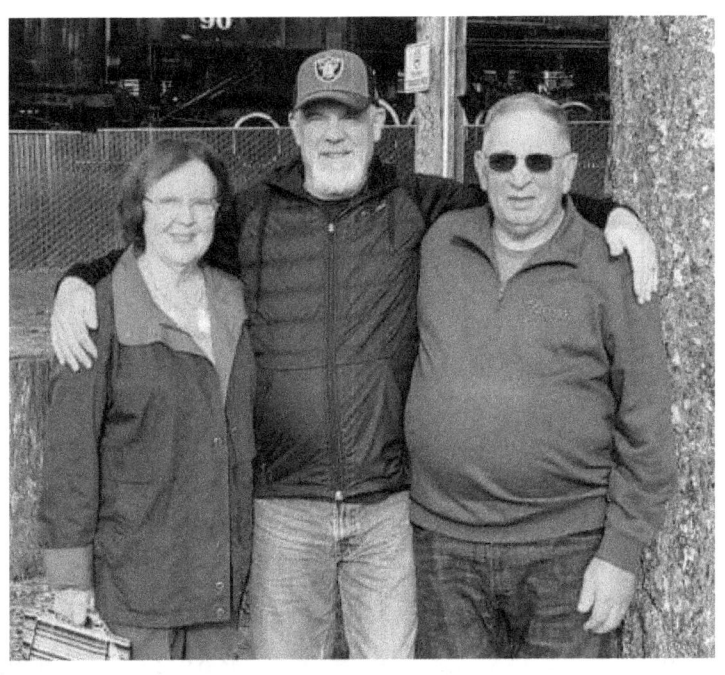

Doug with his parents in 2018

Doug started to do some of the recovery work. His truck got fixed a few weeks later. He decided to stay up at his sister's house. His sister's kids were little at the time. The way he talks about them I can see he loves them very much. All the sudden he was Uncle Doug. Doug always wanted a sister growing up and now he got one. His new family came down to Tillamook to meet his mom and dad and the rest of his family. His birth mom at that time was still not ready to tell Doug who his real father was. He did find out who he was about 6 months ago. He stayed with his sister for a while, he went to meetings every day at noon in downtown Spokane, he got a job at a dairy farm. Doug could do anything when it came to cows, they were really happy with him at the farm. He took care of 60 cows which was easy for him compared to the 400 he was used to take care of. He had a nice routine. He came back one time to Tillamook and met a girl. She went back to Spokane with him. He ended up having to get out of his sister's house because of her Christian believes conflicted with Doug spending a night with a girl when they were not married. She felt this was the wrong example to her kids. They ended up staying in a motel for a while. In December they had a child together. Keenen. He lives with Doug now. For one week he could not find a motel room because there was a big AA convention in town. They ended up going back to Tillamook. This was not a good choice. Doug started to use again, and his life went downhill again very fast. I asked Doug why he think the relapse was? He tells me he forgot where he come from. **"I forgot those moments of incomprehensible demoralization of mind and body"**. He forgot that he hated his life when he was using. He forgot where his addiction had taken him before. He forgot how and why to stay clean. He let his situation get the best of him. He did not want to feel. He did not want to have a kid at that time. He went down the path of addiction again. Doug cannot remember what he started doing when he came back home. His brother Denny was getting sick.

Denny's death

Denny started to spike temperatures shortly after Doug moved back home. It began as 98F, then jumped to 101F, 105F, 108F. They did not know initially what is going on, they could not find the problem. They put Denny in an oxygen chamber. Doctors could not get the fever to stop. Finally, they have run an MRI on Denny's whole body. They found a ½ inch screw in the middle of his lower back that the doctor forgot to remove when they removed the rods. The doctors went back to the surgery note it said that the screw was lost. Denny went into surgery. They opened his back open and there was a softball size of gangrene (dead body tissue) they cleaned out as much as they could but there was no technology to remove that dead tissue. His brother was told that they could send him to Mexico put maggots in there and thy would eat it all down to the diseased tissue. Then the maggots would leave, they could graph and close him up. His brother said no. He ended up contracting meningitis and died. This was in 2005. Denny before his death found out that Doug was an IV drug user and he wanted nothing that he wanted to do with him. His brother would tell him that he was a piece of shit, wasting his life, he had 2 good legs, good parents, throwing his life away and kicked him out he did not want to see Doug. This was the last time Doug saw his brother.

Doug was living in the basement of his parents' house with his dog Mojo. His daily routine was to pick up a little drug here and there. He used up every relationship he'd ever been in, nobody trusted him anymore. In April 13, 2006 he was sitting at a riverbank waiting for his shipment of meth to come over. He is been 4 days dope sick. He was strictly and IV user of meth at this time. He got a phone call that Denny was experiencing renal failure and probably will not survive.

Denny was rushed to the hospital in Portland. Doug chose to sit on the riverbank while his brother went to the hospital and passed away. This is still a very hard memory for Doug. His voice is very emotional. The pain on his face is very visible. 3 days later he went to see his brother in the funeral home. He wrote a letter to Denny saying he loved him and asked him for forgiveness. Doug put it into Denny's shirt pocket. Denny was buried with the letter. From that point of April 13, 2006 to May 8, 2007 Doug had tried to end his life by overdose. He knew if he would end his life he would not go to heaven. He saw the pain his brother's death caused to his parents. He felt responsible. He felt that the pain was also caused by him. He had seen the pain in his mother's eyes. His dad would not look him in the eye. He would just get up in the morning and go out to the field. He had a warrant out for his arrest at that time, he had drug charges of felony possession, failure to appear in court x2, could have been that thrown out of court, but he could not stay sober long enough to go to court. His attorney dropped him. He got a public defender. He made a deal. He wanted his hunting privileges back. His bargain was that if he completed 3 years of formal probation, he would get misdemeanors instead of the felonies.

Getting Clean

May 8, 2007, Doug just went through 11 days of hell kicking the needle and the spoon. He had a little pot. He hated himself, he hated what he was doing to his parents. He smoked a little pot for the nausea. May 8, he came out of the basement. He turned right which was opposite to his normal routine. He picked up the phone and dialed this phone number that he somehow memorized and still knows today. It was his buddy's parent's house. His buddy answered the phone. His buddy was getting ready to go to an NA meeting. Doug asked him to pick him up. He was there in 5 minutes. He was telling Doug that he was 2 years clean that day. Doug cried like a baby- his words. Doug wanted the pain to go away, he wanted to stop hurting. Doug's voice is still emotional talking about this.

He went to his first meeting again. By that time, he been in 100s of meetings before, he started meetings in his county. He would always fall away; he would forget where he came from. He truly believes in his heart today that God used his brother's death as a vehicle to get him sober. He tells me that he should not be here, but he is. He is not sure why. He feels like God thought he could be saved. He started to go to meetings and his first two years he went to every meeting he could find. He got a sponsor. He tells me that his sobriety date should have been May 8, 2007 but he had to learn two important lessons.

He needed to learn to change his phone number and to quit hanging out with people who used.

He one day went to a river with someone. He liked to collect rocks. He tells me he was a rock hound anything shiny he brought home. They went fishing one day. He was 12 days clean he told his buddy he does not want to be around drugs. He told him it is fine he won't bring any. They are fishing and in about 15 minutes his buddy tells him that he thinks he locked his keys in the Jeep. He told Doug he will be right back, and he took off. Doug knew it was not true. He knew exactly what his buddy was doing. Doug went up to him and told him: you better have enough for me. Doug smoked some meth. He hated it. He tells me the way it makes me chuckle: "There is nothing worse than a head full of NA and a body full of meth". Doug wanted so bad to stay clean. He went back to a meeting and admitted his use. Got back on track. He went back to going to two meetings a day. When he had a bad day, he would call his sponsor and spend a day with him at his construction work, so he won't be alone. He would hang out at the job site. He had another relapse in between there.

One of his friends called him to go to the island on the river where they used to go, there is a picnic ground there. He wanted to have crack cocaine. He tells me: you rock up some cocaine and smoke it on steel wool. Doug did not even think about it he met him down there 15 minutes later he is down there on the island, smoking crack cocaine, he is hating life about that time and his mom walks down to the island as they were all sitting there with this crack cocaine. His mom ended up leaving, Doug hated it. This was around June 2007. Doug did not feel comfortable in his own skin. He met with his sponsor a few days later and admitted his use. He picked a new sobriety date. It was the next day June 13th of 2007. Interestingly his brother Denny was born on the 13th and passed away on the 13th and Doug got sober on the 13th he feels now this was all God's plan. Big sigh from Doug, this is still difficult to share, his voice rattles. His mind even goes blank. He forgot what he was going to say next. I reassure him it is ok.

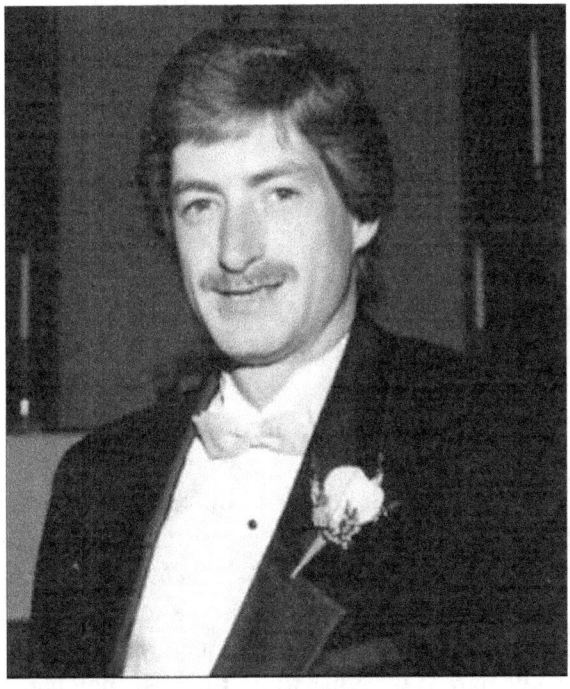

Denny on his wedding day

Doug started to work at a recycling and trucking business in town. It was still hard he would wake up every day and all he could think about is getting loaded. He knew he needed something because all he could think about is getting loaded all day long. He was uncomfortable. Doug started praying every morning. He was praying to remove the desire, the obsession, the compulsion, the thought to use. He used the AA book and read the prayer on page 63 every morning before his feet hit the floor. He did everything his sponsor asked him to do. He did not want to be f***ing be there no more, he was willing to do whatever it takes not to go back to using. He tells me the prayer he started to recite every morning. See prayer below:

"God, I offer myself to Thee - to build with me and to do with me as Thou wilt. Relieve me of the bondage of self, that I may better do Thy will. Take away my difficulties, that victory over them may bear witness to those I would help of Thy Power, Thy Love, and Thy Way of life. May I do Thy will always!"

This prayer become a part of Doug's morning routine. He started to believe a higher power. He did not have a name for it yet. He got involved with celebrate recovery. He shows me some of his tattoos. Doug has a scripture on his back. He got involved in a county program called healthy families and that is where he met Neal again. Doug got invited into the schools to talk to the kids. The idea was to bring awareness to the schools. He has now been doing this for 12 years and he loves it, he goes 3 times a year and talks to 8th grade kids and tell them his story. He had many good relationships with the kids. We discuss going into 6th grade for prevention. We discuss where the problems start. He asks me if I think it starts at home. He tells me he thinks it is one parent families, he seen that a lot in his practice. He feels those kids don't have enough guidance, counseling and supervision. Their parent is trying to do the best they can and working

10-hour days and the kids where are those kids he asks me. No accountability.

Doug got recommended to participate in an educational video that shares his story about meth use with Partnership for Drug Free America. They made 2 anti-meth commercials out of Doug's story. This was around 2011. He tells me about the commercials. Since Doug got clean and sober, he rebuilt the relationship with his mom and dad. He met his wife at a church. His wife is a schoolteacher. He tells me how they met. Very sweet story. It started as occasional texting until one day he accidently hit the call button. He ended the call then she called him back. I burst out laughing because Doug makes these funny sounds like someone who does not know what to say. It went something like this: ah, ba da bah. He shows me a picture of his wife. It is a beautiful picture. Doug does some show and tell with pictures. He shows me some pictures of his son too. He showed me a picture of his wife that had won a first prize on the Tillamook fair. The theme was:" magic in the air with the County Flair". It was the best use of the Fair theme out of all entries. It was quite of honor for him and there is a great story behind the picture related to the little girl who they like to adopt and her love for the wishy weeds.

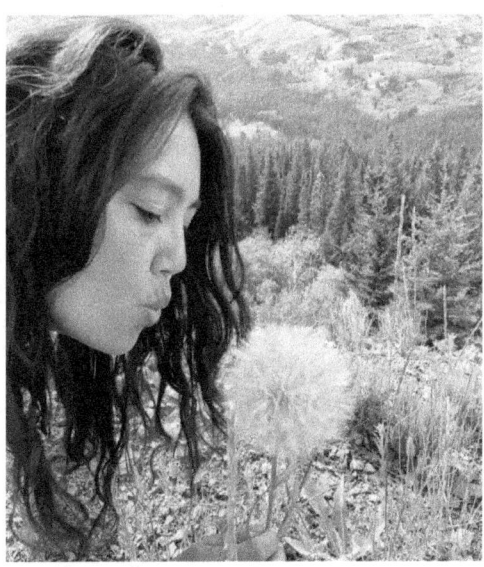

Doug's wife Tiffany in the picture: Magic in the air

Road to current job

"From hopeless Dopefiend to Dope less Hopefiend" - Doug

Doug currently works as a peer support specialist and recovery mentor. He has been helping a lot of people. Prior he was working at the recycling plant. Doug tells me in a horrible tooth pain he had in the first day of his job. He was already labeled as a drug seeker. He was in so much pain. He had remembered prayer; he said a prayer and the pain went away. He got the job. He worked there for 9.5 years. After that he wanted a better job. He met his wife, got married. He wanted more. He wanted to travel and live his life again that would not work from $13.50 per hour. He had a friend call him from Tillamook family counseling she told him about a job as a peers support specialist. Doug did not want to work in an office which was perfect because this was not an office job. He checked out the job and what it entailed. He was not sure first. Then his wife behind his back goes online and applied for him. He had not heard back for a long time he thought they had hired somebody else. He finally got a call for an interview. They offered him a job. He started part time and build up his clients within a year he become a full-time employee. Doug loves what he does. It is a hard job; it can be exhausting. He also gets calls from the community to help out. He tries to leave work at work. This is hard he gets attached.

One of his clients called him last night telling him he got a job. Doug was very happy for him, getting a job was a big deal for him. He has been volunteering at the same place and they finally figured out how to put him on the payroll. Very nice news to get. Doug just could hear his smile and excitement through the phone that he is the member of the work force again. It is huge for him. Doug also works on the ACT team. He co-facilitates a group twice a week. It is an EIRM group. Enhanced Individual Recovery Module it is part of the ACT program. There are about 8-10 men in the group. They meet twice a week for about 2 hours. Doug tells me how rewarding his job is, he feels getting money for it is a bonus. He loves to engage with clients and building trust. He tells me about a client who only comes in to talk to Doug she does not trust anybody else. Gaining someone's trust is so rewarding in itself he tells me. Doug gets up to get coffee. Doug cannot imagine his life being anywhere else then where it is today. Doug made it this far and was able to make a full recovery. He has so much to offer others who are going through similar things he experiences in his life. He really knows how it is because he had been there.

    Doug starts to tell me about his son. About 5 years ago he got endangered custody of him. His mom was living in the woods. They had a lot of police contact and a lot of drug activity. He went for custody and he won. A little sidetrack Neal just texted checking in I had plans to meet with him after and go over things about the book and his story. Doug said just have him come and meet here. Doug wanted to see him. Neal agreed. Neal's wife Karen was one of Doug's high school teachers. Doug tells me that addiction when he was in it took away all his morals and values: "Had me by the balls, I had no way out, it took everything I had". He was happy that his grandmother got to see him clean and sober before she passed. She lived to be 101 years and 7 days old. Doug got to hold her hand when she passed. He feels that through many of the hard times his grandma was his rock. In her will he left nothing for Doug his cousins got the farm. It was not his inheritance anymore.

    When Doug first got sober it was very hard for him to drive by the farm. He likes to work with animals in the farm. There is just something about working with them he adds. He likes to take friends and show them the animals and go to picnic and fishing to the property. Doug tells me that he would love to show me the farm one day. He tells me all wonderful things about his mother. Doug shows me a picture of the farm and tells me about the details where his cousins lives, things about the farm. Showed me where his grandmother used to live and how the roads go. He showed me where his parent's house is. Doug has a big family, when they get together for Thanksgiving, they have about 50 people. Neal arrived. The dogs started to bark. Doug invites Neal in and offers him coffee. From this point on Neal joins us for the rest of the interview. We take a break, have a nice conversation, Neal and Doug catch up, then we start the interview again.

Doug's Birth Family

Doug tells me that about 2 years ago his mom got him an ancestry kit. Doug's birthmother finally opened up about wanting to help locate who was Doug's birth father. Dough's birthmother recalled that his name was Ray and that he owned a hardware store in Spokane. He was thinking there is not enough information to go on and it probably did not happen. He was not sure about doing the DNA kit first. He did the kit and got the results. Doug is not very good at computers and searching pages. He figured out that nobody really close showed up in the match. He would look some of the matches up that were farther away from his DNA, and they were not related. He forgot about the DNA test for a while. He hopped back on the website about 6 months ago and there was a message from a girl who was 3 degrees off from Doug. This would be a sister or a first cousin. Doug sent her a message. He was not even sure that he did it right.

About 3 months ago Doug saw that she responded. She told Doug that who her dad was Ray and she grew up in Spokane, WA. Ray passed away in 2007. He spent the last 9.5 years of his life in a care facility. He never got to meet his birthfather. Doug gained another sister. It is amazing that Doug always wanted a sister and now he has two. Actually 3. There is another sister who was adopted out from another of Ray's acquaintances he adds. She is in Salt Lake City. His sister Sally lives in Seattle, Doug from Tiffany's side have family in Seattle as well. He found out about an aunt in Vancouver and an uncle in Spokane. Doug and Tiffany took a week off and went to Vancouver where they had met his aunt who had all kinds of stories about Ray. Ray was a brilliant artist. He was accepted to the fine arts school in San Francisco right after high school. He did not go; he chose to stick a needle in his arm instead. Now Doug had some answers. Doug had a genetic addiction component that he did not know playing against him. Doug was looking up pictures to show us from his Trip to Seattle and Neal asked him what he thinks how big of a role genetics played in his addiction. Doug said good question, then he got distracted with the pictures. The pictures are from a month and a half ago Doug and his sister looks so happy that they found each other. Doug noticed a lot of similarities with his sister, she can't sit still, moves constantly, her little mannerisms was just like Doug's. Doug's sister was coming down to Tillamook ironically, she had other family in the area as well. It just happened to be Doug's family's reunion, so Doug invited her. Doug met some more cousins who he did not know about.

    There is another component he did not know people he was related to in Tillamook through his birth mother as well he found out he had some cousins. His birth mom grew up in a very religious family. When she got pregnant her dad was not happy, her mother rescued her and took her to Portland to the white shield house to have her baby. She had to give up her baby. Doug was adopted through the Waverly children's home. His birth mom went back to Spokane. While she was pregnant with Doug, she made a little blue knitted heat and booties and his mom had them in a hope chest. When his sister found Doug in 2004, she showed them to Doug. Now it is in Doug's hope chest. Doug's second sister Sally's mom left Ray when she found out how abusive he was when he was loaded. Ray was also using drugs when he met Doug's mom and Doug's mom was also partying. Doug got double genetics leading him toward addiction. No wonder he had such a hard time coming out of addictions. Neal sighs. When Doug first met his birthmother up in Spokane when his sister was not there, he was smoking pot and drinking beer with his mother. He shows us some more pictures. Doug does not know if Ray knew Doug existed. Doug shows me a picture of his mom and dad. His dad looks tough. Neal tells me Doug's dad is a marshmallow inside. Doug looks at me and said: "Today, Gabriella, my Dad hugs me with two hands and tells me he loves me". He showed me a picture of Denny. Silence in the room for a moment. Big sigh from Neal and Doug. Doug lost a brother and gained 3 sisters and a lot of other family he did not knew about.

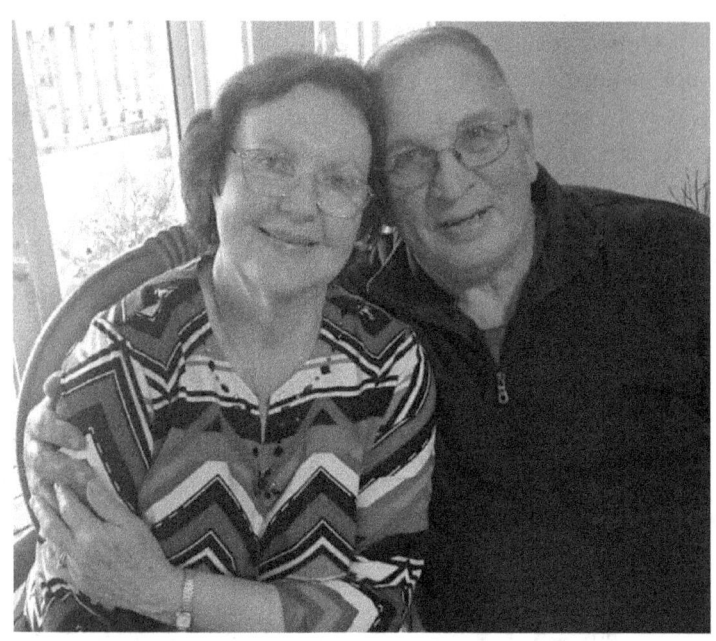

Doug's parents Muriel and Ron on their 60th anniversary

Doug and his son

I asked Doug if he had talked to his son about addiction. He tells me yes; his son knows his whole story. He knows not to try anything. Doug is hoping he will adhere to that. He is so high risk. Doug tells me that his son is so much like him. He is a comedian, center of attention. Doug talks to him about things as they come up and his son tells him: I know dad you don't have to worry. He is a freshman in high school this year. Before Doug got his son, friends were watching out for him and kept telling Doug: you need to get him. Doug hired an attorney. Neal also knows this attorney. Doug tells me initially he thought he made a mistake. The attorney was not nice. He calls her a bulldog.

She would tell Doug: "I could charge you twice of this or you can do some of the f****n work". She would keep telling Doug what to do and how things will go. Doug did what she said. They went for full custody, there was no custody set at that time. This was about 5- 6 years ago. He was keeping notes and writing all things down when he could not get his son. Doug tells me he has PTSD over some ring tones that he used for his ex. Still to this day. He would cringe. She would say bad things about Doug's wife Tiffany. He was not getting visitation time. Then Doug started to hear about all the police contact and the drug use and being homeless. Officially they were not homeless they were living in a tent in the woods. His attorney felt that they have enough to get danger custody and asked Doug if he wants to try it. He said yes. At that hearing they were told that they don't have enough evidence. They had a second hearing after 3 weeks out. During that time, they found out about more things including 911 calls, situations where his mom was putting Doug's son in harm's way, people showing up, cops being called, knives being pulled in the camp. There was a 3rd hearing and it was set to the day for the time when Doug had his son. This way there would be no fight.

    Doug remembers sitting up there at the hearing have his wife next to him and all his friends behind him. His son was at the grandparent's house during the hearing. He did not know any of this was going on. Doug got sole custody of his son. His ex and his boyfriend stormed out saying they are going to get him and f*** this and f*** that. There were 2 sheriffs in the courtroom that day. They called a deputy to go over to Doug's mom's house make sure his ex is not trying to show up there to take him. Doug had his son in counseling ever since then. He is doing great today. He does not want to see his mom anymore.

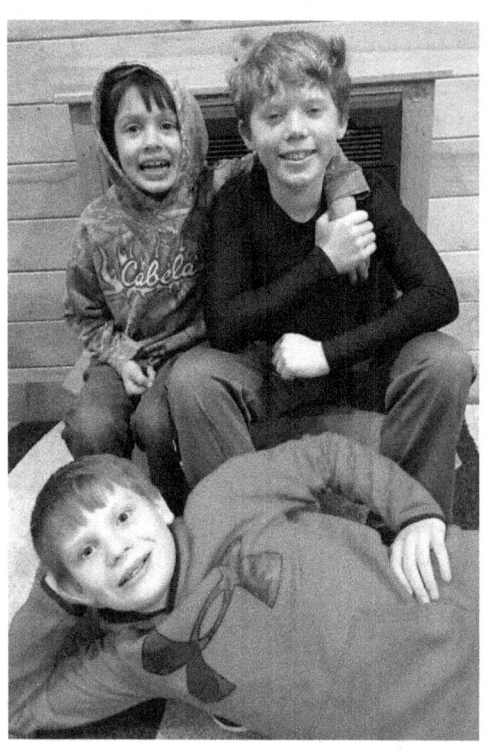

Keenen Doug's son on the front, Carson Tiffany's son and Cody Doug's nephew in the back

He does not want to talk about things that happened to him. He was very defiant for a long time and very angry and destructive. Doug would tell his son that his mom is a good person she just needs to get well. All his son ever knew before was chaos and destruction and if things were not falling apart around him, he did not know what to do. They all have a good relationship now. His son looks up to Tiffany too. Tiffany is a great mom to him. Neal said an important thing that Tiffany chose to be in Doug's son's life. Tiffany also works with difficult kids and has a way with them. She just uses the right words Doug adds.

Doug shows us some more pictures. Makes us guess which one is he in the pictures. He tells us who are in the pictures. Doug had a great childhood. He tells us some stories about his childhood. Neal brings it up how Doug can help people now and how much he can relate to them. Doug tells Neal some of the stories he told me earlier about getting sober. He tells me this is his story and he is sticking to it. Doug first met Neal in the courts. They then discussed what work and groups they did together. They both tell me about a program they were going to teach together, and it did not happen QPR. Question Persuade and Refer. It was a suicide prevention program. Neal tells me that the biggest thing is to ask the question. They did the training together. Neal then tells Doug that he thinks that Doug is one of the chief people in the community for sobriety and addiction. Neal adds that Doug is one of the top 5 people around there. Doug is thankful for those words from Neal.

    Neal also tells Doug how extremely good he is at his job: "You saved hundreds of lives'- Neal adds. Doug is grateful for those words. He will save even more with his story. It is truly amazing to see this friendship between a prior prosecutor and Doug. The relationship started in the courtroom not under the best circumstances. True mentoring and lasting friendship. We have a little side discussion Doug makes me laugh, he tells Neal how he looked me up and expected someone to come in a lab coat to see him. Neal said you change people by telling people another person's story. We discuss the stories Neal shared in his book about mentoring. Now something very unexpected happens. You know the feeling when things just fall into place. Doug all the sudden said thank you. You both being here this morning prepared me for this afternoon's hearing. All we talked about now was fresh in Doug's mind. Neal brings up the need for education and not just putting people in jail. Neal tells Doug he feels that people have a psychological and spiritual wound. It is so painful that the only way they can go through life is to self-medicate and numb themselves. Neal asserts that if people are given the support and the right tools, they can make progress. Doug agrees. Jail is not the place to do this. No treatment centers within 1 hour and 45 minutes Doug adds. The main problem is that once you get people who want to go and get clean there are no beds anywhere. The windows of opportunity close very quickly. People get discouraged and go back to the life of addiction and the life of crime. The waiting list is so long Doug adds. In the rural areas there is just nothing else, he adds. People self-medicate. Part of our culture, Neal adds. We need to change the culture.

35. Criminal Justice System

Albert is a criminal defense attorney. He tells me about cases he saw through his work. He gets the hardest of the hardest cases, it is rare to get somebody who is functional in society and a methamphetamine user for example. He tells me how amazing that so much of his work is related to drug or substance use. Most people he meets though his work tend to have some kind of an addiction problem. Even if he does not see it on the surface when he starts to poke around like: "oh ok you were drunk that night", or "this was your drug history and you are trying to rebuild afterwards". There is a huge impact on the criminal justice system Albert asserts. Growing up in a small town there was a lot of drinking and driving. Albert had a friend who was killed by someone who was driving under the influence and ended up in prison for 7 years. This was rough on Albert and others realizing the seriousness of drinking and driving. We were just dumb kids back then; we did not realize what could happen. They also knew the women who died because of this accident, she was a grandmother of one of their friends at school. Small town, a lot of people know each other. Albert recalls watching drugs taking over the area. When he graduated from high school there were no drugs, only pot and alcohol. Four years later when his brother graduated from high school people were overdosing on pills. Most offenses he sees now are related to heroin or methamphetamine use sometimes both. I ask him how does it make him feel especially with having his children growing up in the same area? He feels it is scary. Many people get started with something like having their wisdom teeth pulled out and getting a prescription. Next thing they are stealing pills. It is scary to think about that. He recalls when he had his wisdom teeth pulled and he got a bunch of Vicodin. Addiction could have happened to him. He sees an occasional gambling addiction. Mostly what he sees is people drinking too much and get in a fight with their wife for example or go driving and do something "stupid" or they are on the street because they cannot stop using heroin. Albert tells me that the people who get arrested and go in and out of jail is about 1% of the community. There are a lot more people out there who are doing it. They stay out of trouble more or less and still function, so they fly under the radar.

Defelonize drugs would be a good idea Albert asserts. The criminal justice system is not the right place for people dealing with addiction it should be more like the mental health system or the health care system so having better access to health care, having better health care instead of using the criminal justice system which is not built for treating addiction.

36. Schools

    Talking to Angel she felt that when addiction happens to one of the kids, and youth she knows at the school it breaks her heart. She loves every single one of her kids and youth. Seeing the potential of what that student could become. Being a teacher gives her more opportunities to be patient with the kids at school who are dealing with addiction issues. Much more than at home. Angel describes that it is easier to be empathetic when it is not her family. The detachment that students are not immediate family, they go home makes it easier for her to have empathy toward them. Angel describes sad stories about "busting" kids at school having Vicodin (normally a prescribed opiate) and the kids are taking it because their tooth hurts, it is infected, and they don't have dental insurance. How is a kid supposed to learn and function like that is school? Angel asks. Prevention and the importance of universal health and dental care for all so kids is essential so can go to the doctor and the dentist when they need too, so they don't have rotten teeth and health issues. Really, how can someone learn like that? Not well. A lot to be fixed Angel said.
    Rory has been working with a kid who started vaping and he is vaping in the school. His mom does not know what to do. Rory feels like teachers allow the vaping in the schools. The schools say they don't allow it, and if people get up to, (he mentioned 2 local high schools) and go to the bathrooms, the fog and the smell of flavors from the vapes are so obvious. He is wondering why the schools are not doing anything about it. Why is there not an adult in the bathroom or at least checking the bathrooms regularly. He is pretty angry about this. He said he is tired of hearing from people that they cannot do anything. He suggests maybe live in a 2000sq home instead of a 4000sq homework one job instead of 2 jobs and spend time with their kids. He feels like a lot of things have to change in the home.
    Fuchsia describes experiences working in the school system with underprivileged children, seeing a lot of poverty, single parents and substance abuse. She had a hard time with it. It is one thing to learn in the books that the parents are struggling, and it is not their fault and there is oppression. It is another thing seeing the little kids and watching them come to school unbathed for days on end, smelling

like cigarettes so bad that the school would buy them their own coats to wear for school. The smoke was making the staff feel sick. It was hard for Fuchsia to see parents showing up every morning high on something. She had a hard time not blaming the parents. The kids were hurting so much. Seeing this firsthand is very difficult. Seeing parents keep dropping the ball. She feels that from an educational perspective a teacher has no chance. There are so many problems with society, that teachers are now expected to be these social workers who can do so many more things then what they are given time and budget for. Kids are coming to school without their basic needs being met. They are going to have a hard time learning, progressing and focusing, they are hungry, tired and not sleeping. It is hard to watch kids not being taken care of very well. Fuchsia feels this is a societal problem. She tells me that when people are in it every day it is hard to step back and see the bigger picture. It is hard not to be protective of the kids. It is painful to see kids suffering. We talk about caring and compassion, then she tells me that people doing this work are so strong, she feels she is too empathetic, and she gets burnt out very quickly. She decided to work for nonprofits that serve this population, and not work with the population directly. She is helping to organize the people who serve the population, this seems to be a better balance for her.

37. Family

Angel describes her emotions toward her brothers as being heartbroken and being pissed off at the same time. How can her brothers make those decisions that impacted them, impacted Angel, her sister, their parents, his children? Angel describes difficulties being empathetic with her brothers. We had a conversation about the emotions and how much stronger they are when it comes to family. Angel kept saying it just pisses her off. There are a lot of emotions going on. Nobody wants to lose any part of their family because of addiction or anything else. We both felt that there is more anger probably because there is more love and emotional attachment to a family member. Makes it more personal. Paige described situations when family does not know what to do with addiction. Her family missed the signs that her stepfather been drinking. Then her mom had no knowledge or understanding how to support him when he was sober. Paige feels that there is a lot of codependency going on between her mother and her stepfather and he does not have a lot of motivation to stop drinking. Her mother does not have the initiative to make that happen either. Paige describes her mother growing up in a dysfunctional family including drinking in the family. Kayla had a similar experience. Her family did not know the signs or what to look for either until the problem of drinking for her father become more apparent. Kayla was away in college when this happened, so she did not see her father all the time. When she would come home for a visit is was "extremely apparent". Kayla makes a great point that addiction can happen to anybody. Her family was really close and still missed the signs. Jason talked about how disturbing it was to see the damage that addiction does to families and the community. It comes down to sadness Jason said, it is just very difficult for the family. It is not something someone can control.

Rory described a situation with a client with his first mental break and psychosis. The client's mother said yes, he was arrested for mushrooms, and he told her it was for his friends. Was it really for his friends? Rory said of course it was not for his friends. He was using mushrooms and he had his first psychotic break. Parents still don't agree, and he won't admit to it. He still said oh, I just had these on me for my friends. A break to the case comes when his girlfriend admitted that he had been using mushrooms for a while before he become ill. Rory asserts that some people use hallucinogens and they never be the same as before. The problem is that mom refuses to hear this, so then what can he do. Rory said: "I can't help them". He sounded very sad saying this. He really wanted to help this family and sounds like there is a lot of denial.

Tracy is doing work related to addictions with families because of the addictions in her family. She has not been able to be honest with her family like she can be with the families through her work. She does not want to hurt her family or hurt them more than they are already hurting because of the addictions. She could do this with other people as her job, she needs to be honest and tell them what is going on and what will happen if they don't try to get better. She feels that honesty and the truth can have a positive effect on the families. It is hard to be honest when it comes to her own family. Tracy describes herself as the black sheep of the family because she turned out ok while nobody else in her family did. She is the odd one because she is not drinking or using any substances. She gets told by her family:" that you are just good, you just think you are better than all of us". This was very hard growing up, now as an adult even though it "stinks" she tells her family:" yes you are right I make better choices then you do". Not easy, not easy at all. It is hard to be picked on and to be rejected by her own family. Family is supposed to be everyone's safety net. Be there for each other no matter what. It is hard to see families pulled apart because of addictions. There is enough struggle in the world already. We just don't need this too. Addiction is tearing people and families apart unfortunately.

Diana from one day to the next from being a grandmother had to be the mother of 3 boys because her daughter could not take care of them. She describes this as a big change in their lifestyle, her husband was getting ready to retire and she was working full time at a clinic. They did it, and it was not easy. All 3 boys turned out beautifully she said. The oldest boy had forgiven his mom for the past. He did not forgive his dad who used to beat him as well as his mother. The youngest of the 3 ended up moving in with mom when he was in high school, they have an ok relationship. There is still lot of blaming going on. They considered grandpa their dad, and they call Diana grandma. Between Diana and her daughter there was a lot of resentment because of the past and the kids. The last 6 years have been ok, and she told Diana that she did the right thing for taking the kids and loves her for that. Recognizing this took a long time. There was a lot of trying to pick a fight situation before. Diana did not respond to those; she would not fight with her daughter. Her daughter still deals with a lot of anxiety and works very hard to please others. Diana keep telling her she was forgiven. Diana also had some difficulties with some outside relatives that criticized her and her husband for adopting the boys at their age. This was quite difficult. For a while the family was split over the issue. For Diana going through all this was worrisome that something is going to happen to her daughter, her job, how to deal with the boys if anything would happen, dealing with resentment toward her daughter, she was conflicted. Diana has an older daughter who is a nurse and she helped Diana a lot to be able to understand what is going on in addition to the body and mind. The boys' father and that family were all abusers. The behavior was learned for the father as well, he was beat up as a kid too. He now wants to be friends with the boys, the boys talk to him, and keep a space between each other. He has been sober for a while. He also has PTSD and a schizophrenia diagnosis. The kids had to attend counseling; it was difficult first, with time it got better. All 3 boys saw the same counselor. Diana also have heard other families hoping that their loved one will break the law so they can get into treatment court and get into treatment. It is very sad to think about it. Breaking the law to get to treatment. Diana asserts that this is very sad, and it happens a lot. Breaking the law to get a warm meal, to get a safe place to sleep and to get treatment. How did we get here? Someone needs to break the law, cause harm to get help. It is a scream. Desperation.

      Michelle describes the difficulties of being disconnected from family as a support system to raise kids. It can be difficult to raise kids on our own. It is nice to have others to be there if needed. In today's society this is not common or expected. It is expected that people grew up and move out. Then everyone is on their own. Michelle described an experience with a group of moms that agreed to watch each other's kids when the others need help, then someone just told her to get a babysitter. It is not the norm, and not everyone can afford a babysitter. Joel feels like her family is very quiet about things when it comes to addictions. She sees things and concerned about things, and don't talk about it. She had some uncles who talked about it a little more. Mostly just keeping quiet about it. Janett shares a story about her aunt and difficult conversations. Her aunt been treating her boyfriend badly and Janett was not sure what to do. She talked to her uncle who advised that since it is a good relationship and they don't want it to end maybe tell her aunt the truth of what she observed. Janett did. To her surprise she listened and was paying attention how she treated her boyfriend. She told Janett specific things what she will do different. They are still together. It was important that they had that conversation. Maybe one day they can also have a conversation about her aunt's addiction. Janett feels like it is hard to talk to someone who is a generation older. Her aunt is very set on her ways and very stubborn. She is the most stubborn person Janett knows. She does not want her aunt to feel like she is judging her. Janett had the experience of telling others in her life before then people still did the behavior, just behind her back. She does not want her aunt to have to hide her drinking when she comes to her house. It is a very fine line with acceptance, watching self-harm, respect and trying to do the right thing. It is difficult to try to phrase something exactly the right way that the person knows that there is a concern about them, and they won't hide it or make the situation worse. Janett is very cautious not to make things worse than they are now. She wants to make sure that her aunt will keep talking to her. Janett feels more comfortable about talking to people who are in her peer group, then family. Janett talks to her mom about this problem with her aunt all the time. They both feel that them saying something will just put a wedge between the family and the closeness would disappear. Janett describes her aunt normally as a happy person who wakes up in the right side of the bed every morning. She describes her as a very stable person normally. We were wondering if there is an underlying problem that causes her aunt to drink. Many other family members have some mental health problems. Janett feels like that for her aunt it is just a habitual thing that become and addiction now.

    Flower talks about difficulties watching a family member deal with addiction to alcohol. The relative is in recovery now and she felt like she was never put in a position to be co-dependent. As a family member she describes her heart going out to them. She is grateful that her family member is doing well in their recovery and they are healthy. She felt like this is a most beautiful thing someone can ever witness. Flower tells me a story of recently traveling on a plane and having a conversation with a woman sitting next to her. She disclosed to Flower that her son had been dealing with addiction and she quit her job for 2 years to take him to the methadone clinic every day. He is sober now, has a family, working for their company. Doing very well now, the family is intact. She had to focus all her energy to support her child in recovery. It was a gift for Flower to have this conversation, working in addictions people don't always get to see the other side. Hear the success stories. The whole family fought for this man to recover. They succeeded. He is in recovery. What about those who are single parents and can't quit their jobs? ***We should all fight for each other.*** If there is a child hurt from addiction, let's come together and support that family and child. Can we do that? Imagine that. That would be beautiful. Flower's heart goes out to people who are suffering from addictions. She feels that every person suffering from addictions needs a role model who succeeded in their recovery. If someone doesn't have one, find one she asserts. People need to know it is possible. People need to know how others did it, how they succeeded. They need to know somebody who walks that walk and did it. Experiences shared in a group can be huge and cannot be replaced, when sharing people pull each other up, Flower explains.

  Fuchsia tells me about an experience watching and supporting her friend with her father's relapse. Her friend's father relapsed to alcohol after being sober for 17 years. Her brother just died a few weeks before. Fuchsia had seen him recently in an outdoor event in town, he was so drunk he could not even stand up, it was hard to watch. Her friend is having a hard time discussing the alcohol use with her father, she does not like confrontations. She recently had a beer with her father at a concert and told Fuchsia later it felt very weird and uncomfortable after. He was hiding his relapse first now he is openly drinking in front of them. She does not want to tell her father to stop drinking. It is his choice, yet she does not want to enable him either.

Her friend is upset by her father's relapse and feels he is going to do what he is going to do she can't control it.

38. Leslie's Story

Leslie is a Registered Nurse; she has a great compassion and kindness toward others. We have our conversation over the phone, and we talk about 1.5 hours. We also had multiple other conversations before and after the interview. Leslie was one of the people who encouraged me to write a book. She is been very supportive through his process and offered me feedback. We start our conversation by her telling me about her mother. Leslie's mother was a very high functioning alcoholic. She had a couple liters of wine a night. She carried on a very successful business until she was 80 years old. She is a hard example because she was so highly functional, that created a denial that she had a problem. Her drinking caused a lot of heartache and a lot of trauma for Leslie who kept hoping that she would quit drinking and smoking. She never did and she never admitted that those things are damaging her at all. Leslie's mother blacked out a lot. Her consumption of wine was enormous. It was agonizing for Leslie to see her mother drinking. She got to a point where she could not go over and see her mother in the evening. Just seeing all the alcohol on the table was so painful. Leslie's mother Rose never agreed that her drinking affected Leslie, her brother or anybody else around her. It was devastating for Leslie. Rose did not start to drink so much in the beginning. Her full-on alcoholism hit around age 40. Rose would drink for the next 40 years. This was a long time for Leslie to agonize over her mother falling down, worrying about if she will burn down the house, her denial. By 9 or 10 pm she would become dysfunctional, she was so intoxicated. At 7 am Rose was up drinking coffee, smoking and doing business. Leslie feels a lot of rage against her mother for not acknowledging how difficult it was for her and her brother to be around her. Leslie gives me an example when they would go to a restaurant and she would drink too much and she would literally fall over her dinner plate. She chuckles. This happened few times. I ask Leslie how she felt when stuff like that happened. She felt horrible and embarrassed, humiliated and angry. The next day her mother would be fine. Rose never admitted to alcoholism or that the smoking is killing her. It did kill her ultimately. It was very confusing; she did not have withdrawal and she did not have to drink during the day. Her metabolism of alcohol was different than normal. She never gained weight and her liver function was always good. It felt like a true mystery to Leslie. Leslie wanted to get an intervention for her mother, and she was looking for others to support her in this process, and nobody would. This was devastating to Leslie. Ask Leslie why she thinks that was? She felt that half of the people who she asked wanted to continue to drink and they did not want to change their lifestyle. Leslie also thinks that people were afraid of Rose that she would become very defiant and hostile. Later, when it was suggested to Rose to go to a rehab place, she did become very angry and defiant. She never went to treatment. Rose smoked 2 packs a day for 50 years. She never got lung cancer but did get COPD (Chronic Obstructive Pulmonary Disease) and ended up dying of respiratory failure. Rose would refuse to have oxygen in her house because then she would have to admit that the smoking was an issue. She wanted to pretend that she did not need it. Her oxygen level was running 88% for the last 10 years of her life. A normal oxygen level is 94%-99%. Leslie feels that it would have been better if she would have got a DUI or had withdrawals or deliriums because then she would be forced to admit that there was a problem, and that never happened. Rose was extremely sturdy physically. Leslie feels that if her mother would have stopped drinking and smoking probably, she could have lived another 30 years. Rose would also play bridge and go to her friends' house and they all would drink too much. Rose's friends from grade school and college all drank too much. Rose never had a ticket in her life, and she was never stopped by police while driving. Her mother was a constant worry that she would somehow harm herself.

  Leslie's father was an episodic drinker. He would drink once in a while every 6 or 7 weeks. He would lose control and drink way too much. When he started to drink it would go on for a while and he was very violent and angry. Leslie was so relieved when her parents got a divorce and he was out of the house. She could never invite friends over because he was so unpredictable. After he left Leslie's mother started drinking and she thought oh my God, not again. She thought: "we just got rid of him let's not start in on this". She was very distressed. Leslie was 17 when her father left. Leslie's father never touched Leslie or her brother. He always hurt their mother. Leslie is not sure why. Rose would not leave her husband for a long time. Leslie describes their relationship as a weird kind of drama. It was a strange chaos between the two of them. There was a lot of attraction. It was just wrong all around. Leslie's mother was quite a bit younger and he was chauvinistic and controlling. One day Leslie's mother got very sick from a virus and just decided she will leave him. He did not take that very well. He could be very cruel. Rose would have injuries like black eye, broken arm and in those days, there was nothing done about it. Leslie's dad had a charisma and was a very interesting men from one side then he had this dark side that was very miserable. Leslie was relieved when he left because he could no longer hurt her mother. He was in the war in WWII. He was a fighter pilot; he killed a lot of people. He could never forgive himself. He was anti-war and anti-United States. He was anti-Vietnam war and the protestor against the American government. Most people felt that the war broke Leslie's father and his drinking was related to the trauma caused by the war. He would never talk about it. He had a lot of rage. He came back from the war thinking that everything we did was wrong. He became unpatriotic and very interested in other cultures. He had friends from all over the world. After her father left, the word from others were that he never drank again, he did go into deep isolation and reclusiveness and died alone. He did want to leave the United States, wanted the kids to visit and live in another country. One time they were traveling through New York to go to South America. They were driving from Seattle to New York and they stopped in South Dakota. In South Dakota there were a lot of young men who he was with in the war and they looked up to him and thought he was a hero. When they heard he is coming they organized a parade for him. Leslie's father found out and he packed up in the middle of the night and left the town. He was not there for his own parade. He did not want to be acknowledged that way.

    I ask Leslie how she was affected by growing up this way with parents drinking. Leslie recalls that she always tried to take care of her father and make him feel good. Leslie thought he was very depressed, so she tried to cheer him up. He was not a nice parent and criticized Leslie terribly. He said horrible things to Leslie all the time about her being worthless. She did not believe it she just thought he was depressed. Leslie sat with him a lot to try to talk him down. Now that

Leslie is older and looking back what happened, she realizes it affected her much more then she thought at that time. Mostly, she is hurt, that her mother never acknowledged that her and her father's behavior was painful. Leslie feels things would have been different for her if either of her parents would have been interested in parenting, she would have had more freedom to do whatever she liked to do. Because of her mother's drinking Leslie always felt she had to stay close to her. All this caused Leslie a lot of anxiety and a lot of other problems. Leslie describes her mother as both a narcissist and a victim. She never acknowledged anything Leslie had done for her. Rose always wanted other people to feel sorry for her and see her as somebody who is self-sacrificing, a wonderful person who does so much for other people. Rose was like from a 1960's melodrama. Nothing ever was ok, there was always some kind of crisis. She wanted a lot of attention. Even at her work she always had to have fires to put out. It was all about her all the time. She would create a crisis then take credit for taking the fires out. If Leslie would tell her mother that she had a bad day Rose would say she had a worse day. Then she would launch into how bad her day was. She always had to be in the center of attention. Rose would complain a lot to her friends about Leslie and her brother. To a point that people would think that they were criminals in jail.

  Rose liked to say that she sacrificed everything for her kids. The worse of it when Leslie would get calls from people who would say: "Why don't you ever see your mother?" Leslie would say, well, I saw her last night, so it has not been that long. In the last 10 years or so she also started to add that she only liked to see her mother during the day because she does not want to drink wine with her in the evening. Leslie told her mom that she cannot be there anymore in the evening and watch her drink. People did adore Rose; she had a great following. She was attractive, funny, had a beautiful house, she was kind of glamorous. People liked the life she lived. Rose would make sure that all those people did not like Leslie. She would tell them that Leslie is taking advantage of her. This was hard for Leslie. She used Leslie and saying bad things about her to get attention. People could never call Rose and hear that she is doing well she would always say oh I am horrible. Leslie makes me laugh because of the way she said this: well, at some point people have to look at the women and say she has a wonderful group of people, a beautiful house, has money. How difficult life could be? How about people who don't have a place to live and don't have a job – she adds. No one could ever talk about their problems because she would stop people to talk about her problems.

    The first time Leslie realized that her mother had a drinking problem they were going to a party on Bainbridge Island and Leslie was carrying things from the car inside and she picked up her handbag and it was very heavy. There was a 1.5 liter of wine in her purse. It was not for sharing. This horrified Leslie that her mom is going to this party and she was not sure if she was going to get enough alcohol. Leslie was around 20 years old at that time. The thing about my mom Leslie adds is that she got away with so much. She smoked up to two days before she died. She died at age 82. She worked until age 80 as an interior designer. Leslie was very angry at her for putting her kids down in front of others. Rose was very generous with other people. Many people got married in her house or had parties in her house. Leslie does not miss her mom at all, not even a little bit. She thought she might have some memories that are good, and she does not have any of those. It is a relief not to have to worry about her every day. Rose would go to the liquor store every week on Capitol Hill and she would buy a case of white wine 1.5-liter bottles about 12 in a case. She would occasionally drink other things, but her choice was mostly wine. Rose was economical. She bought inexpensive white wine. She was conservative with the spending on it. She would have some expensive liquor around the house for some of the bridge club people. Rose was never hung over or sick or vomiting. Rose friends were her friends and did not care for Leslie at all. None of them contacted Leslie after Rose's death. Not even to send condolences.

    Leslie drinks red wine occasionally but does not seek it out. She likes food. Neither Leslie or her brother smoke or drink. Leslie's dad never worked; he never made any money he lived off her mother. Leslie never understood why her mom stayed so long with her dad. When he left Rose had to pay him a lot of money to get rid of him. He never spoke with the kids again. That was hurtful for Leslie. Leslie spent so much time trying to please her father. She felt foolish. He actually tried very hard to take all of Rose's money. He tried to have her institutionalized as crazy. Her dad did a lot of weird things. It did not work. Rose finally got to her senses and realized what he was doing. Leslie forgive him all he had done. Leslie's parents never showed up on a school function or on any occasion. They were too involved about their stuff. Leslie got very sick few times while growing up including a blood clot in her leg, rheumatic fever, and her mom kept talking about how sick she is but would not do anything about it Leslie would have to tell her mom: "I am very sick I need to go to the hospital". Rose somehow lacked the maternal instinct to take care of her child. Rose did not embrace medicine she thought doctors were always wrong.

    We switch talking about society. Leslie tells me she is dumbfounded about all the drugs and alcohol and smoking present in our society today. She finds it daunting and totally overwhelming. It is truly crazy the amount of substances available to hurt people. Leslie just had a friend whose son got a job mostly because no one else could pass the drug test. That is scary. It is so bad she adds. In her generation growing up there were boundaries, there was a line people wouldn't cross. People knew to care about their families and not to ruin themselves. Now it feels like people don't have those boundaries – she adds. It used to be that even if kids were 1000 miles away from their parents, they would not do things that their parents would not approve. That all seems to be gone. Leslie also feels that there been a huge leap from going to the doctor and getting prescription medication to go to the street for illegal drugs. It is a huge switch in thinking to seek out illegal drugs if someone is not getting what they need from their doctor. She is wondering why is it family structure or is it we can't stand the discomfort of life? She is not sure. She feels people have no interest in mental health for example, it is a huge commitment, more needed then getting 15 minutes with a psychiatrist. That is nothing but a drug deal she adds. People need therapy and structure and family and relationships. She tells me about hearing the Guantanamo Bay Cuba takes $40-60 million to run a year for no good reason. To have 22 prisoners who never even had a trial. Just think what that money could do in the community to redirect addicts to something else. Leslie sounds very hopeless about our mental health and addiction situation. She feels that not many people who want to deal with it and actually spend the time that needed to sit down with people for an hour or two and talk about their problems. She adds that we all talk about it but spending the money and doing it is different. She tells me look at Seattle we have the most billionaires and millionaires here, we have so much money and we cannot do anything about the drug problems and the homeless on the streets? Why can't we she asks? It is a great question. It takes way more than throwing socks or food at someone people need treatment, job training, housing, support system. It is complex and it does cost a lot of money. So, what we rather build a wall for our neighboring country? Leslie feels that both the republicans and the democrats need to work together and come up with a cohesive plan otherwise nothing is going to happen. She does not have much faith in the current government. She tells me that nobody can tell her that it is not a huge public health problem having people on the streets not having toilets, she feels it is just like an epidemic waiting to happen. The drugs are so potent and grab people so quickly she adds. She does not know what the answer is. She feels that there is a lack of community and family life. She feels that we can do simple things like being a teacher a very high paying prestigious job, make it competitive, pay them high salary, get the cream of the crop who are very interested in being educators. In the schools have food that does not come in frozen from somewhere. Real food and sit down and eat like civilized people. Have a little gym class to exercise every day and kids don't get to use their phone all day. We need to put resources in our kids. Wearing a uniform might be helpful she adds. Then we have to work on the parents. Make sure that the first 5 years of life for the kids is very good. Not putting so much resources into war, weaponry and the military and prisons. ***Just absolutely treasure the children.*** We need happy teachers who feel rewarded and not at odds with all the bureaucracy. Have a sense of community at school, so if the kids don't have it at home at least they would have it in the school. We should take care of our children. We are the richest country of the world she adds how come there are inner city schools who don't have school supplies? -Leslie asks. Provide hope. She brings up Mexico and how many of the teenagers have a child at age 15. They don't have hope. Nobody is telling them that they have other choices and education to become a professional. Having a goal and purpose is very important for kids Leslie adds. We discuss education and how important it is and how difficult is to get into education. Leslie tells me that she thinks student loans are the crime against humanity. When she used to have a student loan it was 3% that could be the maximum and it never changed. It was a government loan. The current loans are above 6%. It became a business that creates a lot of difficulties for people to try to pay off their student loans. Many people have some kind of student loan that they are still paying off. Predatory loans of all kinds should not happen Leslie adds. Leslie tells me it is just like the prison system they are making more money incarcerating people. Why are we incarcerating all these people? It is a money maker for the owners. It is terrible she adds. She tells me about a news report she heard recently about hiring a private business to detain kids at the border. A private business will have zero incentive to get the kids out. They would get paid to have the kids in there. It is all just wrong. They will also not be going to be providing good services because they are going to be cheap. That should not happen that is also a crime against humanity she adds. It should not happen. Leslie brings up also the cost of drugs. It should not be so expensive that people cannot afford it. It is like withholding care from people. It is embarrassing that lot of people go to Mexico or Canada to get their medications because they cannot afford it in the United States. It is ridiculous she adds. The lobbyist in Washington with the drug companies and the weapons are so influential and they support all these politicians so much that they just buy them off not to make changes. It is just so wrong. Going back to addictions she tells me that there are not enough places for people to go to treatment. We discuss treatment options and the length of treatment. Leslie does not see why we cannot afford to get everyone treatment who want to get better. She tells me that we have to spend so much money on defense. What will this defense do for us if we have a population of uneducated children who become criminals and drug addicts? – Leslie asks. She feels that everyone would like to know what they can do to help this situation. A grassroot movement. Create a sense of community. Have interactions with other humans. Eat dinner with family. Leslie is disgusted with the pharmaceutical companies and the availability of opiates. It is scary. She feels that the American appetite for drugs is so overwhelming. If someone can't find a way to create a good life for themselves here something is really wrong. Leslie thinks about all these things all the time.

39. Happiness and Joy

What is happiness for people? Are people happy? Do they experience joy? What causes joy? Can we be happy all the time? Are people who are dealing with addictions happy? Do they experience happiness and joy? Happiness and joy are an important part of our life. Beth describes happiness as living life the fullest. Being healthy, surrounded by loved ones. Being competent within ourselves, loving ourselves. Sheila thinks people who struggle with addiction at times they are happy; at times we are happy we all have our moments. It might depend on what are someone is addicted to. In addiction using drugs releases the happy cells called dopamine in the brain and make people feel good, feel pleasure, feel happy. Some foods and activities do the same. Examples would be chocolate, bread, cheese, sex and exercise. What causes people to be happy? Some things might be are obvious, and some are not. We might not be even aware of it. If someone has never been a millionaire, they do not miss the private jet flight and private fancy dinner parties. If someone has never been sick, they might not appreciate getting up and walking in the sunshine. If someone has never used drugs or slept under the bridge, they might will not be happy or appreciate sleeping in their own bed under a roof. People can be grateful for what they have. It can be hard if someone has not been without things. It is all about experiences in our lives, and most of the things we know are biased based in our own perceptions. Do we really know what makes us happy and live a good life? Everyone is different and happiness is an individual domain. Someone might think another new shoe, or a better house might make them happy, it can be false perception. It depends what they need to do to get their next "fix" of a new house, shoe, next dose of drugs. Some people might feel that things will get them happy. The things they need to do to get them happy might causes destruction in their lives like using drugs or alcohol. To get the next fix they might have to hurt somebody, steel, sell their body, sell drugs to others.

> *Take a moment to close your eyes, take a deep breath and think about what makes you happy. Open your eyes and write it down. Life is too short; it is important that people practice what makes them happy.*

Could being happy help, to give up addiction? Sheila described happiness as a tough question. It can be just being out and having fun with friends, things in life going well. It can even be when is someone is having a tough time, then the kid comes home, and they been doing something that makes the individual happy. Children, spouse, friends doing well brings lots of moment of happiness. Moments of happiness. Mary describes moments of happiness as well. Collect your moments of happiness and treasure them.

Beth does not feel that people who are addicted are happy. She feels like they are lost. She felt that addiction is controlling the mind, and nothing else fits in. Beth describes that she is grateful every single day that she does not have an addiction even that she had been surrounded by it and feels like people with addiction need to replace the addictive behavior with something positive. Mary describes people who are dealing with addiction as being shameful, feeling that they failed others and themselves, their families. Edward felt that people with addiction might have momentary happiness. When I asked Edward, what happiness is for him, there was a pause that felt like was going on for a long time. Then he said: well, that is a good question. Then he said contentment and pleasure, that creates a more positive attitude, also pleasing. Some people might have originally started drugs for the pleasure and the momentary high, certainly not all.

What makes us experience joy? Everyone would like to be happy and experience joy in their lives. Many people when turning to drugs are not happy and content in their life and they start to look for something else that can make them happy, make them feel good. Edward mentioned to me that he thinks people turn to opiates when they experience pain or have some other issues. Happiness is a state when there is a sense of peace and fulfillment of goals that make people feel that they have done something with their life. It can be as simple as being able to cook a meal for their family or more complex of bringing peace to a country. It can make people happy to see others happy, seeing their children, friends and family happy. Seeing others in a sense of fulfillment, creating and learning something new. Helping others can make people feel happy. Living a good and happy life includes obstacles in our lives that sometimes bring hardships or lessons that help people appreciate things that they have not appreciated before. Examples can be our health, family, friends, the place we live. If people have all these things and lose them, people will be happier to have any of them back and will appreciate things better. If someone endured the pain of not getting to see their friends or family, or not having a place to sleep or not having a meal to eat when they are able to have a meal or see family the appreciation and happiness is greater than before. Are we supposed to be happy all the time? Everyone needs happiness but not all the time, in small doses to be able to function well in their lives.

> *Write down one thing a day that made you smile. Try two things the next day, pretty soon you have so many things you cannot keep up with paper. It feels good to write down good things that happen to you. I advised this to my patients all the time, list the things that make you happy or list the things that made you smile today.*

    Angel been asking the questions on happiness and joy related to her brothers' addictions. Angel has a biology and chemistry background and she firmly believe that there is a point where addiction changes the brain and brain functions. She believes that those changes are permanent because the brain gets re-wired. In deep addiction she felt that people who are dealing with this issue not trying to get "high" anymore, just trying to survive. She believes that they at that point lost the ability to experience joy. Joy in a way she would define it. She gave me examples of being with family, having coffee with a neighbor, having a conversation. She feels that people when addicted to drugs do not have the capacity to experience joy. Looking at her brothers, even though they are in a good place now, they are not the same people who they were before their addiction. During addiction people get lost in a deep dark hole. She believes that once people overcome addiction, they can find joy again. It will be different than before, because the brain is permanently changed.

Kayla felt happiness is a tough topic. She felt that people dealing with addiction can feel happiness. Happiness can be gathering around with friends and drinking alcohol. It can be confusing she said, at what point do we draw the line. Is fulfillment and security happiness? Kayla describes loving to go out and having a beer with friends, yet alcohol is depressing. Kayla asks: "Should there be a regulation on how many breweries are in a 10 x10 town"? We are human beings Kayla said we all feel happiness. Depending on what makes us happy and what people think happiness is. Kayla feels that in order to be happy we have to love ourselves. This can be a struggle for everybody at any point in their lives. She went through it; she feels everyone goes through this and we can be really hard on ourselves. Kayla feels that society makes it very easy to be hard on ourselves especially for young girls and with the presence of social media. She describes that **_some of the happiest people have no belongings and live in mud huts_**. Having a sense of security from friends and family. Feeling connected with nature. Basic needs like that there is a roof over her head, food, have family, a great group of loving friends, this makes her happy. Basic needs need to be met to have happiness. It means something different to everybody. Kayla described a situation from her life moving to a new city and feeling alone and isolated creating a low in her life and affecting her happiness. She feels it is important to be self-aware of a situation like this and self-consciously make choices to meet new people and do new activities. She added: "I think a lot of time people don't take time to think about why the heck they aren't happy". Take the time to figure out what is going on if someone is not feeling happiness, contentment or joy.

Ron feels that once people are deep into addiction, they might think they have joy, and they really don't. It is a symptom after the party ends and people literally look like zombies. It is not much fun and joy. Ron describes an evening where after the party people were walking out on the street and they looked like zombies. He was talking about thousands of people. He said everybody was drunk, used cocaine, meth, and whatever else was available. Bugged out eyes, it was comical and sad the same time. A sea of people. While all this was going on, he loved everybody, he loved the zombie next to him, and it was all a fake sensation. He was just thinking that all these people now will get into their car and drive. Now he thinks how bad this party was. It would take him days to recover and feel himself again. The damage to the body and mind were devastating. He called this event: "pack of wild zombies". He had never seen anything else like it. He was part of this group. This was a huge group, a stadium full of people. This was only one night of a 5-night celebration he attended. At the time it seemed fun. Now, looking back it was horrifying. The world is a very dark place now- Ron adds.

Joel feels that addiction and happiness is a very complicated question. There is the brain chemistry that creates addiction in some people and not in others. She talks about gateway drugs. Balance and happiness is very important to Joel. She feels a little imbalanced now. She feels happiness is hard, she likes simple, she does not like complicated. She describes the importance of quietness and quiet time. She went to a trip to Nicaragua for a mission and there was no cell phone, no sounds except the animals. It was nice. Coming back to the United States after the trip was very overwhelming. She turns down the radio in the car too, it is too much. Joel likes her quiet time in the morning, coffee maybe with soft music sometimes. Her husband gets up and turns on the TV. She does not like the sound of it. She does not like to see it; it is frustrating for her. We talked about how much we pay a month for noise. TV/satellite bill, cell phone bill, Netflix, cable, Hulu, internet bill for example. Lots of money to get more noise in our lives. Easily can add up to $400-500 per month depending on where someone lives. Joel feels like sound can be an addiction too. Happiness for Joel is not having as much noise in her life.

Janett describes that when she was younger, she discovered differences between short term and long-term happiness and joy. Short term might be being in a party dancing. She decided that the long-term low-key contentment and happiness was what she was looking for in life. She is suspicious of short-term happiness. She feels like if people get caught up in a lot of short-term happiness, they might end up doing something they should not. She describes cheating on a spouse as an example. Become addicted to a drug like if someone just seeing momentary pleasure. She describes that having too many momentary pleasures can damage long term contentment. For her family is very important, having strong connections and being close to them. Having a purpose in life, not religion, and trying to good while here on earth. At work trying to do good, better her community, help with what they need. She likes to help people, being a kind person. Having a network of people around her and staying on top of being healthy. Mental, financial and physical health. She does not have a goal to be rich. It is not her lifetime goal.

Albert feels like that people who are in deep into their addiction are not usually happy or experience joy in their lives. People into addictions are not doing well because of other reasons too in their lives. He laughs and tells me he does not think he has seen a real addict who is happy and the two play off of each other. When someone uses substances, they can lose things in their life. When someone is using too much they can try to taper off when things go bad yet often when things go bad people use more to boost themselves up again, it is a cycle. People he sees are in the lowest on the economic level, low education. He feels he has some bias because of this, low social interaction and education. There are people who just really don't know any better or know any different because their parents were addicts too or maybe they raised themselves. Many people he sees don't have a lot of good role models in their lives, barely getting by, then fall into addictions too. Albert describes happiness and joy as having a purpose in life, have family, work people care about, work towards something meaningful. Have a place where people want to be, feeling like they have a purpose.

I asked Dr. Beatty about happiness and joy. He felt it depends on the person, their state of mind at the time if they can experience happiness and joy in their lives. He feels that a person needs to feel some confidence about themselves to experience happiness and joy in their lives. If someone is sad or depressed it might not be a good place or time to be experiencing happiness and joy in their life. He is thinking about all those people he knows who had addiction. They might or might not have joy in their lives. There are the people who have other issues like depression or other complicated problems, and they might also not be able to experience joy in their lives. Dr. Beatty experiences happiness and joy by being able to do something. Going outside for example and interacting with people, helping somebody do something, accomplishing something makes him feel good and fulfilled. He feels joy all the time. He is happy about helping people doing something.

Brenda feels that people deep in their addiction might experience some joy. It is more to the response to what they are addicted too. We get our joy from our relationships and people who overcome addiction are the ones who were able to build some connections and socialization with others. When someone gives up all connections to chase an addiction that cannot create lasting happiness or joy. Maybe moments, nothing that is sustainable- she adds. People in general need people. Happiness for Brenda is feeling positive, enjoying things and positive feelings with others. Someone maybe can be happy in the forest all by themselves, and she thinks that is like living in a vacuum. She feels that happiness meant to be shared because if people share happiness then they receive more happiness back. We talked about people's relationship with animals and volunteering at an animal shelter for example. Brenda feels that having an animal is a safe relationship because animals don't judge.

Dolores feels that life is hard, and it has a lot of challenges even if someone is successful and has a family and job. She feels that people think it should be easier when it is not and justify getting drugs. She thinks a more realistic understanding of what a good life is or what is an ok life is would be helpful. Most people are not going to be wealthy and are going to struggle for money and work and get the stuff they need or want. Letting young people know that struggling is useful, and most people struggle might be helpful. Dolores asserts that these are hard questions. Dolores feels happy when she is around her grandchildren, children. She enjoys work. She has a good relationship that makes her happy. She feels she has a lot of good things in her life. She is generally pretty healthy and feels she is doing ok; this makes her happy. Appreciate what she has. She likes to do arts and crafts, canning tomatoes and pickles. She can be very happy just doing that. Making something makes her happy.

Fuchsia tells me that she had to prioritize happiness after her brain injury and for her happiness is being around her family, being outside, taking time for mental health. She describes that in college she had to choose sometimes to either cook a healthy meal for herself or study more and have a better grade. She questions why we have this college system that so cutthroat. She does not think that people are in their addiction are not happy, they are struggling. She has been thinking about happiness a lot lately. She feels that certain people have a hard time with their own happiness. She feels like that people with addictions get better when they find a sense of purpose and balance that leads them to happiness. Family brings happiness to her, connected to land, nature, plants. Helping others. Someone told her she sees the world in plants.

Bob tells me ideally people should have a better way to pursue happiness. To Bob happiness is to pursue what he wants to do, what is the best use to our time. He feels most people are not doing what they want. They just try to pay bills and fend for themselves and others who depend on them. He feels it is usually it is pretty close, people on average live paycheck to paycheck. This creates a constant stress. How's anyone supposed to have any kind of relief there? In your two-week vacation they might get? That is kind of crazy he tells me. He feels like people just get caught up in the cycle.

40. Stigma

What about stigma? Is it there when we talk about addictions? Beth said yes, of course, she lied to others because she was afraid of what others might have thought that when her brother died of an overdose. Beth felt that by telling people her brother died of an overdose it would make him less than he was; he had a brain; he had a heart. She felt she would be judged, and her brother would be judged. She loved him very much and did not want others to make a judgement. Maybe stigma can be useful to a certain point? It was pointed out in tobacco use and the decrease in the use, it is not popular anymore. New things have come since then so now it is vaping. So, addictive. Could we create an image where alcohol use is not popular anymore, drug and substance abuse not popular anymore? These areas are stigmatized in a wrong way. Nobody likes an alcoholic family member who just causes trouble, violence and problems all the time. Alcohol is still everywhere in our society and it is accepted to drink on many occasions. It is there in the movies, posters, advertisement and in every store. Could we make alcohol unpopular the same as tobacco – at least cigarettes become unpopular? Alcohol is proven to cause cancer; it is a carcinogen. Could we make all the substance and drug use uncool? That nobody would want to do it. Treat the people who have the problem with love, caring and support. What we can do to make things better? Sheila describes that we need to find a way to destigmatize addiction, so people are comfortable to go and ask for help. When I asked her how we can do that she responded probably education so everyone can understand a little more about addiction. Then she said: "Your book". Get people to read it so people understand how addition works. Not just health professionals and people in the addiction world but everyone else too. Thank you, Sheila. Sheila feels that people need to be compassionate. It could have been them who fall into the trap of addiction. Be grateful if it is not you or someone you know. Don't judge those who fell into the trap of addiction. Love them. Every single one and help if you can. We are all in this together. Nobody born wants to be addicted to anything. It happens for whatever reason. Being compassionate toward others is important, we are all connected. One of my long-time friends have a son who is been addicted to opiates for 15 years, she fights every day to keep him alive, friends and family don't understand and faded away. Sheila described stigma through a story about how some alcoholics she knows try to hide their addiction and she felt this make the addiction worse, with less stigma maybe they would not go so far down the path. Would not have to hide it. Have the ability to openly talk about it.

Beth felt that most people make a judgement when they hear that someone is an IV drug user, even doctors. They provide care, and it is special care. Beth describes a situation with antibiotics for abscesses when many times people dealing with addiction leave the hospital earlier then recommended to use drugs to get high. She feels people are going to judge. She felt many times people with addiction do not want the care. She had to choose between them and people who want the care she provided. People will judge others for using drugs and having that problem. Mary asserted that we need to understand that some people do not want to stop. It can take many tries. It can take a person's life. Edward felt like that there is a lack of understanding of others about addiction and that people who are dealing with addiction might lack fortitude and inner strength to overcome it. What could we do? Edward thinks prevention and education can help. Increasing the discussion about addiction at an early age. The discussion has to go farther than saying no. More conversations about addiction.

Dr. Tedd Levin feels that stigma prevents people from coming to the doctor especially if there is a mental health component to the addiction. People in society think of addiction as a moral weakness and it is not as accepted as other diseases. This creates a barrier for individuals with addiction. Angel felt that stigma is just a blame game. It is easier to blame others. It is also uncomfortable, in the mist of addiction people can be unpredictable, scary, hard to relate too. Paige tries very hard not to place judgment. She feels like that the stigma is changing now and people are starting to realize that addiction can hit anyone. She felt that up to a few years ago people using were more looked down on then now. People realizing now that nobody is above addiction it can be anyone's husband or wife. Chief Jason feels like stigma comes from lack of understanding and all the package that comes with addiction like stealing and lies. He feels like keeping people involved, education and awareness about addiction and what comes with it would help decrease stigma with education being the biggest part. Kayla added that addiction is taboo to talk about unless someone is at an AA meeting or a safe place. She does not personally understand why, yet also understand why people would want to be in a safe place to talk about it. To decrease stigma in our society Kayla feels that we need to talk about addiction more, need to say what addiction means, talk about the signs and symptoms of addiction or what can turn into addiction. Let's look at the cause how people ended up using drugs or meth for example and not judge. It is so easy to judge others, and we need to hear the story. Kayla feels like having people's stories told would help decrease stigma against addiction. Talk about experiences they had. Just talk more about it, addictions should not be taboo, acknowledge the existence and understand this can happen to anybody.

Rory feels stigma in general is ignorance. People don't understand. They do not have the knowledge. They blame the person dealing with addiction. Could anyone blame someone with depression? He feels that the American tradition is to blame because they failed somehow, they don't have the moral strength of others to say no to addiction. He thinks there is still a lot of shaming done even by the media through television. He gets into politics at this point. He feels it goes high in the hierarchy of our political structure when it comes to shaming others. Rory asserts he is not ashamed; he will tell anyone his story. It should be stigma free, yet it is not, why he asks? Teach people to have courage, ask for help. He feels like it is another American tradition that we don't ask for help, it is considered shameful to ask for help. He feels this is very unique to our culture.

Diana stated that dealing with the stigma of addiction was very hard for her daughter in a small town. The stigma encourages users to go back to using. They don't want to deal with the ridicule or being shunned. Acceptance had gotten better, and it still needs to get way better. She gives an example of her daughter, when she was looking for a job, her daughter always felt that the interviewer was reluctant to give her the opportunity because of her past. This created a lot of discouragement. "How will I ever pass this?" - she asked. Diana encouraged her, just fight through it, keep fighting. Diana describes an experience about commercials related to stigma in television and how they have been cut off during the past year. Why don't they let them run the whole add to help people with stigma she asks? Good question. Why do ads get cut off? She got really angry about this especially during mental health treatment month last year.

Chloe describes judgements on people that she had seen with alcohol and drug use. She feels that the judgements are there because they have a tendency to hurt other people. This creates other people not wanting to be around them. She describes making judgements every day on people walking by her. She would not say bad things out loud and might avoid people on the street because of their addictions. Janett describes having a lot of respect for people who made it through addictions and she never judges them. She knows that if she would have gone through what they had to go through in their lives or had their genetics she might be in the same place as them. It would be good, Janett thought if we talk more about addictions to help break down the stigma. Share with others what happened to people with addictions. It can go either way. People can be supportive or not, it could cause trouble at workplace. It is ultimately an individual choice to share. Stigma can create a lot of barriers. Janett describes a country where they changed how they are doing counseling and people told families friends about their addictions and they were supportive of them. This helped them become and remain sober because of all the support that surrounded them. Of course, people need to be supportive for this to happen Janett asserts. Could someone tell their boss that they have a problem with alcohol?

Albert felt that he was never judgmental about others. He would sill hang out with people regardless of what others say if that person used alcohol or being perceived as a "bad kid". He never felt that way. It does not mean he had to do what that kid is doing he asserts. Don't have to be writing that person off. He has to empathetic to do the kind of work he does. People do mess up, and it is easy to jump into judgment. There is a lot of stigma in addiction like" oh those meth heads out there wrecking the cars". There are people who are struggling with addiction who are doing stupid stuff like committing crimes that are a real problem. Albert feels it is counterproductive to assume and say things that if someone using drugs, they are a criminal or a scum bag for example. He feels just building a culture like that is not really helpful. Places like safe injection sites could be helpful to bring people out of the shadows.

    Dr. Beatty feels that movies and TV shows, news, commercials can help remove the stigma around addictions and mental health issues. More visual makes more acceptable. Talk about it in a way to promote equality. Treat everybody equal. Can we just treat everybody as a human being no matter where they from what is their background, what color they are, what religion they believe in? We are all human after all, have the same genetic makeup, we are all related. Why then we still treat others as something so different, something so hated? Is it the lack of self-understanding, self-reflection, culture and upbringing? Do we hate someone just because they are different? Dr. Beatty was telling me that California it is very open when it comes to the gay population and gay marriage while other states are not. Same with countries, some countries still do not accept gay marriage. Why do we even need to name things and create different groups to fight for rights? Aren't we all the same? People could be more accepting of each other and not bring hate in their own name or anyone else's name either. All of this comes back to stigma, greed and judgement. Some people and leaders thinking they are better than others.

    Brenda tells me about stigma and addiction. Some people will admit that they have an addiction, they get it, and they don't want to do anything about it. There are also a lot of people who don't want to admit that they have a problem. Brenda feels that part of that has to do with the stigma. Brenda gives me an example with her patients. Patients have more difficulty saying that they have an opiate dependence then saying that they have pain and need medication for it. Trying to have conversation with people and explaining the physiology behind it, the social benefit of recognizing what they have to be able to create a treatment plan. Admitting dependence on something is huge for people, then dealing with how society looks down on them because of it is very difficult. It is another barrier they need to face Brenda asserts. Treating people with no judgement is super important to Brenda. Susan felt like when she went to school others had judged her family based on her brother's addiction. She would defend them.

41. Debt and Consumerism

Flower describes debt and consumerism as an addictive process for a lot of people. We live in a culture that normalizes debt. Debt has been an accepted piece in our society and something that creates addictive behaviors. She feels like this is an unhealthy relationship of living outside of our means and it is destructive. Our culture normalizes it. It is encouraged to keep buying things that we don't need. Lots of advertisements for all occasions. Why do people need to buy a diamond for valentine's day or Mother's Day? Why would anyone need the 15th purse or light set for Christmas? It is so easy to go to the store and buy the next gadget. Do we look at if we really need this before buying anything? Do we need the next fanciest thing because our neighbor or Joe down the road has one? Flower describes an advertisement she just saw that recommends people to pay money to bump up their credit score. She thinks the only reason for this is to get more debt. It does not make sense she asserts it is just so absurd. Flower feels like people don't have an alternative lifestyle that they can imagine. Some people do go to the extreme and move off the grid to decrease debt and be self-sustained, which she agrees with. We have so much access to everything which is so readily available that we just live in kind of an excessive world. Including so much food, so much alcohol, cigarettes, vaping, marijuana, as humans she asserts it is hard to resist that access when we have so much to choose from, it is hard to decline availability.

42. Resiliency and Prevention

Why it is so hard to change? What we can try to do to help break the cycle or support people? How to become a resilient person? Resiliency building is a great tool to gain understanding of ourselves and better our minds, develop essential skills to survive and say no to destructive things and nourish our souls. It has been shown in the research that resiliency skills are very beneficial and preventative, help manage stress and cope with things in our lives. Edward thinks building resiliency would help, absolutely, but not sure how would that look like. We were having a conversation about a little town where there are a lot of shops and restaurants and bars serving alcohol and it can be difficult to find entertainment without alcohol being available. Resiliency training can help to create behaviors that are positive and helpful to our lives, increase caring toward others, motivation, team building and help to work through feelings. Listen better, assume a positive intent, trying not to take things personally, focus on things that the body and mental health needs to stay a focused healthy individual. Show caring and love toward others. Sheila thinks that building resiliency would create less likelihood for people to become addicted. Coping skills might help.

Beth felt like she did not actually know that addiction was a disease until her husband went into treatment. Beth describes resiliency building by stopping a cycle and talking to our children about addiction in a way they can understand it. Teaching coping skills, education. She feels that education is the key to prevention in addiction. This is very challenging in today's society. In the discussion it came up that if she even did not know that this was a disease and she is a nurse; she is educated how about others do they know? How about our children? Angel felt that resilience building needs to start when children are very young and developing their social and emotional skills. The beginning of it is having a conversation and sharing our own experiences. Kayla describes resiliency as connection, involvement, equity, inclusiveness in the community. Making sure that everyone is included. Talk to people, being there for people. Building relationships with people, having genuine conversations with each other in person not with social media.

Rory felt that other cultures like northern European cultures are more connected to each other than Americans. He describes Portugal doing some amazing work in addictions. It is worth to look up Portugal's national strategy. They have different options that might work to fight addictions. Rory feels like the only reason we don't do this in our county because no one had figured out how to make money out of it. All of it is tied to money Rory emphasized. In his mind this is what kills people. Joel felt that we have to create resiliency with each other who are doing the hard work to try to help people and communities dealing with addictions. It is a very hard work she asserts with not much reward and emotionally draining. Providing fair pay would be a start for the extremely hard work. Educating and teaching people is hard, supporting chronic health problems is hard. Janett feels that resiliency and supporting communities to be more resilient would be helpful. More resources in the schools for kids especially who are going through a hard time.

Albert feels like we could do things for prevention he describes the DARE program they had in school, which was pretty much just don't use drugs, he felt it was not really helpful. Some of it was good as an education for why not to do drugs, but he feels it was not enough. Albert thinks mental health issues need to be addressed, having social workers in the schools, who can look at what is going on in a kid's family, why is this kid higher risk at addiction and mental health issues, are the parents addicted? He feels it is all tied together. Just saying drugs are bad does not solve anything. More prevention would be helpful he said and earlier intervention, more education, more support for kids in schools. In schools there is a lot of opportunity to identify kids who are struggling and figure out what can be done to help that child now rather than wait until they are 22 and getting arrested or wait until they are overdosing.

43. Role of Nutrition

Does nutrition play a role of being healthy? What is nutrition's role in addiction and addiction treatment or prevention? Sheila describes that there are things during development that could cause more likelihood for addiction and nutrition could be one of those factors. Sheila mentioned that if someone is eating unhealthy food, they will not feel good and it will be one more obstacle for healing. This is a very likely scenario. Sheila recommends that there are certain things that should only be consumed moderately including processed foods, sugar, salt, fat, especially processed carbs. Eating whole foods, fruits, vegetable whole grains, and healthy source of a protein is important for our health. Beth describes that the body needs nutrients. She feels when people use drugs, that is the only thing they think about and they don't think about what their body needs and all the damage that could be caused by not eating well. With alcohol for example, it is very bad for the body, causes so much damage, the body does not absorb thiamine. Beth believes having a healthy diet is very important. Beth talks about specific foods that are needed if there are preexisting conditions like kidney disease. She describes nutrition as it is dependent on personal needs the condition of our kidneys, our liver. Beth feels that the best thing people can do is have a garden. This might be difficult for people, and even if someone can have some plants in pots where they live that can be helpful. There are also community gardens. Friends and family who has space at their house could let people use a small space for a garden and share the produce. Having a garden, planting things in the ground as well as in pots, barrels. Fruit and nut trees are also beneficial. There is nothing better than a fresh pea pod or a piece of fresh mint, blueberry or raspberry in the morning. Beth describes moderation as an important factor, be good to our bodies. Beth feels that when somebody deals with addictions it might be good for them to take some supplements if they can because she feels they might not get what they need through diet. At that point in their lives diet is not where their focus is. At least until they are healthier, she describes changes she has seen in people's eyes and skin when they are dealing with addiction. Even when somebody becomes sober again it takes a while for the body to recover from addictions.

Mary describes the importance of access to healthy food for everyone. She talked about food allergies that have been emerging in the US. It didn't used to be like that. She had lived her whole life without having to see people with allergies. Now gluten, grain or any other allergies emerged, and she felt like food became so adulterated and so industrialized that it feels like not even real food anymore. Even seeds are bio- engineered. Mary feels that a lot of misery and pain in our bodies comes from poor nutrition. We don't have access to growing our own food and understanding where our food is coming from. Cooking fresh foods allows us to prepare healthy meals. The more people can learn about nutrition and nourish their own bodies by eating healthy food the better. Knowing where the food comes from is empowering, people feel better about taking care of themselves. Mary recommends avoiding things that are processed, people just don't know what is in the cans, packages. Avoid fast foods. Discussed sugar, Mary feels like it is important to know that food also have and emotional component and a birthday cake, a cookie or a slice of pie can be a very meaningful exchange between people. She cautions about total elimination and reminds us to the emotional component of food, and the community component of food. She tells people to avoid foods that makes them feel bad when they eat them. If it makes us feel bad don't eat it.

Angel describes that people have to be physically healthy to be mentally healthy and vice versa and nutrition plays a huge role in addiction treatment and prevention. The body is one big connected system. Addressing the poverty and income disparity is the bigger issue behind nutrition asserts Angel. Poverty is a huge factor. Angel describes when she and her husband were making minimum wage, and everything was canned and boxed in their house. They got what they could whatever was cheap. Now she does not have canned anything at her house unless they made it themselves. Families especially young families when they start out usually do not have the financial resources to eat well. Discussed healthy eating with no processed foods from the store and eating as healthy as possible with the fruits and vegetables people can grow. Angel also mentioned the roles of big food corporations that started in the depression era pushing foods that were processed.

Now, 70 years later we have a very unhealthy population. We also talked about grassroot movement for health and nutrition. Angel asserts that we have to be more cognizant about what we buy and where we spend our money. Encouraging to buy healthy foods and on the other hand making healthy foods more affordable to everyone. Also talked about food banks and the food they provide. So, if someone is dealing with addiction the last thing, they need is highly caffeinated or high in sugar foods. Angel talked about a radio show she heard recently that recommended to be conscious that if people donate something to the foodbank, donate things they would feed their family. Paige talks about her stepfather and how much nutrition helped him in recovery when he followed guidance from counseling and AA it really helped him with his cravings.

Kayla said: "WE are what WE eat". When we eat better, we are more likely to feel better. In recovery there is a lot going on with the body, trying to get through the physical addiction. Kayla feels that nutrition can transform the way we express ourselves and it can play a neat role in recovery. Eating nutritious foods will make the body feel better. Kayla shared something that she called a farfetched idea: **_When we wake up and feel like we empowered enough to care about ourselves and the more likely that we want to care about ourselves the more likely that we will not continue using or being addicted to whatever our substance is_**. Express ourselves through cooking, learn a new skill Kayla recommended. She feels cooking can be a great distraction when people are trying to recover from addictions. Throw ourselves into learning a skill, make something yummy. Kayla also clarified the confusion about process foods. Once we pick something from our garden and cook it, it is processed. So not all processed foods are bad. Staying away from processed food would mean only eating raw things we pick from our garden. She recommends eating whole foods that are from the earth, from the ground, processed minimally so they don't have a lot of package and preservatives, sodium. What people are eating should go bad in a week. Tracy feels she does not know much about nutrition but in recovery it would be a huge part. Meet the needs of the body in healthy ways.

Joel has a different spin on nutrition. She describes basic needs not being met for people and people might be using drugs and alcohol to forget that they are hungry. She feels that basic nutrition is very important for our brain to function. She thinks that if the brain not getting what it needs from nutrition it will start to look where the needs are met. Healthy or unhealthy to curb the need. She talked about food, chemicals placed into food that can change the needs of our brain and brain chemistry. High fructose corn syrup for example. It is in almost everything. Artificial flavoring of chips, soda pops, that might create a need and wanting more.

Janett describes her brother and that nutrition is very important for him. He and his wife try multiple diets, vegan, vegetarian, gluten free for example and being very conscientious about what they put in their body. Janett had some nutrition education in high school. She thinks that nutrition education could be helpful when it comes to addictions. It is one piece of the puzzle; other supports are also necessary like mental health support. Some of it is just where someone is from, she said. Flower feels like the role of nutrition is huge, she recommends the book Seven Weeks to Sobriety by Joan Matthews Larson. It fights alcoholism through nutrition. She feels through the hospital there is not enough being done when it comes to nutrition. The program has a 74% success rate which is a huge success. She decided to read this book. Prevention, health and wellness is important when it comes to relapse. She felt this sounds like a program with great success that should be looked at more. In the hospital system we got caught up so much with acute illness, we don't promote wellness enough. Brenda feels that nutrition is underestimated in all of our chronic morbidities. Many people who deal with drug addiction have nutritional deficits. In other addictions it is also a problem she adds because people set aside nutritional need to meet the needs of their action whatever it is. Besides working with at her clinic she had not thought of how to bring nutritional needs to the forefront when it comes to addictions.

44. Homelessness

Sometimes, things just don't work out. My mom lives in an area in Hungary where the soil is very sandy. She tried to plant different plant. Many died because of the sand or the hot summer and the lack of rain. There is only so much watering she can do, water is expensive, and it just runs down on the sand. She changed tactics. She put tomato plants in big pots buried the pots with the plant to hold some moisture. Topsoil can be added as another solution she would need a lot of it to have enough to prevent the sand just filtering through the water but not providing nutrition. How much support and topsoil would a homeless person needs to create roots and become part of society again? To re-create broken family connections, friendships, find a job, feel like a productive happy person in their skin? Can we just add topsoil? Or do we need to dig deep and remove the sand first? How do people feel like when they see someone living on the streets? Under the bridge? Squatting in an abandoned house? There is a video called Seattle is Dying addresses some of these issues. Homelessness is a problem. Homelessness came up in many conversations I had with people. Bernadette describes frustration with the homeless problem in her county. She feels like the situation has changed a lot in the last decade. She feels that mental illness is scapegoated a lot. Tracy mentioned earlier that she felt that homelessness and mental health are linked.

    Bernadette thinks that the people who are homeless now maybe have some mental illness, and the main problem is addiction. She feels a major problem in the USA is that people don't want to give back. She gives an example that part of her emotional health is giving back to others, she feels that many of the homeless people we have now don't want to give back. They want to take. They want to get high all day, she does not agree with this. She feels when she first moved to Clatsop County, Oregon the majority of homeless people were severely mentally ill. She feels the problem now has been talked about for a decade and nothing been done. She does not think the rest of the people who live there fear this. She does not like to be harassed for money all the time and see littering on the sidewalk. Defecating on the sidewalk. She feels addiction is the problem. She does not know what the solution is. It is bad for business and it creates an unhealthy downtown. Her view about this issue just changed in the past few years. She sees homeless people more in their addiction less as a victim and more as people dealing with addiction and harassing others. Not a simple situation. What can we do? Can we send people to rehab by a court order? It would benefit society in a long run. Problem is there is not even enough room for people who want to be clean. She feels this would only happen if it is mandated. She sees so much lying and manipulation on the streets. Long term rehab might help.

How about people's rights? Is putting a needle in the arm causing harm to self? Could treatment be mandated for this? She feels hopeless about the issue. Lot of putting band aids over the issue that won't fix the problem. Is it fixable? Bernadette recalls knowing students from Portland, Oregon who were homeless and shooting up heroin. Then they go to a hotel with their pimp and the pimp sells them out to other men and they can't leave the hotel and now they are prostitutes, still shooting up. Then she said:" F***, then until they go to jail, and can clean up they just can't get out". She does not want people living in the streets and also don't want them living in tent city either. She gives an examples in Portland, Oregon where the camp was in Chinatown and a lot of those businesses had to close. They were open for decades before. Homeless people are not seen in the rich white neighborhood she adds. They were in Chinatown where Asian people have businesses. She feels this is institutionalized racism. F***, she said how is that ok? Where are the business owners' rights she asks? They are just trying to make a living too. Provide for their families. What about their rights? She feels like the homeless are not victims anymore and they are in an environment that allows them to continue using. It is not ok, she said, it makes her mad. She is truly mad I can hear in her voice. She thinks the solution could be to make everyone go to rehab and make them stay there for 16 months.

Another view on homelessness. Diana recalled a news report where a neighborhood decided to keep the homeless people agitated by playing loud music 24/7. Why would anyone do this Diana asks? These people need to sleep. Why people are being so cruel and try to get them away? Disturbing them and making their mental health worse by having to listen to this crazy music 24/7? Bill tells me a story about getting breakfast sandwiches one morning to give to people by McDonalds in Astoria to prevent them getting a ticket for hanging out in an area they are not supposed to be. Just to see that the truck before him did the same thing. Then he decided to drive into downtown area and give away the 6 breakfast sandwiches to people who were hungry that morning. He said: "looks like you could use a breakfast sandwich". He did not ask why they are there, why they have nothing to eat. He was just kind. He gave what he could. Without being asked, without wanting anything in return. Those 6 people had a breakfast that morning. With the good deed by the truck driver 3 other people had breakfast in Astoria that Sunday morning. He did not tell me the story to show off or put himself in a good light, he just did what needed to be done. He wanted to help the three people by McDonalds, so they don't get into trouble. He ended up helping another 6 people.

    Flower talks about the homeless problem, she feels that a lot of the homelessness is connected to addictions and mental illness issues that are not being addressed. She feels like we have to come up with a better solution, something that actually helps. Not just move people from camp to camp. Identify and assess the actual reasons for homelessness to come up with a solution. She does feel strongly about people using the streets for a bathroom, she does not think this should be allowed and there can be better solutions. She feels that we as a society need to take the responsibility and look at homelessness. She feels that there are people who are down on their luck and providing support is great and purposeful but to tolerate that this is an issue is not a solution. Flower tells me a story about something she saw last week at Northgate in Seattle. There is a sign for cars stating littering will hurt. Meant for cars. Just across the street the City of Seattle was there with Police and people from transportation to clean up a prior homeless encampment. They had an excavator to clean up all the litter and the trash. Huge amount of trash. She found it ironic that there are no consequences for people in that case but right across the street it states litter will hurt. She feels like it is a double standard for sure. There are two different standards for people, and she thinks, no, it's not right we should come up with a better solution so the city would not have to come with an excavator to clean up all the trash. People could have a safe place to be, offer them treatment services and mental health services would be a biggest intervention of all. We talk about difficulty getting into treatment and treatment only being available for certain types of addictions. She knows that they closed down a quite few Medicaid services and opening some for pregnant women. How about the men who are the partners for the pregnant moms? How about other women and men? Flower feels that the more we can do to support people the better outcomes we are going to see. Making it less difficult to get into treatment if people don't have insurance. It is a perpetuating problem. Sometimes people get better in jail because they can't get stuff in jail, but there got to be a better way. There need to be a better solution for this.

45. Reproduction

Bernadette describes herself as a feminist who believes in pro-choice all the way that is the way she votes. She said there is no other way around it. But she adds that is someone is an addict and they have a baby and that baby comes out altered that person should be sterilized. She really believes this. She has seen too many kids in foster care. Who then are being abused by their foster parents. Then they have their own trauma, then they become addicted. Then they are in the system. She breaks with another feminist on this. She knows the history of sterilization in this country with Native Americans, Puerto Ricans, Black women, poor women, she knows, still she firmly believes in this. She is asking why the baby who is born with heroin in their system is less privileged then the mom to have another baby. She feels this is a serious matter, she breaks with progressives on this, she breaks with feminist about this, she just has seen too many babies suffer. She has seen moms putting needles in their arm when they are pregnant. She feels it is just such a vast problem that harms so many kids. It is not their fault and it is not fair. Otherwise she asks where it stops. The mom might not be at fault she might have been abused by a stepdad, and where does this end. She talks about evolution and evolution works the way that people normally want their child to have a chance at a good life. She feels like addiction is counterintuitive to evolution. Are we slowly killing ourselves with addiction?

46. Jail

Bernadette talks about her brother in law who was a very bad crack addict for years, he could not get clean. He finally robbed a bank and ended up in jail. She said this was the best thing that ever happened to him. His system had time to recover from the drugs, they cleared out and he became sober. He is alive now because of it. The family was grateful when he was in jail because then they knew that he was alive. He was in jail before too because of breaking into his ex-girlfriend's house to steal her stuff for crack. He used to lie all the time. They would know because the story was just too long. He is still clean today and doing good for the first time. It was prison that did it. He just had another baby. A little boy. He abandoned his first kid. The second baby was born when he was in prison, he is clean now and has become a good dad. He shows up and he is there. He was not able to parent the first kid, he was gone, he is keeping in touch with his first born now. There is a lot to say about atonement she adds. Be grateful, remain sober and live a productive life. People got to make up for the shitty stuff they did before, be better, want to do better. Addiction s****, it hurts everybody, the person, the family, kids, job, community, everything. It is so bizarre she feels, it is what it is.

Albert feels that even if people were sober in the jail many times they get out and there is a cliff, no support and they go back to what they know, where they used to hang out, do the same things they used to do. He feels that the hand off is not really clean often times. There are some places that are trying to start treatment in the jail. People fall back to the same trap or habits they done before. Some jails now are trying to start treatment in the jail and continue to move people into services when people leave. That would be great he said. He describes people getting out for example Saturday night, now the jail sentence is done so good luck. If they want to go to the health care clinic down the road they can, except that they are closed until Monday. Then they might need to wait 2 months to get in. Even when jail is a good thing for people Albert explains they might not be able to use it as one because of the lack of follow up after they get out. Great step would be starting medication assisted treatment in the jail with immediate follow up after release with connection to services like housing. We discussed improper MAT use as well, Albert had seen people on Suboxone 5 years with high doses and he asserts that does not make sense either. Suboxone as a solution and use it responsibly. Albert states yes, people are supposed to start with Suboxone then taper it down because if it is not administered properly it can be just as bad as other drugs. Albert mentions studies had shown that when it is done right it can help people, and if it is not done correctly then it just leaves people now "doped up" on something else. Same thing with methadone, people go to clinic and use it as a base line then use other drugs on top of it. He laughs.

47. Neal's Story

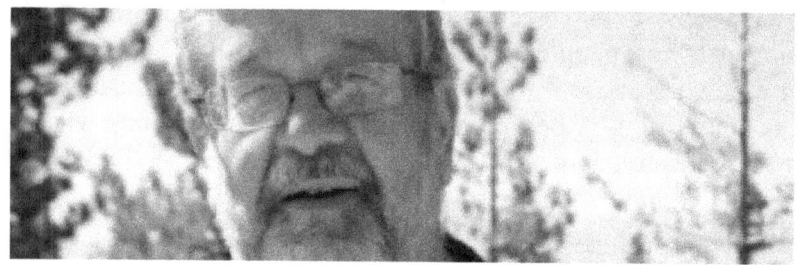

    A mutual friend recommended for me to reach out and talk to Neal. We arranged our meeting via e-mails, and I met Neal in Seaside, Oregon in a coffee shop. We had a wonderful conversation. It was a nice summer day. When I walked into the coffee shop and looked around, I knew exactly that it has to be him. He was having breakfast at a small table reading a book. Neal has a very kind and friendly face. After introductions we moved to a little quieter place in the coffee shop by the windows. We talked about an hour about the plan for this book, we also talked about, him, his books and some world views, then decided to move to the library, the coffee shop got really busy. At the library we talked for another 2-3 hours. Neal is a writer himself; he wrote multiple books one of them is about mentoring boys and men. Neal has been working in the court systems for a long time. He is a mentor, support and father figure for young men in trouble. He is a wonderful person to be around. We need a lot of Neals in this world.

    Neal tells me about his experiences in addiction and his life. He grew up in Tillamook, Oregon, his father was a physician. He had talked with his father about a lot of situations and medical, psychological problems that people had in the community. He helped out in the office for the while and met different patients who had medical and mental health problems. This was in the 1960's before Tillamook had a mental health clinic, AA and NA in the community. Neal felt that his dad's office was kind of a mental health clinic. He studied psychology in school, got a degree in political science. He decided to go toward a law degree, while in school he become a resident assistant and counselor in the dorms. He took some more psychology and sociology classes. During college he had seen a lot of drug and alcohol abuse. During law school he ended up being a counselor in his class. Students in the class would come to him and talk to him about their problems. Neal is very easy to talk to. He helped some people to get into counseling and treatment and did some suicide interventions. Once he got his degree he moved back to Tillamook and opened up his own practice. He noticed that his clients had other things going on like depression, alcoholism, family problems like divorce, addiction. He noticed a trend in the families as well. Neal did a lot of networking with the social workers, the counselors in his community, the mental health clinic to help his clients.

    He ended up specializing in working with clients in the legal community who had addiction, mental health and psychological problems. It is a small community, he adds. He learned about mental disorders and diagnoses. After about 5 years Neal become the district attorney. He tried to focus on how to get people into treatment and what are the things that are going to work. He did collaboration with the sheriff, the jail, the mental health clinic to improve services. There was a struggle personally and professionally trying to help people with addiction and mental health problems. I ask Neal why he thinks there was a struggle. He tells me that he was supposed to be this mean prosecutor. He tells me: "I am supposed to be Mr. Law and Order". Instead he was trying to help people and not throwing them to jail or prison. He was trying to get them help and treatment. He wanted to help the people change their lives around. This become politically controversial. There was a lot of resistance to this way of trying to help people. Neal tells me that there was also a lot of struggle to try to get the support people needed like counseling and therapy. He had dealt a lot with sex offenders and there was no program in the county. People had to go to Portland to get help. Neal wanted them to go to treatment, he felt just throwing them in jail without treatment is not going to help, without treatment they will just go out and reoffend once they get out of jail. Neal got defeated by another prosecutor in the office and he went back to private practice. He became a traffic court judge for Tillamook and Clatsop counties for a while. Later he got a full-time judgeship in Tillamook. Neal tells me that running for judicial office, people are not supposed to be political, but he was in a sense of advocating for people with mental health and addiction problems to get services. He was on the board for the women's crisis center, on the board of AA and the mental health clinic.

As a judge he had a lot of diversion programs and referred people to get help. He had worked with a lot of minors who had possession of alcohol and marijuana. He created workshops for the first-time offenders. He describes Tillamook at that time as a logging, fishing community with a lot of drinking that was part of the culture. He was trying to change the culture. He was advocating for change. Working as a judge and working in the community people turned to Neal for help with their kids. He was a resource for: "I got trouble with my kid what do I do". I asked Neal what he talked to the kids and parents about? He talked about unconditional love, compassion, empathy, healthy father figure in their lives. He was active in men's groups. Neal realized that in our society we do not do a celebration for adulthood like in some other cultures. In some cultures, a whole village might come together to celebrate. Neal feels those transitions are important to make young people feel valued, celebrated and honored. A lot of adolescents today don't have a place and a role in society. Neal thinks because of this ritual and coming of age ceremonies for youth are important.

Neal tells me a story about a young boy who was 14 years old and been involved in small crimes before. He was sitting in his room with a pistol and was threatening to kill himself. His mom called Neal. He was trying to get mental health support from the local mental health entity to go his house, but no one was available. Neal decided to go over. He was not sure what to do. Neal had a choice to go or not to go. He thought if he does not go, he might kill himself, if he does maybe he won't. He knew this boy from before and they had a trusting relationship. He kind of turned into being a crisis worker. It resolved favorably, he was just angry and in the end of his rope Neal explains, he did not know what else to do. He still had the gun in his hand when Neal got there after a few minutes Neal told him he felt uncomfortable with the gun, the boy pointed it away then gave it to Neal after a few more minutes. He did not really want to use it. Neal unloaded the gun and put it away. It was all about anger for his dad who called him worthless, he was also lost and self-medicated with drugs and alcohol. Neal was able to take him to the counseling after and he talked to a counselor. Neal was sitting in on the sessions, he would not talk to the counselor without Neal being present. Neal feels that just like that youth, others also need some adults who support them in their lives besides their parents. Someone who creates a positive influence who can tell them that they are important, have potential, they are worthy. we have a conversation about fragmented society. Neal thinks that people are really isolated, and they think that they don't matter or that they are not important.

    Neal is passionate about helping young people to start out a better life, to know that someone cares for them, to know that they matter. Neal also had two foster sons and helped guiding their lives. Neal tells me that when people feel that someone cares about them then it might switch the thinking from, I don't matter to I do matter. Neal feels that then people can move on and start talking about what is going on. The story with the boy and the gun ends well. He went back to school, did counselling and called Neal a few years later and told him he met the woman of his dreams and was asking Neal to officiate at his wedding. Of course, Neal did. Neal felt like he cried more than anyone else. This made me chuckle. I can hear in his voice he was very proud. It is like one of his little ducklings now all grown up and ready to be on his own in the world. He still friends with him and talks to him occasionally. What a wonderful story of being able to turn someone's life around. He was really there for this young boy. The substance abuse went away once he realized that he is angry and depressed he got therapy and once the rejection, depression and anger was worked out he realized he does not need alcohol and marijuana and other stuff. He figured out he was self-medicating. He was able to work through it. He had some great insight, desire to change his life. That experience really changed Neal. He felt that we need to do a lot better in society and need to get to kids before they have a gun in their hand. Neal talked in schools, talked to counselors, the police to get the community more engaged. Neal worked on connecting the police officers with counseling to share information and skills like emphatic listening. 20 years ago, it was not a part of training now it is. Back then the police officers were not trained on how to deal with mental health or suicide or substance abuse problems, just put people in jail if they caused a disturbance. Neal feels like he was influenced a lot by his wife who was a teacher at that time to educate and effect people that way. Neal had a friend who invited him to go out to the youth prison and work with youth who did not have families or fathers to help with socialization and to teach them about friendship. Neal started to go and listen to their stories. Neal did this for about 8 years. He would go 3 times a week. There was a little canteen where he would get coffee and candy bar for them and listen to their stories, play cards, play a guitar. Most of these young boys did not know how to have a conversation or play a game. It was a lot to take in what happened to some of these boys and Neal had to figure out how to process this at 8:30 pm at night when going home. It was really heavy stuff, horrific stories of neglect and cruelty. He would go home and write down the stories. This is how the book about mentoring young men come about. His wife would read the stories and cry. Then they would talk about that others don't know what these boys went through. Neal expressed that many people might just think, of well they are just a bunch of sex offenders, lock them up and throw away the key. He felt that the world needs to hear their stories. Now people can read about them. Neal feels reading these stories could help others who went through bad experiences. Neal would share some of his own stories with the boys, be there for them, he did different exercises and he tells me about one that is called the trust walk.

The trust walk: You go out the back yard. You tell the person: I want you to know I care about you and you are important to me. I want you to blind fold me and lead me around the back yard. I will trust you. Neal did this with his foster son who really enjoyed. Then they switched roles and have positive affirmation and supportive sentences. His son loved it. It took about 20 minutes. - Neal

---

Neal tells me a story of how his foster sons come into his life. I heard the story before when we were sitting in the coffee, I asked him to please tell it again. Neal's wife was a teacher and she thought an improvisational drama English class. She had their future son in her class, he was very verbal, very bright. He was struggling. One week he was just crashing and awful depressed. She talked to him to find out that his mom kicked him out of the house, the only thing she gave him was a toothbrush, he had a friend who was working at the gas station and he was sleeping there on the floor. He did not have breakfast maybe some school lunch, no dinner, no place to be. She asked him where he would live, he had no one. That night she went home and asked Neal:" Do you want a kid?" He said this with such a great voice that we both busted out laughing. It was a sad situation for this young boy and laughter was a good release. His mom was bipolar. The stepdad he had was abusive to his mom and physically and sexually abusive to him.

    Neal found out from one of his new mentees that one night the boyfriend of his mom took him crabbing to the bay. He realized that there were no crab pots on the boat. He got alarmed. The guy made him get out of the boat, he told him: "I don't want you anymore, I want you to drown tonight". In the middle of the bay he pushed him out of the boat. He started his boat, went back to the land and left him in the water in the middle of the bay. The tide was coming in. He was a good swimmer. It took him about 2 hours, but he swam back to shore. This was about 10 miles from Tillamook in Netarts bay. A young boy in the middle of the night left in the water to die. No words, just emotions that are screaming. How can someone do something so awful to a child whom they supposed to protect? Luckily, he was a good swimmer. He swam back to the shore and had to walk 10 miles back to the house soaking wet. The guy never got charged. Neal's young mentee never believed that anyone would believe in him that this happened, and he felt worthless. He felt that he is disposable if someone can just do this throw him off the boat. He kept what happened inside of him for about a year before he told Neal. He went back to the house after this, he also had a younger brother and he was worried about his brother. In a way he was kind of relieved when mom kicked him out of the house, because this way he was away from the abusive boyfriend as well. He did not really have a choice where to live had nowhere else to go home even after a horrific attempt to drown him. We had a conversation about this person who attempted to drown Neal's young mentee. He is still around Tillamook, was never charged, the young boy just wanted to forget him and now it is too late anyway. It is difficult for Neal to see this person around Tillamook and know what he had done. The boy is now doing very well now. He works in California, have a very nice girlfriend. He teaches others and, he has his own business.

Neal's son's younger brother also eventually come to live with them. He got involved in the criminal justice system, went to jail for 2 years. He had problems with Alcohol. Neal would go to AA meetings with him. Neal was the sober 'dad". He is doing well now, he is married, he is a dad, he has a good job. After he was released and was on parole, he did not know what to do. He loved to cook. Neal hooked him up with a culinary school in Portland and he went through the school, graduated. They are still close. Neal is very proud how well he has done. Neal enjoyed going to the AA meetings with him, enjoyed the process and the support they received. Neal's 2 adopted sons motivated him to keep on with things and help others, he saw the value of having someone in their life who shows up and cares. He tells me this sounds simple and Pollyanna, yet it is incredibly important for someone to show up in our lives. Sometimes the simplest things can be the most meaningful. Being there for someone when they need it is extremely important. Building basic trust, it is the beginning of everything.

I ask Neal if he is willing to share some more details from his work experience. He does. He tells me that a lot of people went to his court and it is a small community, there is criminal court, family court, juvenile court, traffic court. In a small town Neal tells me it is all mixed up. He saw people with different problems and the same fundamental issues including lack of education, deep psychological wounds that were not getting addressed. Alcohol, drugs, violence all mixed up. Neal saw all this happening in the court room and started to think about how to address these issues and work on improving them. The idea was to try to do something that helps and supports people, so they don't repeat the cycle and keep ending up in court. Neal feels that a lot of people go out, commit crimes and mess up so they can go back to jail. Jail is safe, clean, secure, there is medical care, the jailers care about them in some way, there are 3 meals a day, no drama. It is better place then what they have normally in the outside, they don't have to struggle to get a job. There is a lot of reasons to go back to jail Neal asserts and if people are desperate jail can be pretty compelling. It is kind if a safe place. Many people told Neal it is the best place they ever lived. Neal was trying to figure out how to break this cycle how not to spend the jail resources on someone again and again and again. Neal found it helpful to share some of his own personal experiences, and to plug in some resources. Tillamook county is one of the ones in the state that still does not have a drug and mental health court. No treatment at the county jail. He is telling me about the huge heroin, methamphetamine and opiate problem now, how to break the cycle with the resources the county has? 60% of jail inmates are on mental health medications. Neal feels like we have to figure out a different way to do what we are doing now. No halfway house after someone gets out of jail, no safe residential program, no job placement program, no GED program in jail, no literacy. He feels those things are needed to help break the cycle and be successful. Neal is retired now; he still goes out and mentor people in different ways. He is involved in a number of nonprofits, he is a band, monthly open mike, the grange to get together, one of Neal's vision is to have a healthy place for people to get together to have a healthy sober community. A place to get together instead of a bar. We certainly need more of those sober, healthy places in our society. Neal is trying to make this happen in his community.

    Neal feels this is kind of radical. He asks the question ***how we build a community without having it surrounded around a bar?*** All the fraternities in his town have bars. Big community events have alcohol. Neal tells me that he drinks occasionally, and it should not be the center of life and the center of socializing. There is a huge misconception and cultural norm about this. People feel that when they go out and do something they have to drink. Neal agrees. Why do we do that Neal asks. Why do we sell alcohol almost every event? Can't people just go out and have a good time without drinking? Neal tells me that in his professional life he dealt with a lot of this. 90% of his caseload was alcohol and drug related. I asked Neal that based on his experience what addiction means to him, how he would define it. Neal feels addiction is a response to something inside of people that is very close to our soul. Neal is looking for the right words for a second and trying to define what addiction means to him. Then, Neal tells me that he has wounds inside of him. Some of the wounds are from childhood, some are from adulthood. He feels that some of it is genetic, he is interested in the trauma studies that been coming out now. I ask him if he is thinking of the ACE studies. Yes, he was referring to those. Neal feels that trauma and the wounds people experienced, and the wounds of people's parents and grandparents experiences stays with the individual. It is an infected gaping wound. Neal feels that one of our tasks in life is to recognize those wounds and start healing them. We are all interconnected and the closer we are to somebody the more we can feel their pain. Neal feels that until we heal those wounds through love and compassion and other tools it is tempting to self-medicate. It is so psychologically painful to people. It is hard to bear the hurt and the agony. People want to feel better, so society says, have a drink or smoke a joint, have a toxic relationship or whatever it is. It will mask the wound, it will make it feel better, yet it will not go away. The addiction will be there until the wound is cleaned and can start healing. As a nurse I seen many wounds and some heal slow, some heal fast depending on how deep it is, how big it is, how good is the person's immune system, how the person is supported in the healing process. May times it needs a whole team, individual, family, nurses, doctors, specialists to help heal a complex would. Just as with addiction, people cannot do it alone. Most people need help. Neal feels that addiction is this tension and drive to medicate so people don't feel the pain. To help healing people have to go and find the source of their pain and heal that source. Neal had his moments when he self-medicated too. He been destructive before. He is not proud of it. It is real. Neal feels this probably happens to all of us. He tells me: "Then I have to get my ego out of the way and go deal with this stuff". Neal repressed some things in his life, just like many people. He is thinking about this, it is like a self-discovery happening at this moment right in front of my eyes. He tells me it is like just too much happening at this moment if he locks it up for a while, it is in a box. It was interesting we both sad this at the same time. It is in the box. He tells me he can deal with the box in the basement, it is just a locked-up box. If he opens it up, oh my God, now I have to deal with it. It is like of pandora's box, right?

Yeah, he said. In collage, in law school he tells me he drunk way too much, he had been vicious, and angry in some of his relationship with others. He struggled in his marriage with this. His wife struggled with this too. They both had childhood issues that they ignored and placed in the box in the basement. He felt this was one of the reasons they found each other. They helped each other deal with it. Neal gets emotional here and tells me that he realized in the last couple years one of his wounds. His tells me a story about a male relative that was physically violent with him when he was a teenager. He also had a classmate when he was 10 years old who sexually abused him. Neal put those experiences in a box in the basement. Then he tried to ignore the box in the basement. Neal tells me about his male relative, he was like cherished in his in the community, and everybody thought he was a wonderful kind person. He was, yet he also beat Neal. The rest of the community did not know that side of him. This created a conflict. I asked him how often it happened. It happened 3-4 times. He was angry at Neal. Neal talked back when he was a teenager. He punished him by beating. When Neal was raising his stepson and foster sons, he wanted to be a very good parent. Neal describes that when his sons would act out, he had the "old tape" from childhood how to take care of a kid if they misbehave. It was to take of his belt and beat them. He actually almost found himself falling into that pattern too. Then he realized:" Holly crap, no". He realized it is not the right way to go, and that was his programing in his brain. That is what he learned from the male relative. It was terrifying for him. He realized he wanted to change and wanted to do things differently. He wanted to be a good dad. He did not want to be like that relative of his. He broke the cycle. We discussed behavior and actions that are learned in families from generation to generation and how people can break that cycle. How we realize that it is not the right thing to do when it is what we learned? When it is what someone seen and learned from their parents? Behavior change is very difficult. Neal asks me how does this work? He is still thinking about this process. How do we break the cycle?

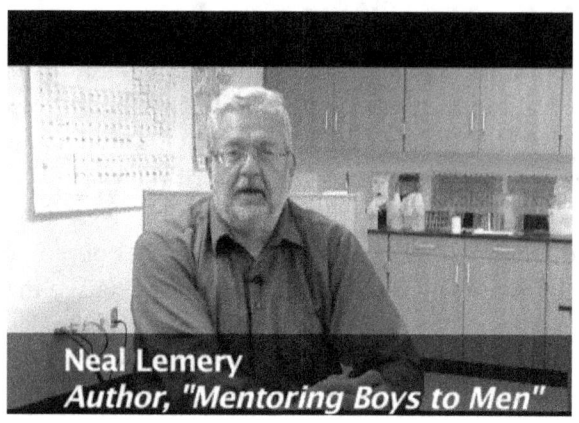

When it comes to our individual and societal responsibilities Neal thinks: "get it out on the table, here is the topic, here is the issue". We need to talk about them the solutions the remedies, the issues. Have conversations. Talk about how we parent a kid, we don't teach parenting he tells me we don't talk about parenting. Neal thinks that it is not only the parent's responsibility to parent a child. It takes a whole village. we should all look out for each other and everyone's kids, they are the future generation. This was a motivator for Neal to go out and help mentor others, he felt like people who live in his community, he wanted them to be healthy. Neal then tells me a story about a murder case where a child saw her mother murdered. He was 9 years old. Neal recognized right away that this kid needs support and counseling and contacted a counselor. The kid got therapy that he needed, and Neal received a bill. The county declined to pay the bill, he had to find money through a grant to pay this counselor. The kid grew up to be a wonderful young man, Neal seen him recently. It was great to see the good outcome. Neal never understood the commissioners not feeling this child important enough to spend money on. He tells me that society and our attitude need to change on what is important. The struggle he tells me to pay the counselor, really? I ask him about healthcare, and he started to laugh. Neal believes that healthcare especially preventative healthcare is a fundamental human right, we should have a single payer system and just do it. He tells me about a meeting he went to yesterday. He found out that 90% of healthcare costs are for preventable conditions. We talk about prevention, treating the whole body doing preventative testing like checking A1c levels for diabetes. Neal compares it to an oil change. Focusing on prevention not treating the disease. This would help the population be healthy. We talk about the concept of getting paid if the population is healthy not when they are sick. He would definitely increase the prevention efforts. Neal believes in preventative healthcare and educating kids about trauma, addiction, mental health, depression, make it a universal educational goal. Provide knowledge. Neal tells me about a person in his community who come out and told people in social media about his depression. He made himself vulnerable to help others. I ask Neal about the government's role. He lets out a big sigh, then he tells me it is a public health crisis. He feels that the government should be able to get involved and be a leader in public health. Not this administration he tells me. Obama's administration, quite a bit. Neal feels that government should provide leadership. We are all in this together, we are all affected by this, here some words of wisdom, sympathy and encouragement. He recalls Reagan's promise when mental health hospitals were closed that we will have community mental health. We really don't have that he said, it is grossly underfunded. Neal feels we need to have a commitment for that. He feels the mental health clinic in his community is the jail. People with drug addiction get hauled off to jail, which is not a very effective method. Neal feels that there is a public demand for change and to do things better. We as a society do not know how to deal with anger and rage. He feels society needs to address this and the role of government can be to convey people to address solutions. Have a nation-wide conference and let's talk about this, addiction is also a spiritual and human crisis as well. He tells me about empathy, compassion, listening, caring. He tells me he feels my book is very timely and highly needed.

48. Humanity/Nationality

What is humanity? What is nationality? Does it matter where someone was born? What makes us human? Are we alone as humans in this universe? How is our humanity connecting to addiction? Is addiction to things are just part of who we are? What are our responsibilities as human beings? Fuchsia is an American citizen, and she was not bon in the Unites States. She came as a child, yet she never fully felt she belonged here. She was born in Japan. She does not fully feel she belongs to Japan either. She is not accepted there. She is white, not Japanese. She feels she has a different perspective. What it means to be American to her is different than a lot of other Americans. I ask her what does it mean to be an American to her? Big sigh. She tells me she does not know. Then she tells me it is a place where she lives. She appreciates freedom of expression. This what was the reason they moved back to the US. Good connection to nature in smaller communities. She likes the diversity, yet she feels it is not protective enough. She does not identify with American food as comforting at all. She feels patriotism is interesting. She thinks that a lot of people are very proud of this country and everything we've done, and it does allow a certain amounts freedom. She lived in other places where Americans are pretty hated. She gives me an example when she lived in Japan on Okanogan island, she tells me 30% island is American because there is a military base there. When she was walking around people were very hostile until they realized she was not part of the military. Then they were very friendly and very warm. She saw American military people trying to talk to Japanese clerks and got mad when they did not understand them. When people are in someone's else's country and they are mad because they don't understand the native language, she felt this was very backwards.

Ron believes that we can do a better societal and emotional path for ourselves as humans through raising some consciousness and clarity focusing on love, families, jobs, creating a better world, that is simple where coping mechanisms like turning to alcohol and drugs is not needed. Ron believes in one unified government and one world unified government. Stop borders and walls and passports and nationalism. Then he shares his dream. He warns me that this will sound like he is totally cuckoo. Ron believes that aliens exist. He believes in the military industrial complex as an evil. Shadow government where all the corporate money is. All the research and technology are there. He believes that the earth had energy and medical technology that far surpasses anything that we know. He talks about free energy we had since the early 1900's. Instead of using coal, oil, wires, telephone poles. Medical technology to cure diabetes, cancer, HIV, but not profitable to be out for the public. He believes in the out alliance which is basically an intergalactic council. He believes all this exists, he had read and seen lots and lots of stuff. He recommends the Gaia channel which is a network of well-done documentaries and series on spiritualism and conspiracy theories, 11, area 51, JFK, and other things on health and science. He watches a lot of these documentaries and having a lot of conversations. He is just waiting for what they are calling the disclosure to happen. Disclosure is other worlds beyond ours and now there is a concept that we are not doing well and the intergalactic presence are worried and feeling that they will need to step in because if earth and people keep going the way they are with climate change and industrial espionage and wars and everything else, they feel that in not too much longer we are done. They are stepping in. That is the disclosure project. Ron thinks this will happen within our lifetime. He thinks we will see when enough is enough. He is excited for this. He would like this to happen as soon as possible. Release all the files and patents to save lives. Take down walls. It is all about money, power, resources.

49. Possible Solutions

Solutions are not easy. Cucumbers and squashes are most of the time easy to grow. Just like kids, most of the time there is no problem. The cucumber and squash are very healthy for people, it grows, it grows many people pick it, eat it raw or cook it, make it into a salad. It makes a cheap healthy food option. Normally, that is, plant the seed, water, pick the vegetable. That does not happen all the time. Moving to a new area about 5 years ago and trying to grow cucumbers, squashes and zucchini that normally grows crazy, the vines did grow crazy, but as soon a little squash appeared when it was less than an inch it started to rot. The garden is not huge, and the vines took up a lot of space with no results. It was not a good environment or not the right seed. Genetics give us a predisposition to things those are our seeds that we come with as a person. Then the environment, like the soil, rain, sun for the squash, housing social economic status, parents, food, education, support, love for a child. Then we all get what we get. For me it took 4 years to be able to create a change for my squash and cucumbers to be happy. And it was not just me. I gave up and gave seeds to a friend who started to grow them in her green house, then another friend mentioned she grows her mini squashes climbing up instead on the ground. My friend asked me every time if I want to take and try some cucumbers and squashes after all they are my babies, my seeds. I said no many times before deciding ok. One more time, will try this new method. Just took a few plants, created strings, trained the vine to go up instead on the ground. Watered, watched. The vine grew. Then cucumbers and squashes appeared. A lot of them. And they were happy. It took others to care, it to me to keep being open and try, it took my friend keep encouraging me when I was ready to give up. Kids need the right environment to become happy, healthy adults and not to turn to drugs and alcohol or games or to any other addictions to be happy, just like my squashes and cucumbers. Still, when they are in trouble a child, youth, or and adult person need someone to get that string and help train the vine to go up, stand toward the right direction instead of laying down and rotting on the ground.

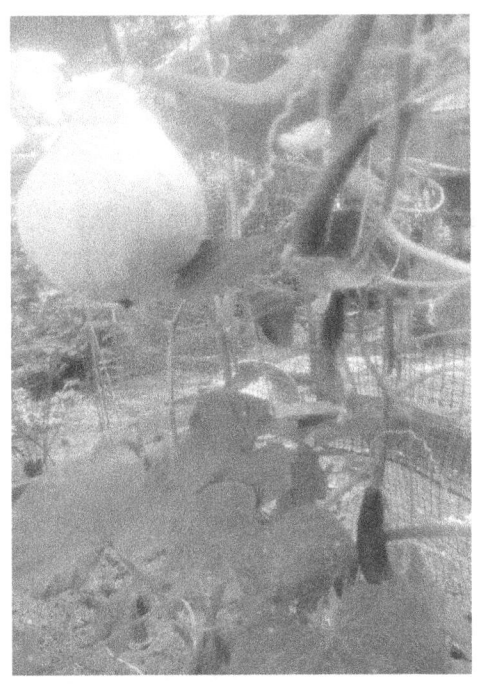

Squashes and cucumbers in my garden summer 2019, Oregon

One of my squash become a 16.3 lb. giant. The biggest squash I had ever grown. What could be possible solutions for addiction? There are so many problems embedded in our society. Can we fix some of those issues? Could we tilt the scale? Can we create a more positive and caring world? Education? Trainings? Free care? Kayla told me she thinks it takes *a multi-dimensional approach* to treat addiction. Nutrition is one of them, it will help us feel better. *We want people to care about what they put in their body* said Kayla. If they learn to care, then they might decide not to put drugs like cocaine int heir body anymore. Beth believes in *education*, education, education. She is always about education. *Getting the word out there, advertisement, radio, education, billboard signs*. Education and support. *Do not enable the person who is addicted*. AA, NA, ALNON, provide resources and maybe create something new, a more up to date group, a group that is more modern, a group for tomorrow. More resources and get people there. Beth was asking me: how do you get people there? It is only once a week. Not enough. More advertisement where the meetings are so they can be found easier could be one solution that Beth recommends. Less pot shops she said. Educate in grade school what is right and wrong to put in our body. Would more education help? Would less pot shops help? Exactly what type of education and whom to educate? Addicts? Their family? People before they become addicted? Youth? Parents before they become parents? Sheila describes that having people to talk to been helpful for her. People who are friends or dealing with similar issues and are non-judgmental, understanding how others feel. They won't put others down if they fail and have to restart the recovery process. Treatment. Beth told a story where we can see treatment can help, it helped her husband. It was too late for her brother unfortunately. She emphasized to me that she will not support the habit of addiction and she made this clear to her nephew. Beth does not believe in relapse. She puts it this way: Relapse is just another excuse to die.

> *"I do not believe in relapse. Period. I had made it clear to my husband and I made it clear to my nephew. I do not believe in it. Relapse is just another excuse to use and another excuse to die". - Beth*

When Beth went into treatment with her nephew a counselor told her it is ok to relapse. She got really upset. Shae said: "do you realize that this kid is using heroin?" It's not ok. Talking to Beth was really emotional. She felt that with relapse her husband and her nephew could die the same way her brother died. In her mind she decided this is not ok, it cannot happen. Beth believes we need more mental health and education in schools about addictions. When I asked Beth what one thing she would change, she would make it that Narcan be more easily available. She was a little unsure, if it would be a good thing or not. She feels like if Narcan would have been available for her brother he could have lived. It could have saved her brother. Beth emphasizes that no matter who the person is or where they go, they will know somebody with addiction. She was wondering if drugs would be harder to get would that help, if alcohol costs more maybe. Getting to the root of the cause and dealing with the disease. Beth believes that the best thing to do is being educated about addiction. Also talk with our children. Talk to them about peer pressure.

"own your own mind"- Beth

Even if someone could do drugs it does not mean that they should. Be mindful the mind and what other things using substances can cause. Think about the money that can be saved. Beth likes the security of money. She grew up poor. Beth once tried to tell a patient how much money he could save by stopping smoking. The patient got very angry; she does not do this anymore. He patient was very mad at her. When we get stressed out:

"count backwards, take a walk, try mediation, try other things, other coping mechanisms before you have that cigarette or drink alcohol next time". - Beth

Beth stresses the importance of adequate education, more addiction treatment services, more information out there. She was uncertain if it is even possible, maybe educating young people. The next generation. Live by example, set a good example. Spreading the word, start a conversation. She said:" buy this book and share a story". Education is a huge part in prevention, intervention and understanding of addictions, its causes, learning coping skills.

I asked Mary what she thinks a solution could be, she laughed and said, well abolish capitalism. There are wonderful changes happening in the world regarding LGBTQ populations and being more open. Mary describes other movements like black life matters and Me-too movements, she feels that the more that people feel empowered and say this is enough. The more people are willing to collaborate and talk about hard things, reducing shame and support self-regulate one and other, connection, collaboration. Meet people where they are at. Some people might want to use the harm reduction model, then support them, offer people opportunities for hope. Rehabilitation while learning skills and be with other people like working on a farm, while rebuilding the mind and body. Learning people's own capabilities reconnect to one and other and to our earth were some ideas we talked about. Even if someone might not be able to do farming, they can find some way to build connections. Help other people like a peer support model. We are a social species we need these things to prevent suffering she adds. **_There is hope if we can continue to support a movement of connection and collaboration between human beings and fight against separation and oppression._** Mary feels like addiction is a disease of loss hope, it is a disease of despair so showing a way to people that they can somehow contribute provides hope, maybe creates a willingness of change and have a purpose.

    Edward described genetics testing as a possible solution and letting people know that they have a genetic predisposition to addiction. Education about avoiding certain chemicals. Edward also suggests that doctors need to know this information as well. It might help subscribe fewer opioids and prescribe pain killers in a different way. He feels that maybe we can do a little and can't solve a problem. It is not an easy situation. Working on prevention with any disease is the key. Once the disease is there, we can work on the treatment options. It is much more difficult to cure something as complex as addiction, would be better to prevent it. Addiction is so widespread; we have to work on both prevention and treatment. Looking at the genetic predisposition could be a preventative method just like we use it for any other diseases like cancer. Edward also describes just being supportive of people who are trying to be sober from alcohol. If they don't want to drink don't ask why, just let it be and respect their decision. I asked Edward what he would personally do if he meets someone dealing with addiction what would he recommend for them. He thought professional counseling would be the way to go. Have a clinical intervention, let the professionals decide what is the best.

I asked Dr. Tedd Levin what he think we can do to prevent addiction. He said it is a great question and a very difficult question. He describes programs like AA and NA being there to prevent relapse, not to prevent addiction. Dr. Levin feels that we would need a lot **_more education in the school system_**, peer group support, targeting people according to risk factors, make it a routine for preventative health maintenance. One of the problems is the dysfunctional health care system where the doctors are really rushed. I have heard this from multiple people. Fifteen minutes is not enough to address major problems. Why is the big rush? Is it just to make money? Could health care providers see less patients and spend more time?

Talking to Angel she felt that **_coping skills should be thought to kids from preschool._** The first 3 years of life is when kids develop the social emotional skills that helps us to be healthy people. It has to start at the very beginning. Angel feels that as a parent we have to empower our kids to feel things, figure out things, have the power to know that they can fix things, and every tiny experience can help. She gives an example when a mother was trying to fix a seat belt for her 14-year-old son in a go cart. Angel told him to let him be he will figure it out. It might seem small, the only way kids will learn, parent want to provide guidance and they cannot be there all the time so teach kids how they can figure things out. Empower children, so they can be strong in the world and they can believe in themselves. Be there as a safety net of course. Sometimes they have to fail, which can be difficult to see as a parent. Angel asserts it is ok to fail sometimes. This is how they learn. This will create the power to get up and start over again.

> _Empower our children, so they can get up on their own when they fall down._ Life is going to knock you down and make you start over again, that is just the way it is. - Angel

Life can throw people down on a path that they had no idea how and where they will end up. People have to have the strength and ability to get through tough times. Angel believes that all parents generally want their kids to be happy and healthy. They might not think that how their current action might affect their kids as adults. Treatment is not accessible for people who do not have insurance or money, in a rural county it is very difficult to get help. - asserts Angel. **_Make treatment affordable and available_** to people regardless to where they live. Stop blaming, not helpful. **_Teach kids that it is ok to struggle_** sometimes, not everything will be great all the time. Work on **_removing stigma_** from metal health conditions like bipolar, anxiety or depression for example. People should not have to hide their mental health issues from other people. Ultimately, **_there is a lot we need to do and a lot we can do_**. What is it that we can do? I asked. Having conversations, she said, having conversations like this is the first step. Make our own self a little vulnerable, uncomfortable and volunteering, supporting people and organizations that are doing good work. Putting pressure on our politicians: "this has to be a priority and we need to take care of each other". – Angel. Engage and talk about addictions. Help whatever the help looks like. Stop kicking the can down the road thinking that someone else will fix this, it is not going to happen. Teaching our kids how to be healthy, how to eat heathy, how to take care of themselves because the body is one big interconnected system. Be empathetic and just be there for those people who are dealing with addictions. Let them know that people are there for them. Don't blame, nobody makes this choice. Help each other it makes us better as people.

      Paige thinks we need more mental health services to be available. Services should be quicker, when people are ready. Have counseling available. Paige feels that time laps makes people feel like they are not worthy. Keep talking to kids, keep telling them real stories. Not just one story, but many. Stories will tell kids that even people who were stubborn and thought they were super strong got taken by the drugs. Tell them how it started. She feels the stories could tell kids don't even try it does not worth it. There might not be a simple fix, but definitely need to have more discussion about addiction. Telling stories can be very powerful. Giving examples what happened to others can send a message to watch out, be careful, don't try to fit in by using substances it really is not worth it.

Chief Jason felt that having more readily available treatment options for any type of addiction is very important. Additionally, supporting people, not judging people, having the understanding that addiction is a sickness. Find the humanity inside, separate their actions from being who they are. People with addiction might do horrible things like stealing, robbery or assault. They are also someone's daughter, son, family or friend. They are controlled by the addiction no matter what type of addiction it is. Jason mentioned gambling, alcohol and drugs. Jason stated: "treat the beast that is inside them, that is not who they are". Do not feed into it. He saw that sometimes families either ignore what is going on or being enabling by giving money to their loved one who is dealing with addiction. He cautions families not to fall for lies when their loved one said they need it for food it is probably not for food but to buy drugs or alcohol. Jason recommends that if a family member is asking for money buy them what they need or go with them to the store. This is what he did with his mom. Then families will know that they are actually buying food or hygiene items for example. Create support by strengthening education, building stronger families, building stronger influences at the schools, teachers paying more attention to things going on behind the scenes. Kayla described solutions that can include enough mental health care providers where people can actually go and talk to, having more education and awareness about addictions. Have healthcare. Urgent care for mental health and addictions so people can go and talk to someone if they need to talk to someone. Kayla also felt that there is not as much information out there as there should be about where people can go if they need help. She does not know about the resources, and if she does not then maybe others do not know the resources as well.

Rory compares solutions to a measles outbreak, even if it is deadly there are still people who do not vaccinate. Even with evidence that there is no risk there are people who don't vaccinate, and their kids get sick and die. He feels we are not going to change people's minds. He said quite frankly we are not. He describes family culture of use that goes back generations. He describes people's parents as heavy drinkers for example. It is just what they do. It is very hard to change these cultural norms. He brings up smoking as an example as not a lot of success because now the young generation just uses a new product. Honestly, he feels that these things just live on an assigned wave, they peak then go down, peak and go down again. Maybe try to get messages out ahead of time before the next peak, he did also feel that he does not have any answers. Is there a solution? Do we just let it be? Is it just part of a cycle? What about other diseases? Do we just let them be? Rory feels that we should just do what feels right no matter what it is. If it is the just say no campaign or the DARE to be off drugs, good. Whatever it is. He describes an experience when he was working on the AIDS project. Trying to convince people to use condoms. He said: "just put a baggie on it". They would not do it. For lots of reasons he said, and he had to respect that, had to respect their choice. We had a conversation about at what point it is someone's choice and at what point it is not because the "brain is hijacked" by the drugs or alcohol. It is very fluid and changing Rory felt. Complex issue for sure. No simple solution but it is certainly interesting what different people come up with. Maybe we can all find solutions together. It is certainly not a one size fits all problem. We are all unique individuals with a unique set of issues and past. There is no golden ticket.

 Tracy felt that education is a key. Education at an early age. Having resources out there. The person also needs to want the help. Tracy does not think we can help someone who does not want the help. Have places where people can get help with addictions. Make it accessible, affordable. It is not affordable now- asserts Tracy. Tracy has clients who would like to get help, and their insurance does not cover the help they need. Making help more accessible and friendly for moms and families. Tracy brings up the example where would the children go if mom needs to go to treatment? Sometimes there is no other family member who can take care of the kids. There might be programs now, and still it does not look at how the whole family is affected by the addiction. Tracy gives the examples of parents going into treatment and how that affects the children, grandchildren and spouses. Having a system out there that is more supportive for a whole family unit would be helpful. Housing for recovery where families can stay, and therapy that is built in. Help people getting connected to jobs. There are some programs like that out there, not many.

Diana feels like people need more programs where they can go by choice. Allow people to talk about their addiction, listen to them. Sometimes law is the only way. Having trained people to help with addictions. I asked Diana if she could make one change to help people with addiction what it would be. She said start with the drug companies. Restrict who they are selling to and what they are selling. Diana feels that the schools need to talk more in their health classes what drug addiction is, how to prevent it, be upfront with the kids. Don't circle around it. In the end Diana said: "**we basically all need to take care ourselves**". It helps if people have the tools to do so, if there are family and friends who support the person dealing with addiction. If someone is already deep in addiction this can be really hard because the brain just not working right. Chloe feels we can only help people if they want to be helped. Some people don't want the help, they want to keep their addiction. If someone does want to stop, help them or guide them toward support. She gives examples of being there for someone and clearing their house from alcohol. Allow the public to have better facilities for treatment of addictions, easy access to reach out when they need help.

    Joel talks about finding out the vulnerability that is causing the need for people to turn toward addictions and have a multitude of approaches for prevention and support. What are the stressors, that are helping people to make the decision to use substances? Joel thinks our culture is very fractured and we need to find out the causes that drive people to hide out in a video room or use alcohol or drugs to feel better. Joel feels that maybe admission is the first step and the recognition that whatever it is the cause it is making people to turn unhealthy ways to try to feel better. Provide universal health care of course she adds. It is a right; it should not be based on how much money we make. Fundamental right. Joel also talks about advertising and how when companies are trying to sell something get into our brains that now we think we need to have this thing whatever it is. We don't really need all those things that are advertised to us and we might think we need them. Then our conversation ventured to trees, planting more trees instead of cutting them down. Trees, especially evergreens produce a calming chemical for our brains. Spending time around nature and trees can be very helpful to create a balance in life.

Creating quiet spaces where there is no constant buzzing in our environment.

Janett likes to be proud of the fact that she made a conscious choice not to do what her mother or grandmother did. She had the opportunity. She describes herself lucky, maybe she did not get the addiction gene. She was very aware where substances could lead her, and she worked very hard not to go down that road. Janett only drinks if the occasion is very special, it is difficult or awkward sometimes for Janett and her mom to go to parties where there is alcohol, and everybody is drinking. She describes people bringing a bottle of wine when they moved into their new house. Then what we do when we end up with 5 bottles of wine for our housewarming party and we don't drink. She brought it up that I asked her about her dietary restrictions before bringing something to her house. Others don't and people just think it is ok with everyone to bring wine. Well, it is not. Not to any house or place where anyone struggled with addiction before.

One solution can be is just to be mindful about others, be mindful what we take to someone's house. Ask before. Try to bring something healthy. Something that everyone would want to eat, drink or feed children with. Janett recalled her wedding and other weddings where they just have champagne for the toast, and they don't have anything else. She instructed people at her wedding to put 2-3glassess of sparkling apple ciders on the tray too, it did not happen of course. They did not do what she wanted. She was 3 months pregnant and not drinking and they gave her champagne. She asked them for the sparkling cider, they did not bring any out. She tells the story to illustrate that things like this happen all the time. No other thing is offered in an event just alcohol. She made sure at her brother's wedding they had a sparkling cider for her mom so she can have a toast.

Bernadette thinks teaching emotional intelligence at schools with coping skills can help. Having more social workers, nutritious food and yoga classes in schools to support the next generation. Bernadette does feel hopelessness around this topic of addictions. Uncertain what could be the right solution. Here is so much that we can't control. Can't control what people do at home. She feels many people do not want to get better. Providing safe jobs, safe and affordable childcare for women could help. Support parents better. After my magic wand discussion with Chelsea, some laughter, she asserts this is not realistic she feels. Stopping drugs, changing brain chemistry and genetics would be her wish. Making education and mental health more part of daily life not something that is weird and have to go seek it out.

Bill feels the needs for affordable housing. He had met people who are struggling to get on their feet and have no options for housing. He does not want to be in the housing business. He still does want to help people in this need. He gave me an example of a carpenter who lost everything because of addictions, except his truck and tools, now he is better he got his job back. He does not have stable housing. He feels like housing is the natural next step for this person to feel as a contributing part of society and have his self-esteem back. He tells me we all have to look at ourselves and see what is it that we can do to help. He wishes he could offer more than what he can now. He feels that when it comes to people who are on the streets begging give or don't give it is up to each individual. If someone does not want to give or can't then treat that person with respect and at least say hello, wish them a good day. Give respect, a smile or wave, whatever we can give. Give the gift of resect. He talks about hospitality. Just be kind. If someone can buy a breakfast sandwich to somebody who need it, do it. Without strings attached.

Albert feels that making possession of drugs a felony does not help. Oregon is better, they did change the law most single dose drug possession is not a felony or at least not at the first time. It can become eventually. He feels that stigma follows people a long time and it makes hard for people to get jobs. Once someone is a felon, they cannot get certain jobs, can't get into certain apartments, can't get into schools, hunting, fishing things people like to do, it can mess with people. It can really stigmatize them and kick them out of society. Keep them on the edge of society. Sometimes people can get felonies removed, it is depending on what was the charge. Usually a person has to have 3 to 10 years of staying out of trouble, sober time before a felony can be removed. Albert feels this creates hopelessness, why even try? There has been in some progress making drug possession misdemeanors or making them less prosecutable for certain possession crimes, he feels that we should do more of that. The felony tag really hurts people a lot.

      Brenda thinks education can help. Reaching kids early in elementary and middle school. Before the drugs reach the kids. Helping them understand the choices they might be faced with. Helping kids understand how quickly they can become addicted to substances whether that is including meth or alcohol for example. Reaching out and teaching kids how to cope with anxiety in life. Now, Brenda tells me kids get out of school and they have no coping skills. It is easy for them to fall into drugs and addictions in order to cope and get some life satisfaction. Brenda grew up in California in San Diego area the police went out to elementary schools and talked to kids about saying no to drugs, this could be one element that could help. Health care workers, people well known in the community, movie starts need to pick up the prevention piece and support their community. Maybe it can be done in community forums. There is a lack of funding, maybe through grants. ***Thinking out of a box with new ideas.*** We need to go out of the box on this one and use every tool we have in a box as well as invent new ones to prevent addiction and help those who are already addicted. In her community if Brenda would have a magic wand, she would collaborate with people including businesses build a small collaborative and brainstorm how we can get this message best received in the schools and start with the elementary schools. Go out do programs, small giveaways, help kids understand that it is positive to be drug free, fill them with positive things, teach them how to say no and deal with their emotions. It needs to start young Brenda asserts because by junior high or high school they already having to make that choice. Brenda feel that if they are not taught how to say know they will just fall right into it. Not giving up on people. Build connections and support around people. People might fail but is important to be there and support them, so they keep coming back. Providing persistent support for them.

      Bob feels like education could be helpful for people to learn more about addiction prevention. I asked him where he would see it if the education existed. He felt there could be marketing and events, organized series of events to interest people, incentivize people, make it like a social thing. What a good incentive would be. He thinks for a while. Then he said maybe just the event itself, maybe it could be something like a concert, a place people would want to go. Work the education into the event. There is stigma about addictions. Need to get people to want to go and do something find a compelling reason to want to go and get informed. Were he would advertise it? Social media, snap chat he adds.

50. Self – Preservation

It is very important to take care of ourselves to be able to take care others in our lives or work. This can be hard sometimes when people are caring and compassionate. It can be hard to say no. It can be hard to take care ourselves when we are so used to taking care of others. My kids and friends remind me of this all the time. They say it is ok mom, do something for ourselves. I had seen throughout my work in addiction and in the community how difficult can it be on family and friends when they have someone whom they love trapped in the addiction cycle. Beth said:" I just don't go and cannot be around and hang out with people if I know they use anything. I just can't." She described separating herself to prevent herself from being drawn into their drama. Beth does not trust someone with an addiction problem, she does not trust the behavior, she describes a line between drinking a little occasionally which she finds acceptable, she would not hang out with someone who is drunk. Beth feels she cannot help somebody who won't help themselves. She describes a friend growing up who got into drugs and she was trying to do everything she could for her, then she had to make a decision to separate herself from it, she did not want to be like that. She did not want to use drugs. She felt like people who use drugs have a separate world where everybody uses drugs. She had to separate herself and make a decision who does she want around her children. Beth describes that having children changes everything.

Mary described frustration sometimes when trying to help others. She is not the only one. Following through with something is important to Mary, if she said she will do something she will follow through. She describes this as a core value. Also seeing potentials that others have and watch them sabotage themselves and see them in pain has been hard. Angel mentioned that sometimes it is easier to put someone at arm's length because of all the craziness that is going on with addiction. Angel describes the difficulty her parents had to go through to be there for her brothers and also protect themselves financially and emotionally while still being supportive. Sometimes they had to make hard decisions. Paige had to decide to move out of her mother's and stepfather's house as being with them was not a good place to raise her family related to the drinking that was going on in the house. Originally, they moved together to save money. She had to make a decision to protect her children and herself. It is to a point now that she just cannot be around them a lot. This hurts her and her mom, it is very hard. Her children are also embarrassed by it, her youngest picked her stepfather up once when he needed a ride and he was so drunk that the car reeked of the smell of alcohol for hours after he was gone. Her husband saw him recently and he was bumping into walls. It has been very sad for Paige, and she just can't be more involved, she is protecting herself and her family from the pain that this addiction causes. Paige feels sad and frustrated about the whole situation. She wants to be helpful and also not want to push her mom away either. It is a very fine balance. She talked to her mom and told her that if she needs help and wants to leave or if he wants to go to treatment, they will be there for her. She will not bail them out of financial problems that is caused by the drinking. Paige's feeling had been hurt so many times that she has difficulty to be understanding and she has to be careful how much time she spends with them because it causes more hurt and pain. On her father's side there is a dangerous situation that involves heroin and drug use to a point that Paige cannot even be involved with that part of her family at all. She describes that part of her family as doing toxic and despicable things. Paige feels bad about people who are addicted, she describes deep rooted problems. Tracy had to pull away from her family. It has been really hard to deal with all that is going on, it is too much. Ironically, she works with other families with similar problems. She got out of it somehow while others did not.

51. Creating Change

Creating change is not easy. Going to a school for my doctorate degree we had talked a lot about social change. There are a lot of things that can improve in our society, addictions, homelessness, war, money and the way people use power for example. Creating positive change is very important for everyone. If we all do a little on our part, we can create positive social change. We are the people. Dolores said that we need a grassroot movement to create change in addictions. How can we do that? Make enough people interested. Get attention. Speak up. Share our voice. Be a role model. Make small miracles happen. Mentor kids and youth like Neal. Talk to someone. Care about someone. Care about ourselves keep ourselves safe, healthy. We all matter. Everyone matters. Ron talks about our civilization and how old it is, he asks why do we do things like dog fighting, cage fighting? Are we still barbarians? Why are we competing? Why can't we just play for fun? Why are we spending money on a few people when we could spend the same on millions of people? Who are our role models in society? Who are we putting on the pedestal? Ron asks where is the farmers parade? Where is the teacher's parade? Why there is such and access and greed? Ron knows that there is a lot of good people out there. What is visible to most people is bad stuff in the media. Ron follows the good news app. To get good news not just bad. Albert if he could make one change to make things better it would be universal health care. More people would have contact with a system without worrying to be bankrupt. The biggest thing we can do to make a difference, universal health care. Be open and more supportive of one and another would be a good idea. Albert feels instead of "othering" people and pointing fingers to good guys or bad guys. People are not that different from each other no matter which are they live in.

People are people we should not be treating people as "other" just because we don't know them. - Albert

---

It is humanity for better or worse we are all in this pot together called Earth. Just be nice to each other. If we could just do that that would help, he said. He told me laughing: "if you figure it out, let me know I will sign up". For some reason at this point we just both had a laughing fit. It was a nice way to end the conversation. Laugh as much as we can, enjoy happy moments. Flower told me that she hopes this book will be a light to a lot of people to continue a conversation among people no matter what place people come to the table from. Keep the hope of healing and potentially we can do a better job in our society. She was not sure how that would look like, but at least this is part of the discussion and that is where it's kind of begins

Dr. Beatty was very excited about me writing this book. He was recently in a conference with university institutions and the number one topic was addictions in college campuses. It is a major concern. It was not supposed to be the number one topic, but it turned out to be. The biggest problems that the deans and school presidents had was how do we deal with addiction. How do we deal with mental health problems. Dr. Beatty was sitting in the audience thinking that there is no resource for the students on how to cope with addictions.

52. Final Thoughts

One of the greatest joys in creating this book is all the wonderful conversations I had with people. Conversations went in all kinds of directions. They become very personal sometimes. I enjoyed writing too. Sometimes it has been emotionally hard. I had to step away for a few hours or days here and there. Some people had to reschedule multiple times because of issues that happen in life. I want to say thank you for everyone sharing their experiences with me. A while back I was thinking of addiction and had this image in my head: ***One small drop in the sea can change the color of the water.*** It really can't, but many drops can. Just keep adding drops. Depending on also how strong of a color of the drop is, and how big is our water. It has been years since this thought come to me. Change takes time and it would come slowly. One action, one support class, one person can make a difference and change something that gives a spark of hope in recovery. It will take time. Dealing with addiction is a difficult journey. It is possible. Since our minds are a wonder with a lot of unknown properties; every little action or seed can make a difference, because every action is stored in our unconscious mind even if we are aware of it or not. This would be our glutamate system in our brain that is keeping our memories. Addiction to anything in this world is not a choice that an individual makes for themselves; it is a disease, a very bad disease. It might seem like and easy choice to sop what harming us, and it is not. Our brains and emotions are very powerful. ***Addiction is a deadly disease.*** Addiction is a disease that kills and claims millions of lives every day. One drop of a drug can change the way of a person thinks acts and lives their life. There is so much more to learn about the neurobiology of addiction and any other type of disease. Positive reinforcement can go a long way. I would like to say thank you for reading this book. I hope it helped some way. It helped me writing this book. It has been a joyful and difficult journey. I met wonderful people on the way. It has also been very painful and sad to hear the experiences people had. We shared sadness, tears, anger, laughter and joy together.

Finally, I like to share some thoughts with you. One day during the summer of 2019 when I was visiting a friend in Seattle and was just in the beginning to make the decision about continuing to write this book. I woke up and was thinking about some points, some ways I want to live my life. I felt this was important, so I wrote them down. Here they are:

1. Be good.
2. Do no harm.
3. Help when you can.
4. Breathe.
5. Love.
6. Forgive yourself and others for their mistakes.
7. Don't blame others.
8. Reach out.
9. Ask for help when you need it.
10. Advocate for yourself and for those who cannot advocate for themselves.

I had a recent conversation with Mike who is a pastor and EMT. He told me that a lot of people get stuck at number 6. Forgive yourself and others for their mistakes. It is not easy. It can be very hard. Assume good intentions. We are human. We make mistakes. I believe that we are all connected to everyone and everything. The better we do, the stronger the connection is. I imagine connection strings between me and others I get in touch with, colors can be blue (healing), pink (caring, love), gold (protection). These are the colors for me, it might be different for you. I believe that all living things are connected. The better we do the stronger the light of love shines in us. I see it in light pink and gold. The connections can go dark and become damaged based on individual behavior, intentionally causing pain to others including our environment hurts everyone and everything. Connections can turn gray and black. Basically, be kind, do good, don't hurt others, love everyone and everything that is living as we are all connected. Show empathy and compassion toward others. Save all you can. We can all do our part. Pick up trash. Don't create more trash and harm. Help one another. Take a walk in the forest. Enjoy your life. Smile. Laugh. Grow vegetables and fruit if you can. Have good intentions. Do the best you can. When you mess up ask for help. And please don't put people in a box. It is ok if not everyone fits into a checkmark or act differently than others. Help and provide support when you can. Remember no borders, no state lines, no country lines when it comes to a disease, loss, sadness or joy. Be there for others. We are all in this together. Wishing everyone lots of joy in their life.

53. QUESTIONS

Some of the guiding questions I had asked people that had helped to build this book during our conversations included, but not limited to these:
What has been your experience in addictions at work? Or at your personal life? Or both?
Do you know anyone who is dealing with addiction?
What do you think addiction is? The way you think about it not a dictionary definition. What does addiction mean to you?
What do you think our individual and societal responsibility is related to addiction?
How do you think we can help people who are addicted to any substance?
How do you feel about people who are dealing with addiction?
What role do you think nutrition plays in addiction and recovery?
How important you think nutrition is to our health and wellbeing? Why?
What change could be made by society related to addiction?
Based on your experience what would you recommend to people who are currently dealing with addictions?
What foods would you recommend avoiding?
What one change could you do to help people with addiction?
What you think the healthcare role is related to addiction? or should be?
Government role?
Do you think people deep into addiction are happy?
Why? What do you think happiness is? What do you think Joy is?
Do you think addicts have a right to be cared for?
What do you think about stigma and addiction?
What do you think about resiliency and addiction?
Anything else you can think of or would like to add or share that I did not asked you about?
    I did encourage people to tell me if down the road in a few days or weeks they think about other things that they want to include or someone who they know that I should talk to about their experience in addictions. Additionally, did ask people how different stories or

examples they gave me made them feel. Asked details about personal experiences and asked them to share stories with me from their life experiences. Conversations went to all kinds of directions based on the stories shared. I did not ask everyone all the questions; it was kind of depend upon their story to and which way I felt that they want to go with it what was important for them. I also made up a lot of questions on the fly based on what we talked about. I would like to say thank you again for all those who volunteered to be part of this book and shared their stories with you. Thank you for your encouragement and support. Thank you, I am grateful for you.

54. Media, Web and Book Recommendations

If you are tired of bad news all the time, I recommend the good news app for you. It's just called good news. You can find it in your app store. Additionally, there are some books, websites and media I would like to recommend as a resource:

- Gabor Maté, MD: In the Realm of Hungry Ghosts- close encounters with addiction
- Neal Lemery: Mentoring Boys to Men: Climbing Their Own Mountains
- Sarah Wilson: First we make the beast beautiful – a new journey through anxiety
- Martha Beck: Finding Your Way in a Wild New World
- Emma Young: How Iceland fixed its teen substance abuse problem you can find this article on the blue zones website which I also highly recommend. www.bluezones.com
- Richard Leider's guide to unlocking your purpose https://richardleider.com/wp-content/uploads/2018/08/Power_Of_Purpose.pdf
- I recommend this nutritional website of Michel Greger, MD; they have a weekly newsletter with new scientific info that you can get every Sunday and lot of videos. www.nutritionfacts.org
- Forks Over Knives – movie and book, there is also a cookbook
- Michel Greger, MD: How Not to Die book and cookbook
- Rosemary Ellsworth Brown, PhD - Addiction Is the Symptom: Heal the Cause and Prevent Relapse with 12 Steps That Really Work
- John Dewar Gleissner - Get Tough & Smart: How to Start Winning the War on Drug Addiction
- Centers for Disease Control and Prevention (CDC) Alcohol and Drug use website up to date research and articles: https://www.cdc.gov/publichealthgateway/didyouknow/topic/alcohol.html
- CDC Treatment and recovery resources: https://www.cdc.gov/rxawareness/treatment/index.html

- CDC collected resources from the CDC, White House, SAMHSA, and NIDA about drugs, substance abuse, addiction, and communities at risk:
  https://www.cdc.gov/pwid/addiction.html
- SAMHSA's (Substance Abuse and Mental Health Administration) National Helpline – 1-800-662-HELP (4357); Website https://www.samhsa.gov/
- NIH National Institute on Drug Abuse – Resources https://www.drugabuse.gov/publications/principles-drug-addiction-treatment-research-based-guide-third-edition/resources
- Public Health Addiction Resources https://www.publichealth.org/resources/addiction/

www.ingramcontent.com/pod-product-compliance
Lightning Source LLC
Chambersburg PA
CBHW072026230526
45466CB00020B/937